Food Addiction, Obesity, and Disorders of Overeating

Claire E. Wilcox

Food Addiction, Obesity, and Disorders of Overeating

An Evidence-Based Assessment and Clinical Guide

Springer

Claire E. Wilcox
Mind Research Network
Albuquerque, NM
USA

ISBN 978-3-030-83077-9 ISBN 978-3-030-83078-6 (eBook)
https://doi.org/10.1007/978-3-030-83078-6

This Springer imprint is published by the registered company Springer Nature Switzerland AG
The registered company address is: Gewerbestrasse 11, 6330 Cham, Switzerland

Introduction: Obesity, Eating Disorders and Food Addiction: Towards a Synthesis

The biology regulating human appetite developed through natural selection during conditions of nutritional scarcity, and, as a result, it favors the consumption of high-calorie foods which more efficiently provide the body with energy for day-to-day functioning. Unfortunately, in the current environment, there is an overabundance of this energy dense, highly palatable food, especially high-sugar, high-fat, and industry-designed foods. Furthermore, people eat not only for hunger or nutrition but also for pleasure, in modern cultures [1–4]. With our preexisting evolutionarily-based tendency to overconsume these foods, it is no wonder that so many of us humans of today overeat, and why, also, rates of overweight, obesity, and eating disorders (ED) associated with binge eating are so high.

This textbook is written for providers of broad training backgrounds and aims to help those who care for people with EDs, overweight and obesity provide evidence-based treatment. The goal of the book is to offer these providers a straightforward resource summarizing the current standard of care. However, it goes further by also introducing the concept of food addiction (FA) as a model to understand some forms of overeating. By considering the possibility of FA in our patients, we may be able to increase our ability to treat them and improve their outcomes, because it makes it possible for us to consider some new ideas and innovative treatment approaches.

This book is suited for both medical and mental health practitioners, including physicians in primary care or psychiatry, nurses, psychologists, social workers, medical students, and medical residents. It may also be suited for science- or medicine-savvy people who struggle with these kinds of disorders too, although it is not a self-help book. The book could also be used in educational settings, such as upper-level college coursework, by students in master's and PhD programs for clinical psychology, medical school, and residency training. Finally, it could be utilized by researchers in obesity and ED fields, stimulating ideas for future research and study design.

In the first chapter we will review the mechanisms of homeostatic feeding, which is the process that regulates appetite and hunger-motivated food-seeking, and which involves multiple organ systems in the body, including the brain. In the second and third chapters we will provide overviews of the standard approaches to assessment of obesity and EDs associated with binge eating [e.g., binge eating disorder (BED) and bulimia nervosa], emphasizing their multifactorial etiology (including the neurobiology), and their negative consequences on mental and physical health, if left untreated. We will also provide an overview of current evidence-based treatment guidelines for obesity and these EDs, discussing the evidence base behind current dietary recommendations, medications, physical exercise, behavioral interventions, and surgery. We also will highlight that, at present, the treatments for both obesity and EDs associated with binge eating overlap in some of their approaches, but are also often distinct in some of their goals: weight loss is usually the primary aim in obesity treatment, but reducing disordered eating and improving body shape over-concern is the focus of bulimia and BED, while weight loss as a primary goal is discouraged because restrictive eating can trigger worsening eating disorder status. However, despite the fact that there are excellent well-studied treatments for both categories of overeaters, the two treatment fields also both still have a long way to go. People who suffer from these disorders often do not get well, despite receiving state-of-the-art evidence-based care, indicating that more effective treatments are needed.

In the remaining chapters we will focus on the concept of FA, which, if embraced by clinicans and researchers, has the potential to improve our understanding and treatment of some (but not all) people with obesity and EDs associated with binge eating. The FA model to explain some forms of overeating has garnered more widespread attention and acceptance over the last decade, which has increased our focus on brain-based mechanisms of overeating as well. Although BED and bulimia are in the DSM-V, obesity and FA are not, although there were both seriously considered for inclusion [5, 6], and it is possible that FA and/or obesity will be included in future editions as the evidence base grows.

We will begin our discussion of FA by reviewing several of the main ongoing controversies associated with the construct. Then we will review both the clinical and neuroscientific evidence that some individuals' eating behavior mirrors that seen in substance use disorders (SUD): i.e., their relationship with food appears to be "addictive." We will also discuss how many of the mechanisms known to underlie SUDs (e.g., tolerance, withdrawal, downregulated dopamine systems, sensitized reward systems, impulse control difficulties, emotion dysregulation, cue-reactivity, conditioning and learning, neuroinflammation, oxidative stress, changes in the serotonergic and endocannabinoid systems) appear to also drive overeating in animal models and humans. All of this will support the argument that the construct of FA has validity. Finally, we will argue that thinking about the similarities between the brain mechanisms of addictive disorders and overeating behavior has the potential to open up new avenues for current treatment and treatment development. It will provide students, mental health providers, primary care providers, and researchers some new ideas for interventions and solutions that may be utilized to help individuals recover, both in the nutritional realm, in the behavioral realm, and maybe even extending into other realms like neurostimulation, for example.

While doing so, we will stay rooted in the evidence. We will be careful to question for whom embracing the FA model might improve patient outcomes, and for whom it might worsen their outcomes or for whom the concept might be especially triggering (e.g., patients with high levels of restrictive eating). This book will discuss the pros and cons of embracing FA and review the evidence for and against the validity and utility of FA (evidence for and against, both science and clinical). By doing so we will come up with a new "middle ground" approach to help people with obesity, BED, and bulimia nervosa plus FA symptomatology who also want to lose weight. Finally, given the fact that overeaters are a highly heterogeneous group (often with wildly different reasons for overeating, and therefore meriting different treatments), we will emphasize that researchers should consider using FA status as a "treatment matching variable" (i.e., to see if it will help identify in advance which treatment a person will more likely respond to). This aligns with federal funding pushes for more "precision medicine" studies [7].

There are important several areas which we will not cover in this book in great detail. For example, although we will certainly mention numerous studies done in adolescents and pediatric populations, we will not be discussing adolescent obesity or pediatric overeating in any focused way. Although we mention prevention and global health in a few places, this is also not a major focus area of this book. Furthermore, we do not review the literature on the assessment and treatment of anorexia nervosa, avoidant-restrictive food intake disorder, or several other EDs, rather focusing on the two primary EDs that also have binge eating in their diagnostic criteria (bulimia nervosa and BED). Moreover, when we discuss psychiatric comorbidities, we do not mention borderline personality disorder (BPD) or other personality disorders frequently. This is because although BPD has a high comorbidity with EDs, adding the diagnosis can be stigmatizing in some settings but often does not help much in terms of treatment planning. Dialectical behavior therapy, which targets dysregulated emotion, is a mainstay of treatment for BPD, and it is also often utilized during ED treatment regardless of whether a patient meets criteria for this disorder, since emotion regulation is a trans-diagnostic treatment construct [8]. Finally, we want to highlight that the two chapters in which we review the treatment of obesity and EDs are, admittedly, simply overviews. For a provider to feel truly comfortable implementing some of the treatment recommendations, it will likely require accessing references and/or existing manuals, dietary and physiotherapist support, and expert training in some of the behavioral interventions, for example.

Finally, by way of orienting the reader, we want to mention that in addition to the individual chapters we have also included at the end an appendix in which we have included some definitions for frequently utilized terms. We also include a list of potentially helpful books and resources, including excellent review articles, manuals for treatment providers, textbooks and self-help books.

Claire E. Wilcox
Mind Research Network
Albuquerque, NM
USA

References

1. Blanco-Gandia MC, Minarro J Rodriguez-Arias M. Common neural mechanisms of palatable food intake and drug abuse: knowledge obtained with animal models. Curr Pharm Des. 2020;26(20):2372–84.
2. Davis C. Evolutionary and neuropsychological perspectives on addictive behaviors and addictive substances: relevance to the "food addiction" construct. Subst Abuse Rehabil. 2014;5:129–37.
3. Carter A, Hardman CA Burrows T. Food addiction and eating addiction: scientific advances and their clinical, social and policy implications. Nutrients. 2020;12(5):1–4.
4. Carter A, Hendrikse J, Lee N, Yucel M, Verdejo-Garcia A, Andrews ZB, et al. The neurobiology of "food addiction" and its implications for obesity treatment and policy. Annu Rev Nutr. 2016;36:105–28.
5. Gever J. APA: obesity rejected as psychiatric diagnosis in DSM-5 MedPage today. 2010. https://www.medpagetoday.com/meetingcoverage/apa/20381. Accessed Dec 8 2018
6. Adams RC, Sedgmond J, Maizey L, Chambers CD Lawrence NS. Food addiction: implications for the diagnosis and treatment of overeating. Nutrients. 2019;11(9):2086.
7. Dishman E. Precision medicine. 2018. https://www.nih.gov/precision-medicine-initiative-cohort-program. Accessed 2018.
8. Sloan E, Hall K, Moulding R, Bryce S, Mildred H Staiger PK. Emotion regulation as a transdiagnostic treatment construct across anxiety, depression, substance, eating and borderline personality disorders: a systematic review. Clin Psychol Rev. 2017;57:141–63.

Contents

Contributors

Pamela B. Arenella, MD Dalhousie University, Halifax, NS, Canada

Shannon Bedford, PsyD Nova Scotia Health Authority, Halifax, NS, Canada

Matthew J. Eck University of Southern California, Los Angeles, CA, USA

Danielle C. Farrar, MD, PhD Department of Psychiatry and Behavioral Sciences, University of New Mexico School of Medicine, Albuquerque, NM, USA

Claire E. Wilcox, MD Mind Research Network, Albuquerque, NM, USA

Part I

Standard Approaches to Clinical Assessment and Treatment of Obesity and Binge Eating Disorder (BED)

1 Determinants of Body Weight: Metabolism and the Homeostatic System

1.1 Energy Balance

Body weight is controlled by a number of factors, the most basic being energy balance (EB). EB is the difference between energy intake (food consumed) and the total daily energy expenditure (TDEE). If the calories consumed exceed the calories expended, then the individual gains weight. The two primary factors that determine TDEE are resting energy expenditure, which depends on resting metabolic rate (RMR), and activity-induced energy expenditure which has to do with the amount of physical activity in which someone engages [2, 3].

Resting energy expenditure is determined by body size and body composition (more muscle, male gender, and younger age are associated with higher resting energy expenditure), RMR, genetics and other environmental factors [4, 5]. Higher fiber diets can promote weight loss by reducing RMR (in addition to reducing energy absorption) [6].

Activity-induced energy expenditure is more variable within a day and between people than RMR, and, as the name implies, depends on the kinds of and amount of activity performed. It refers to both deliberate exercise and "working out", and non-exercise activity thermogenesis (NEAT) such as walking from room to room, or engaging in activities like gardening and even fidgeting [4]. NEAT accounts for about 100 to 800 calories used daily [4, 5].

Thermogenesis is another contributor to energy expenditure and is defined as the dissipation of energy through the production of heat. Thermogenesis occurs in brown adipose tissue, and accounts for less than 10% of our TDEE [3–5]. Thermogenesis also refers to the energy dissipated through food processing (e.g., digesting, absorbing, transporting, and storing the food consumed), otherwise known as diet-induced thermogenesis (DIT) [4, 5, 7]. High-protein diets may help promote weight loss because dietary protein leads to a markedly higher DIT than carbohydrates and fats [7].

Adipocyte (i.e. fat cell) biology is complex. Adipocyte function and the ratios of the different adipocyte subtypes can also affect body weight and in particular energy expenditure [3]. For example, white adipocytes are involved in fat storage and secretion of hormones. Brown adipocytes are involved in thermogenesis and caloric expenditure. Beige adipocytes are transitional adipocytes that in response to various stimuli can turn from white to brown and could be protective against the obesity, enhancing energy expenditure. The conversion of white adipose tissue to beige adipose tissue is a potential new therapeutic target for obesity [8]. Early work indicates that whole grain consumption might have beneficial effects on adipocyte biology and cell-type ratios too [6].

C. E. Wilcox, *Food Addiction, Obesity, and Disorders of Overeating*,
https://doi.org/10.1007/978-3-030-83078-6_1

1.2 Metabolism

Metabolism is the process by which the body converts the calories in what is eaten and drunk into forms of energy that the body can utilize to function [7, 9]. Understanding the complex processes underlying metabolism also helps to understand body weight, since different macronutrient components will affect metabolism processes differently.

Glucose is the primary molecule used for energy by the human body. This molecule is absorbed from the stomach into the blood, where it then travels to tissues all over the body. It is stored in muscle and liver as glycogen, which can later be broken down to produce glucose. Or it can be directly metabolized to carbon dioxide, water, and adenosine triphosphate (ATP), the primary energy source for cells, through the process of glycolysis [10]. If oxygen is in short supply, anaerobic glycolysis occurs, during which glucose is only partially burned and then gets converted into lactic acid, producing sore muscles, like after vigorous exercise [11].

Glucose comes from many dietary sources including simple sugars like sucrose and fructose. Sucrose (table sugar) consists of one molecule of fructose linked to one molecule of glucose, and, like glucose, fructose can be absorbed by the gut and metabolized to carbon dioxide, water, and ATP. However, fructose metabolism is slightly different from glucose metabolism. Excess consumption of fructose (through over-consumption of sucrose or high-fructose corn syrup) can be especially problematic for health: fructose enters glycolysis at a step that bypasses regulation by phosphofructokinase allowing for unimpeded conversion into cholesterol and triglycerides that can raise blood lipid levels and increase body fat [11].

Dietary triglycerides are absorbed through the gut as lipoproteins, which are complexes of protein and fat, and can then be stored as adipose tissue or broken down to produce fatty acids, which are used for energy. The end-products of fatty acid metabolism are glucose, carbon dioxide, water, and ATP. Combustion of fatty acids to these products requires glucose; otherwise, ketones are produced [10, 12]. Triglycerides are also mobilized for breakdown or combustion as described above through stimulation of cells in adipose tissue by various hormones including epinephrine, a hormone released under stress [12].

Gluconeogenesis is the process by which glucose is synthesized from fat or protein for use as fuel, rather than the process by which energy is created from the direct consumption of carbohydrate. Ketogenesis and gluconeogenesis are similar in that they are both chemical processes that provide energy to the body when an inadequate amount of carbohydrate is present in the diet. However, ketogenesis differs from gluconeogenesis in that it produces ketones to be used as fuel, rather than glucose. On a keto eating plan, too much protein may result in gluconeogenesis preventing ketogenesis [13]. Although some people in the keto community express concerns that eating too much protein and switching from ketogenesis to gluconeogenesis will impede weight loss, evidence indicates that both increased gluconeogenesis and ketogenesis reduce appetite and increase satiety [7] and gluconeogenesis slightly increases TDEE [13]. Therefore, eating high amounts of protein while on a low carbohydrate is probably a reasonable option for people wanting to lose weight, regardless of the fact that higher protein intake might impede ketosis [7, 14].

1.3 Why Weight Gain Is So Easy and Weight Loss So Hard

In 1962, the "thrifty genotype hypothesis" was proposed, which surmises that throughout human evolution, the constant pressure of famine led to the natural selection of genes that imparted a tendency towards efficient energy storage and metabolism and selected against genes that encouraged energy expenditure. Although this particular genetic makeup may provide a clear reproductive advantage in a food-sparse environment, it has led to the explosion of the obesity phenotype in many of the environments of today, in which food is plentiful, highly palatable, and in some cases engineered by scientists in the food industry to trigger its own overconsumption [15].

The human body is fixed with numerous counterregulatory systems, involving every organ system in the body, which vigorously defend body weight. These systems are activated when someone tries to diet [2, 3, 16]. When there is a fall in body mass, say due to deliberate dieting, there is a counter push within our systems to reduce energy expenditure, increase appetite, and reduce satiety, all of which make it very difficult to continue to lose weight [15–18]. Unfortunately, a diet-induced reduction in resting energy expenditure appears to persist indefinitely as long as the reduced weight is maintained, resulting in a situation where the individual must reduce energy intake and/or increase energy expenditure through exercise indefinitely to sustain weight loss [3, 16].

The theory of allostasis applies to this phenomena and describes how biologic systems have generally evolved to achieve stability through a dynamic response to external stimuli, the allostatic load, that "achieves controlled variability around a homeostatic mean" [3]. Trying to lose significant weight with diet and exercise alone is so difficult because it requires stepping outside of our allostatic range, going against our biology [3]. Homeostasis is another term to describe this property of biological systems that allows an organism to maintain and regulate the stability and constancy needed to function properly [9, 15–17].

1.4 Homeostatic Feeding Mechanisms

1.4.1 The Hypothalamus

The brain is a primary regulator of homeostasis, and the hypothalamus is a key player as the primary regulator of food and water intake in response to the body's energy needs [9, 17]. Hypothalamic lesions cause decreased eating and drinking behavior, whereas electrical stimulation of the hypothalamus increases intake [17]. Figure 1.1 shows a schemata of the homeostatic feeding system as a whole.

The hypothalamus receives input from numerous sources, which affect its output. In addition to receiving neural input from other brain regions, neurons in the hypothalamus are sensitive to blood levels of several dietary constituents, including glucose, free fatty acids, and amino acids, are affected by sympathetic and parasympathetic neural afferents from multiple organs, including the gut, and respond to signals from several appetitive and satiety-affecting hormones released from various organ systems in the body [15].

In particular, the arcuate nucleus of the hypothalamus is the primary food intake regulating center. It contains two types of neurons: those that produce orexigenic (hunger-inducing) neuropeptides and those that synthesize anorexigenic (satiety-inducing) neuropeptides [15]. Specifically, they produce and release either neuropeptide-Y (NPY) or agouti-related peptide (AgRP; a melanocortin receptor antagonist) which trigger hunger and promote appetite, or they release proopiomelanocortin [POMC; a precursor for α-melanocyte stimulating hormone (MSH)] and cocaine and amphetamine regulated transcript (CART) which cause increased satiety [15, 17]. The arcuate nucleus neurons project to three other regions of the hypothalamus: the paraventricular nucleus, the ventromedial hypothalamus, and the lateral hypothalamus [1, 15, 19]. The paraventricular nucleus of the hypothalamus generates an anorexigenic and catabolic program by causing increased expression of corticotropin-releasing hormone (which increases cortisol, which increases glucose mobilization for use in a stressful situation), thyroid-stimulating hormone, and oxytocin all of which lead to increased satiety and energy expenditure. The ventromedial hypothalamus suppresses feeding behavior through the release of brain-derived neurotrophic factor. The lateral hypothalamus stimulates the search for calorically dense food and promotes locomotor activity to do so through melanin-concentrating hormone (MCH) and orexin A and B [1, 15, 19] and via projections to the hedonic eating system (Chap. 9).

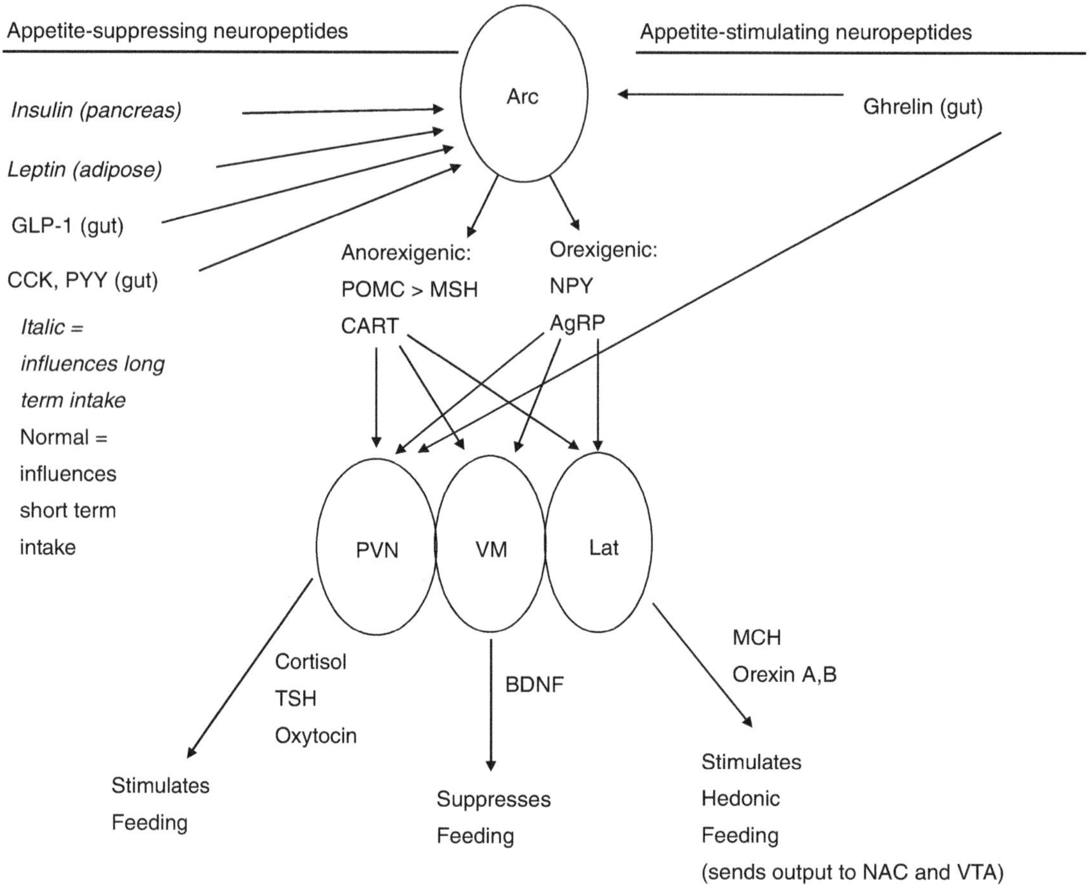

Fig. 1.1 Schemata for homeostatic feeding system centered on the hypothalamus, the primary coordinator of appetitive drive. Circles are drawn around hypothalamic nuclei defined below. Output from the arcuate nucleus can either be anorexigenic (appetite-suppressing) or orexigenic (appetite stimulating), and projections influence what is released from paraventricular nucleus, ventromedial nucleus, and lateral nucleus of the hypothalamus. Arc arcuate nucleus of the hypothalamus, Lat lateral nucleus of hypothalamus, PVN paraventricular nucleus of the hypothalamus, POMC proopiomelanocortin, MSH melanocyte-stimulating hormone, CART cocaine- and amphetamine-related transcript, NPY neuropeptide Y, AgRP agouti-related protein, GLP-1 glucagon-like peptide 1, CCK cholecystokinin, PYY peptide YY, TSH thyroid-stimulating hormone, BDNF brain-derived neurotropic factor, MCH melanin-concentrating hormone, NAc nucleus accumbens, VTA ventral tegmental area

1.4.2 Key Neuropeptides

The glucostatic theory states that short-term hunger and satiety are regulated by blood glucose levels and highlights the importance of glucose uptake and utilization by specific brain regions (like hypothalamus) for appetite regulation. By contrast, long-term mechanisms are primarily dependent on lipostatic factors (e.g., the amount of adipose tissue present in the body and blood lipid levels which also provide feedback to the brain) [20]. Although useful, the glucostatic theory probably underplays the importance of these long-term mechanisms and the hormones and neuropeptides that are released from the brain and other organs in the body which tightly regulate appetite, satiety, and food intake behavior. We will provide an overview of these hormones and neuropeptides below.

The body weight regulating hormones can be appetite-stimulating or orexigenic – e.g., ghrelin, NPY, AgRP, MCH – or satiety-promoting, and anorectic - e.g., leptin, insulin, POMC, CART, glucagon-like peptide-1 (GLP-1) - all of which either bind to hypothalamic receptors and/or are released by the hypothalamus [9, 15–17, 21–24]. Others include orexin A and B, which are orexigenic and appetite-stimulating [15, 25], and cholecystokinin (CCK) and peptide-YY (PYY), which are satiety-promoting [15, 16, 23, 26, 27]. Some of the hormones dominate short-term food intake (CCK, PYY, ghrelin), acting in concert with blood glucose levels and primarily affect meal size and duration [15]. Leptin and insulin dominate long-term food intake, their influence spanning several meals or days [15, 23, 28].

Ghrelin is an appetite-stimulating hormone that is primarily released from cells in the gastric mucosa [9, 29] and binds to receptors in the arcuate nuclei of the hypothalamus and ventromedial hypothalamus [21]. Blood levels of ghrelin normally rise in association with increasing hunger prior to a meal and then fall during and after eating, its release suppressed after ingestion of macronutrients [29, 30]. Ghrelin also causes release of NPY and AgRP from the hypothalamic arcuate nuclei, further mediating its appetite-stimulating effects [17, 18]. Finally, ghrelin decreases energy expenditure [1, 19]. In addition, ghrelin appears to influence hedonic feeding systems (discussed more in Chaps. 8 and 9), increasing food cravings [31–33] and stimulating the reward circuitry to promote feeding behavior [32, 33].

Leptin is a hormone secreted mostly by fat cells [9, 22], and leptin levels reflect the amount of stored body fat [23] in that circulating levels are proportional to fat mass [16]. Leptin levels increase when fed and fall during food restriction and dieting [9, 15, 17]. Leptin binds to arcuate nucleus receptors in the hypothalamus, where it inhibits the orexigenic neurons and stimulates the anorexigenic neurons, pushing the balance from the NPY/AgRP hunger system to the POMC/CART satiety system [15, 17], inhibiting the former and stimulating the latter [9, 16, 23]. Leptin influences levels of orexins and melanin-concentrating hormone (MCH) to induce satiety and reduce food intake [15, 17, 22]. Finally, leptin also stimulates heat production and increases energy expenditure [1, 19]. Genetic mutations in the leptin gene result in obesity in mice [15]. However, this is not the case in humans, where obesity is characterized by elevated leptin levels and *resistance* to leptin's satiety effects, a phenomenon not dissimilar from insulin resistance [15].

Insulin is released following a meal consumption from pancreatic islet cells to promote glucose uptake and storage in peripheral tissues [9]. Insulin also suppresses appetite and further food intake by stimulating receptors in the hypothalamus and also by binding in other brain regions [23, 34]. Like leptin, insulin levels correlate with and reflect the body's total adiposity and energy stores [23].

A few of the other hormones merit more detailed discussion too. AgRP is an orexigenic (hunger-inducing) hormone, but it also influences the foods consumed, increasing consumption of fat and sugar-enriched foods [15, 23, 24]. Orexin A and B are orexigenic/appetite stimulating, but they also play a major role in wakefulness and energy expenditure and appetite [25]. α-MSH is, as we mentioned previously, a product of POMC and acts on the melanocortin 4 receptor in the hypothalamic paraventricular nucleus to induce satiety [27].

Additional important peptides released by the gut which induce satiety include CCK, PYY, GLP-1, enterostatin, amylin, apoliporotein-A4, glucagon, PYY, and some peptides in the bombesin family [23, 26, 35]. These peptides also regulate other important bodily functions other than appetite. For example, CCK also regulates gallbladder function, and GLP-1 promotes insulin secretion, suppresses glucagon release, and inhibits gastric emptying [15, 16]. How these hormones affect appetite is likely multifactorial and may include effects on the hypothalamus and direct effects on other brain regions. For example, a study showed that both GLP-1 and PYY infusions into normal weight participants reduced energy intake, and food-cue-induced neural activity in the insula, and that when administered together, their effects were additive [33, 36].

1.4.3 Other Factors

Several neurotransmitter systems influence satiety and appetite via effects on the homeostatic system including the cannabinoid system and the serotonergic system (Chap. 9). Furthermore, neuroinflammation, the gut-brain microbiome, and oxidative stress will impact and are impacted by many of these appetite-regulating hormones as well, influencing food intake, and body weight (Chap. 9).

What one eats can directly influence this system too, although much more work needs to be done in this area to confirm the optimal diets for weight loss, since, so far, human data regarding the best macronutrient components for this purpose have been, on the whole, inconclusive (Chap. 2). That said, some dietary constituents appear to help suppress appetite to some degree (if not robustly so in all studies), such as dietary fiber and protein, whereas fat, sugar, and highly processed foods do the opposite (Chap. 11) [7, 23, 37–41]. Greater consumption of protein and fiber may aid weight loss in obesity via their effects on these hormone systems. For example, fiber increased PYY and total GLP-1 and reduced leptin and insulin in one study [6]. Protein also affects gut-derived hormone release (e.g., GLP-1, CKK, ghrelin) in ways that promote satiety [7].

1.5 Neuropeptides, Obesity, and Disordered Eating

Weight loss and maintenance of weight loss after dieting is extremely difficult, in part because these hormone systems were designed by natural selection in food-scarce environments to prioritize maintenance of higher body weight [9, 17]. For example, with dieting and weight loss, increases in ghrelin and decreases in leptin, PYY, and CCK occur [42], which then stimulates appetite and reduces satiety. However, circulating ghrelin levels are decreased and leptin levels are increased in obese individuals [43], so at some point, these hormone levels stop favoring weight gain. But the system is unfortunately tipped towards putting weight on and keeping it on.

Medications targetting any one of these hormone systems have failed and will likely continue to fail to have much impact on body weight or disordered eating, due to the complexity of these systems. The leptin system is especially complex. For example, loss-of-function mutations in the leptin gene cause obesity in mice, but exogenous leptin administration does not induce weight loss in humans [15, 44, 45]. Rather, human obesity is characterized by elevated leptin levels and resistance to leptin's satiety effects (in fact hypothalamic resistance to both insulin and leptin have been measured in obese individuals) [15]. Hyperleptinemia may, in fact, contribute to obesity directly, desensitizing leptin receptors in an analogous way to insulin resistance. In fact, early research in animal models indicates that reducing leptin levels to half (partial but not complete reduction) reverses leptin resistance, which then protects against weight gain and *promotes* weight loss whereas complete reduction of leptin levels *induces* weight gain [44, 45]. Furthermore, dieting may not sufficiently reduce circulating leptin levels to the threshold required for restoration of hypothalamic leptin receptor signaling [44, 45]. However, by contrast, bariatric surgery appears to reduce leptin levels through enhanced release of GLP-1 which occurs following roux-en-Y-gastric bypass and vertical sleeve gastrectomy procedures [44, 45]. Antagonists at the cannabinoid- 1-receptor, like rimonabant, might reduce appetite by reducing this leptin resistance and partially reducing leptin levels, interestingly [44, 45].

Unhealthy eating patterns and binge eating can also cause important and difficult-to-reverse imbalances in these neuropeptide systems. For example, binge eating increases fasting glucose and insulin responses and alters the diurnal pattern of leptin secretion [34]. Irregular meal frequency has been found to increase peak and total insulin release in response to a test meal after a period of irregular eating patterns [34, 46]. It is also clear that particular foods (e.g., highly processed, high sugar, high fat) can cause imbalances in this system, leading to a vicious cycle that adversely affects appetite and satiety systems and promotes weight gain (Chap. 14).

1.6 Conclusion

In summary, the homeostatic system is a complicated and has many layers of feedback that tightly regulate food intake. Unfortunately for many, the system inherently favors weight gain rather than weight loss: dieting promotes activation of counterregulatory systems that prevent further weight loss. Medication development targeting this system is also not straightforward, given its complexity and multiple feedback loops.

Despite these barriers to treating and/or changing overeating behavior, through improved understanding of these systems, it has become more clear that what we eat might be equally as important as how much. For example, as we've mentioned above, increasing protein intake prevents a decrease in resting metabolic rate with weight loss, minimizes lean muscle mass loss, helps reduce appetite through promotion of ketogenesis and/or gluconeogenesis, and restores gut hormone levels to a more weight loss promoting state. We've also mentioned that increasing fiber intake through whole grains or fruits and vegetables increases the resting metabolic rate by reducing energy absorption and restoring neuropeptide levels to be in a more favorable state for weight loss promotion and additionally may also promote satiety by its effects on the microbiome [37]. Finally, reducing fructose intake lowers the risk of triggering inflammatory processes that might further promote weight gain [11, 15, 47] (Chap. 9). But more research is needed. More about the importance of food quality will be mentioned in future chapters (Chaps. 2, 11, and 13).

There are important positive changes in physiology that occur with weight loss, which counters insulin resistance, reduces metabolic syndrome measures, and decreases inflammatory processes, so it is essential that we continue to work hard to find other additional ways to help people lose weight and keep weight off, in light of the fact that our tightly regulated systems that are biologically designed in favor of retaining body mass and weight.

References

1. Kinasz KR, Ross DA, Cooper JJ. Eat to live or live to eat? The neurobiology of appetite regulation. Biol Psychiatry. 2017;81(9):e73–e5.
2. Grigolon RB, Brietzke E, Trevizol AP, McIntyre RS, Mansur RB. Caloric restriction, resting metabolic rate and cognitive performance in non-obese adults: a post-hoc analysis from CALERIE study. J Psychiatr Res. 2020;128:16–22.
3. O'Rourke RW. The pathophysiology of obesity and obesity-related disease. The ASMBS textbook of bariatric surgery: Springer https://link.springer.com/chapter/10.1007/978-3-030-27021-6_2?s... internal_7078_20200917&mkt-key=42010A055067 1EEAA2988DEEB95A0F3A; 2019.
4. Westerterp KR. Control of energy expenditure in humans. Eur J Clin Nutr. 2017;71(3):340–4.
5. Staff MC. Metabolism and weight loss: how you burn calories. Mayo Clinic [Internet]. 2020 21 Mar 2021. Available from: https://www.mayoclinic.org/healthy-lifestyle/weight-loss/in-depth/metabolism/art-20046508.
6. Wu WC, Inui A, Chen CY. Weight loss induced by whole grain-rich diet is through a gut microbiota-independent mechanism. World J Diabetes. 2020;11(2):26–32.
7. Moon J, Koh G. Clinical evidence and mechanisms of high-protein diet-induced weight loss. J Obes Metab Syndr. 2020;29(3):166–73.
8. Rossi F, Punzo F, Umano GR, Argenziano M, Miraglia Del Giudice E. Role of cannabinoids in obesity. Int J Mol Sci. 2018;19(9):2690.
9. Karasu SR. Gravity of weight: the daunting science of weight control. Washington, D.C.: American Psychiatric Publishing Incorporated; 2010.
10. Peluso MR. What are the products when carbohydrates and fats are metabolized? SFGate [Internet]. 2018 21 Mar 2021. Available from: https://healthyeating.sfgate.com/products-carbohydrates-fats-metabolized-5772.html
11. Peluso MR. Glucose & fructose metabolism. SFGate [Internet]. 2018. Available from: https://healthyeating.sfgate.com/glucose-fructose-metabolism-6981.html.
12. Peluso MR. What are the metabolic pathways to metabolize fats? SFGate [Internet]. 2018. Available from: https://healthyeating.sfgate.com/metabolic-pathways-metabolize-fats-5747.html.
13. Dolson L. Gluconeogenesis on a low carb diet. Very well fit [Internet]. 2019 21 Mar 2021. Available from: https://www.verywellfit.com/gluconeogenesis-2242007.

14. Gershuni VM, Yan SL, Medici V. Nutritional ketosis for weight management and reversal of metabolic syndrome. Curr Nutr Rep. 2018;7(3):97–106.
15. O'Rourke RW. The pathophysiology of obesity and obesity-related disease. In: Nguyen NT, Brethauer SA, Morton JM, Ponce J, Rosenthal RJ, editors. The ASMBS textbook of bariatric surgery. Cham: Springer; 2020.
16. Apovian CM, Aronne LJ, Bessesen DH, McDonnell ME, Murad MH, Pagotto U, et al. Pharmacological management of obesity: an endocrine Society clinical practice guideline. J Clin Endocrinol Metab. 2015;100(2):342–62.
17. Blanco-Gandia MC, Minarro J, Rodriguez-Arias M. Common neural mechanisms of palatable food intake and drug abuse: knowledge obtained with animal models. Curr Pharm Des. 2020;26(20):2372–84.
18. Ahima RS, Antwi DA. Brain regulation of appetite and satiety. Endocrinol Metab Clin N Am. 2008;37(4):811–23.
19. Ross RA, Mandelblat-Cerf Y, Verstegen AM. Interacting neural processes of feeding, hyperactivity, stress, reward, and the utility of the activity-based anorexia model of anorexia nervosa. Harv Rev Psychiatry. 2016;24(6):416–36.
20. San-Cristobal R, Navas-Carretero S, Martinez-Gonzalez MA, Ordovas JM, Martinez JA. Contribution of macronutrients to obesity: implications for precision nutrition. Nat Rev Endocrinol. 2020;16(6):305–20.
21. Cerit H, Christensen K, Moondra P, Klibanski A, Goldstein JM, Holsen LM. Divergent associations between ghrelin and neural responsivity to palatable food in hyperphagic and hypophagic depression. J Affect Disord. 2019;242:29–38.
22. Morin JP, Rodriguez-Duran LF, Guzman-Ramos K, Perez-Cruz C, Ferreira G, Diaz-Cintra S, et al. Palatable hyper-caloric foods impact on neuronal plasticity. Front Behav Neurosci. 2017;11:19.
23. Onaolapo AY, Onaolapo OJ. Food additives, food and the concept of 'food addiction': is stimulation of the brain reward circuit by food sufficient to trigger addiction? Pathophysiology. 2018;25(4):263–76.
24. Davis C, Curtis C, Levitan RD, Carter JC, Kaplan AS, Kennedy JL. Evidence that 'food addiction' is a valid phenotype of obesity. Appetite. 2011;57(3):711–7.
25. Li SB, de Lecea L. The hypocretin (orexin) system: from a neural circuitry perspective. Neuropharmacology. 2020;167:107993.
26. Woods SC, D'Alessio DA. Central control of body weight and appetite. J Clin Endocrinol Metab. 2008;93(11 Suppl 1):S37–50.
27. Higgins GA, Zeeb FD, Fletcher PJ. Role of impulsivity and reward in the anti-obesity actions of 5-HT2C receptor agonists. J Psychopharmacol. 2017;31(11):1403–18.
28. Ryan KK, Woods SC, Seeley RJ. Central nervous system mechanisms linking the consumption of palatable high-fat diets to the defense of greater adiposity. Cell Metab. 2012;15(2):137–49.
29. Jeynes KD, Gibson EL. The importance of nutrition in aiding recovery from substance use disorders: a review. Drug Alcohol Depend. 2017;179:229–39.
30. Al Massadi O, Lopez M, Tschop M, Dieguez C, Nogueiras R. Current understanding of the hypothalamic Ghrelin pathways inducing appetite and adiposity. Trends Neurosci. 2017;40(3):167–80.
31. Chao AM, Wadden TA, Walsh OA, Gruber KA, Alamuddin N, Berkowitz RI, et al. Effects of Liraglutide and behavioral weight loss on food cravings, eating behaviors, and eating disorder psychopathology. Obesity. 2019;27(12):2005–10.
32. Malik S, McGlone F, Bedrossian D, Dagher A. Ghrelin modulates brain activity in areas that control appetitive behavior. Cell Metab. 2008;7(5):400–9.
33. Schlogl H, Horstmann A, Villringer A, Stumvoll M. Functional neuroimaging in obesity and the potential for development of novel treatments. Lancet Diabetes Endocrinol. 2016;4(8):695–705.
34. Sinha R. Role of addiction and stress neurobiology on food intake and obesity. Biol Psychol. 2018;131:5–13.
35. Moran TH. Gut peptides in the control of food intake: 30 years of ideas. Physiol Behav. 2004;82(1):175–80.
36. De Silva A, Salem V, Long CJ, Makwana A, Newbould RD, Rabiner EA, et al. The gut hormones PYY 3-36 and GLP-1 7-36 amide reduce food intake and modulate brain activity in appetite centers in humans. Cell Metab. 2011;14(5):700–6.
37. Sievenpiper JL. Low-carbohydrate diets and cardiometabolic health: the importance of carbohydrate quality over quantity. Nutr Rev. 2020;78(Suppl 1):69–77.
38. Karl JP, Meydani M, Barnett JB, Vanegas SM, Goldin B, Kane A, et al. Substituting whole grains for refined grains in a 6-wk randomized trial favorably affects energy-balance metrics in healthy men and postmenopausal women. Am J Clin Nutr. 2017;105(3):589–99.
39. Adam CL, Gratz SW, Peinado DI, Thomson LM, Garden KE, Williams PA, et al. Effects of dietary fibre (pectin) and/or increased protein (casein or pea) on satiety, body weight, adiposity and caecal fermentation in high fat diet-induced obese rats. PLoS One. 2016;11(5):e0155871.
40. Schoeller DA, Buchholz AC. Energetics of obesity and weight control: does diet composition matter? J Am Diet Assoc. 2005;105(5 Suppl 1):S24–8.
41. Luhovyy BL, Akhavan T, Anderson GH. Whey proteins in the regulation of food intake and satiety. J Am Coll Nutr. 2007;26(6):704S–12S.
42. Perrault L. Obesity in adults: dietary therapy. 2021 Jan 1 2021 [cited Jan 1 2021]. In: UpToDate [Internet]. Wolters Kluwer, [cited Jan 1 2021]. Available from: www.updtodate.com.
43. Tobore TO. Towards a comprehensive theory of obesity and a healthy diet: the causal role of oxidative

stress in food addiction and obesity. Behav Brain Res. 2020;384:112560.
44. Zhao S, Zhu Y, Schultz RD, Li N, He Z, Zhang Z, et al. Partial leptin reduction as an insulin sensitization and weight loss strategy. Cell Metab. 2019;30(4):706–19 e6.
45. Hankir MK, Seyfried F. Partial leptin reduction: an emerging weight loss paradigm. Trends Endocrinol Metab. 2020;31(6):395–7.
46. Farshchi HR, Taylor MA, Macdonald IA. Regular meal frequency creates more appropriate insulin sensitivity and lipid profiles compared with irregular meal frequency in healthy lean women. Eur J Clin Nutr. 2004;58(7):1071–7.
47. Lustig RH, Schmidt LA, Brindis CD. Public health: the toxic truth about sugar. Nature. 2012;482(7383):27–9.

2 Obesity

2.1 Definition of Obesity

Obesity is defined by having a body mass index (BMI) of ≥30 kg/m^2. A waist circumference of ≥40 inches for men and ≥35 inches for women is defined as abdominal obesity and is a marker of elevated cardiometabolic risk [1]. Normal weight is defined by a BMI between 18.5 and 24.9, underweight by a BMI of <18.5, overweight by a BMI of between 25 and 29.9, and morbid obesity by a BMI of ≥40 kg/m^2.

2.2 Epidemiology

In 2003, obesity was declared a global epidemic by the World Health Organization [2–4]. In 2016, 39% of adults worldwide were estimated to be overweight and 13% to be obese [3]. Also, in 2016, rates of obesity and pre-obesity in the United States exceeded 60%, indicating most Americans are obese, and excess weight reached 9% of the US gross domestic product [5]. The increased availability of highly varied, palatable, and fattening foods is a major contributor [3]. Obesity now appears to be a greater threat to the burden of disease than smoking [3, 6–8]. The COVID-19 pandemic, and its associated isolation, will likely only serve to worsen these numbers [9–11].

The physical and psychological effects of overweight and obesity are well documented and include, but are not limited to, an increased risk of diabetes mellitus, hypertension, cardiovascular disease, metabolic disease, atherosclerosis, and some cancers; osteoarthritis, joint dysfunction, and back pain; nonalcoholic steatohepatitis (NASH), cholelithiasis, asthma, atopy, allergic disease, endocrine problems, and cognitive disorders; and depression, anxiety, social isolation, poor treatment by others due to stigma, low self-esteem, fatigue, and insomnia [3, 12, 13].

2.3 Assessment

During the history and physical exam, providers should measure body weight and waist circumference. Providers should also ask about and explore for related factors and consequences [e.g., reduced levels of high-density lipoprotein (HDL) or elevated levels of low-density lipoprotein (LDL), elevated triglycerides, elevated fasting glucose or diabetes, obstructive sleep apnea, cigarette smoking, NASH, symptomatic osteoarthritis, and cholelithiasis] and screen for depression and impaired quality of life. The coexistence of several diseases, including established coronary heart disease, other atherosclerotic disease, type 2 diabetes mellitus, and sleep apnea, places patients in a very high-risk mortality category [1]. Providers should also screen for evidence of secondary causes of obesity on physical exam [e.g., thyroid goiter from hypothyroidism; proxi-

C. E. Wilcox, *Food Addiction, Obesity, and Disorders of Overeating*,
https://doi.org/10.1007/978-3-030-83078-6_2

mal muscle weakness, purple striae, and osteoporosis from Cushing's syndrome; and acne/hirsutism from polycystic ovary syndrome (PCOS)] [1].

2.4 Causes, Contributors, and Risk Factors

Two primary causes for the growing rates of obesity worldwide are linked to our time in history: namely, a growing tendency towards more sedentary lifestyles and increasing amounts of high-fat/sugar foods in our diets, the latter of which contribute to eating more than calorie expenditure (overeating) [14]. The food industry's processing of food to increase palatability is a clear and important related causal agent as well [4, 12]. There are a number of other risk factors that deserve mention, however, and secondary causes and contributors to obesity that providers should be aware of, especially since some might be preventable or reversible.

Several demographic factors are associated with a higher risk of obesity. Women have more percent body fat than men from puberty onward, gain even more fat during adulthood, and may experience modest but adverse increases in body weight and fat distribution after a first pregnancy that persist [1], and menopause is associated with additional modest weight gain risk [14]. Obesity is also more prevalent in lower socioeconomic groups and African American, Native American, and Hispanic populations [14].

In terms of early prenatal influences, high pregnancy BMI, gestational weight gain, diabetes, and smoking in the mother [14, 15] predispose to later weight gain. Neuroinflammation and epigenetic modification (e.g., changes to the genome post-fertilization), as well as effects on the hedonic reward system, may mediate these effects, causing weight gain in the child and on into later life [12, 16]. Starvation in the mother during gestation also might increase risk of later obesity and metabolic syndrome via epigenetic modification (as seen in studies of the "Dutch Hunger Winter") [12]. Childhood food insecurity [17], childhood adversity [18], and childhood trauma [6, 19] also predict later adolescent and adult obesity.

Other than a more sedentary lifestyle, other lifestyle factors also contribute to weight gain. Sleep deprivation contributes to increased body weight, which may in part be mediated by decreases in leptin and increases in ghrelin, which lead to increased hunger and increased craving for calorie-dense hyperpalatable food (Chap. 1) [14, 20–23]. This may also be caused by the fact that sleep debt makes the brain hypersensitive to images and sounds associated with rewarding food [24] and reduces general self-control [25]. Obesity also causes poor sleep, contributing to a vicious cycle [20]. Smoking cessation is another cause of weight gain, with recently quit smokers having an odds ratio for developing obesity which is twice that of non-smokers [14]. Although nicotine acutely increases metabolic rate and reduces appetite, in the long run, it also causes downregulation in the cholinergic system, so that smoking cessation and associated withdrawal causes the opposite set of symptoms to occur (reduced metabolic rate and increased appetite) to a greater degree than they would have been in a never-smoker; quitting smoking is associated with a weight gain of 1–2 kg in the first 2 weeks and 4–5 kg over the subsequent months on average [14]. Finally, acute alcohol consumption can increase cue reactivity to high calorie food cues and reduce global impulse control [3] and thwart weight loss efforts.

Several disease states can increase the risk of obesity and should be considered during initial history and physical exam. These include hypothyroidism, hypothalamic obesity (e.g., brain tumor), Cushing's syndrome, growth hormone deficiency, other brain tumor, brain injury, and a past history of brain radiation [14, 26]. PCOS is also associated with obesity, but cause and effect are not well understood [14, 26].

Many medications and classes of medications can cause weight gain, and whenever evaluating someone with obesity, seeking opportunities to switch people to alternative, less weight-gain-promoting medications should be prioritized. Weight-gain promoting medications include (but are not limited to) oral contraceptives, antipsychotics (especially clozapine, olanzapine, quetiapine), antihistamines, tricyclic antidepressants, lithium, paroxetine, valproate, gabapentin, some of the antihyperglycemics (insulin, sulfonylureas, thiazolidinediones, and glitazones but not metformin), beta blockers, glucocorticoids, and antiretrovirals [14, 26–28]. Histaminergic and serotonergic effects are posited mechanisms by which many of the medications, especially the antipsychotics, cause weight gain [28].

Psychiatric contributors and causes may include depression, anxiety, eating disorders (ED), and attention deficit hyperactivity disorder (ADHD) [26, 29]. Unhealthy attachment styles, emotional eating, alexithymia, impulsivity, emotion dysregulation, and impaired attention and self-regulation are often seen in people with obesity and are believed to contribute to weight gain [30–33]. Relatedly, social isolation is a very important contributor to weight gain and obesity, and is, of course, also a cause of obesity, contributing to a downward spiral for many [9–11, 34].

Finally, some emerging mechanisms believed to underlie obesity and weight gain should be mentioned. These include inflammation (especially in the brain and gut), the quality of the gut microbiome, and imbalances in the endocannabinoid, serotoninergic, and stress-regulating systems [hypothalamic-pituitary-adrenal axis (HPA)] (Chap. 9). Finally, food addiction (FA), the focus of this book, is likely an important contributor to obesity and weight gain for many individuals.

2.5 Genetics

Studies of twins, adoptees, and families [35, 36] indicate that obesity has a high heritability, with estimates of the amount of risk attributable to genetics ranging from 40 to 90% [35–37]. This has been demonstrated through twin studies finding that there is only a marginally lower risk of obesity in twins raised apart compared with those raised together and that BMI correlates much more strongly with that of the biologic rather than adoptive parent [36].

There are likely thousands of genes involved in obesity risk, however. A combined meta-analysis of genome-wide association studies (GWAS) (n = 82) and Metabochip studies (n = 43) in nearly 340,000 individuals identified 97 loci associated with BMI [12, 38], which accounted for only approximately 2.7 percent of the variation in BMI. The fat mass and obesity-associated (FTO) gene on chromosome 16 has one of the strongest genetic associations with obesity [36] and may account for up to 15 to 20 percent of common obesity. The products of this gene are involved in thermogenesis and in changing adipocyte types from the energy utilization (beige fat) to the energy storage (white fat) subtype [36]. Melanocortin receptor 4 (MCR4), which mediates the effects of leptin in the central nervous system (Chap. 1), represents another important locus, and 90 polymorphisms affecting obesity risk have been identified within the human MC4R gene locus [12]. Other important gene clusters may predispose individuals to develop obesity via affecting fat absorption or brain inflammation [15, 39, 40].

There are genetic factors that contribute to the link between psychiatric disorders and obesity as well. For example, depression is known to increase the genetic susceptibility to high BMI, and both depression and a tendency towards leptin resistance may actually share genetic roots [41, 42]. Studies also show evidence of clustered chromatin domains harboring risk sequences for both schizophrenia and elevated BMI [43].

Several rare syndromes which have known genetic bases are also associated with hyperphagia and/or obesity (as well as often with behavioral and cognitive problems) such as Prader-Willi syndrome, Bardet-Biedl syndrome, Cohen syndrome, Alstrom syndrome, congenital deficiency of MCR4, mutations in the gene encoding the proopiomelanocortin (POMC) gene, and several others [12, 26, 36]. Leptin-deficient mice develop obesity, but leptin mutations are not a common cause of human obesity [12, 36]. Finally, several genes involved in dopamine signaling and dopamine receptor function appear to be involved in both disorders associated with overeating and substance use disorders, but we will discuss this in more detail in later chapters (Chap. 9).

2.6 Management

2.6.1 Overview of Treatment

The goal of obesity therapy is to help promote and maintain weight loss, prevent, reverse, or ameliorate the complications of obesity, and improve quality of life [44, 45]. The greater the weight loss, the greater the reduction in morbidity, mortality, and health risks, including type 2 diabetes, hypertension, dyslipidemia, and coronary heart disease [44, 46]. Weight loss of as little as 5–7% of body weight carries numerous health benefits and should be sought as an initial weight-loss goal [44].

Patients should be evaluated for secondary medical causes of and contributors to weight gain, as discussed above [47]. Stopping medications that cause weight gain, or changing the medications to more weight-neutral ones, should be considered [47]. For antipsychotic-induced weight gain or to prevent antipsychotic-induced weight gain, metformin, topiramate, and samidorphan have shown efficacy [47–49].

Because excess weight and hormonal changes (e.g., leptin elevations) can cause or make worse a variety of psychiatric conditions, and because obesity leads to stigma and social isolation and reduces self-esteem [41, 42], and because underlying mood and anxiety disorders can trigger emotional eating [26, 31, 50], providers should have a low threshold for referring patients with obesity for mental health treatment or support. Treatment should also address body shape negativity [51], as shame and self-esteem which will only contribute to further weight gain through emotional eating. Consideration for supplemental behavioral treatments to target emotional eating and increase body acceptance and body image might be useful [52–55].

Patients seeking weight loss support can be categorized into one of several risk categories. Low risk refers to individuals with a BMI of 25–29.9 kg/m^2, or who do not have risk factors for cardiovascular disease (diabetes, hypertension, dyslipidemia), or other obesity-related comorbidities, and these patients should receive counseling on prevention of weight gain with dietary habits and the benefits of physical activity. Moderate risk refers to individuals with a BMI between 25 and 29.9 kg/m^2 and with one or more risk factors for cardiovascular disease or with a BMI of 30–34.9 kg/m^2, and these patients should be provided information on weight loss interventions (diet, physical activity) and also be considered for treatment with behavioral modification and possibly pharmacotherapy. Individuals with a BMI of 35–40 kg/m^2 are at high risk, and those with a BMI above 40 kg/m^2 are at very high risk from their obesity. Individuals in the highest risk categories should receive the most aggressive treatment (comprehensive combined dietary, physical activity, and behavioral interventions, with consideration for pharmacologic therapy and bariatric surgery) [44, 56].

Obesity is a heterogenous condition. Although the mean effects of many treatments are often small in clinical trials, some individuals experience large amounts of sustained weight loss, and this doesn't come through in the outcomes [57]. Future work should try to identify for whom particular diets, medications, or behavioral interventions are likely to work best so that providers can match treatment recommendations to individuals for whom they are more likely to be effective.

2.6.2 Comprehensive Models and Behavioral Weight Loss Therapy

Comprehensive obesity treatment interventions (basically the same as behavioral weight loss therapy programs) are the mainstays of obesity treatment. These programs involve dietary components, physical exercise, and behavioral aspects, the latter of which promote adherence to nutritional and exercise regimens and include regular self-monitoring of food intake, physical activity, and body weight. The Diabetes Prevention Program (DPP) subsequently used in the Look AHEAD trial is an example of a comprehensive lifestyle intervention [44] (many useful manuals and materials are available at this website - https://div12.org/treatment/behavioral-treatment-for-obesity/). The two major goals of the DPP lifestyle intervention are a minimum of 7% weight loss and a minimum of 150 minutes of exercise per week (such as brisk walking) [44]. The program also includes general and individualized behavioral self-management and adherence strategies, training, and support from individual case managers in both group and/or individual session [44]. The LEARN diet is also an example of a behavioral weight loss program and has a self-help book associated with it [58].

2.6.3 Dietary Component

Not surprisingly, a principal determinant of weight loss appears to be the degree of adherence to the diet, which is why the behavioral components are so important [46, 59]. Tailoring the diet to the individual, rather than focusing on the macronutrient composition of the diet in a "one-size-fits-all" approach, is considered better [44].

Classic approaches to obesity treatments assume that the most important component of the dietary aspect of treatment is that the energy taken in through caloric intake is less than energy expended ("calories in < calories out") [44, 60]. On average 22 kcal/kg is required to maintain a kilogram of body weight in a normal weight adult with a variability of ±20%. An average deficit of 500 kcal/day should result in an initial weight loss of approximately 0.5 kg/week (1 pound/week) [46]. Further caloric restriction or increased caloric expenditure (e.g., through increased activity levels) may be required for weight loss to continue after 3–6 months on a diet due to loss of lean mass [46].

Typical basic recommendations in almost all dietary programs include removing drinks with high sugar and calories, significantly limiting intake of processed foods, practicing portion control, self-monitoring of food and caloric intake, and finding a program that will be feasible for a long-term approach to changing one's eating habits [46]. Experts place emphasis on reductions in refined carbohydrates, processed meats, and foods high in sodium and trans-fat; moderation in unprocessed red meats, poultry, eggs, and milk; and high intakes of fruits, nuts, fish, vegetables, vegetable oils, minimally processed whole grains, legumes, and yogurt [46]. Almost all dietary guidelines recommend reducing the daily intake of fat to <30% of energy intake [46]. It is also generally recommended to keep one's energy consumption above 800 kcal/day: A comparison of 400 versus 800 kcal/day diet formulas showed no difference in weight loss, presumably due to slowing of resting metabolic rate [44, 46]. All adults will lose weight when fed <1000 kcal/day [44] regardless of their previous dieting history so there's no reason to go lower than 800 kcal/day.

Through extensive study, it has become clear that many kinds of nutritional programs produce modest weight loss. These diets include balanced low-calorie, low-fat/low-calorie, moderate-fat/low-calorie, and low-carbohydrate diets, as well as the Mediterranean diet and the Dietary Approaches to Stop Hypertension (DASH) and popular commercial diets such as Atkins, Ornish, Zone, Weight Watchers, Jenny Craig, fasting approaches, and low or very-low carbohydrate ketogenic diets [44, 46] (Box 2.1). The big take-home message is that no single diet is probably the best for all people seeking to lose weight [44, 46, 61] and that rather than any particular diet being better than another, reducing energy intake is the main driver of weight loss [60]. No diet has emerged a clear winner from the adherence perspective, either [59]. Also, the importance of how frequently one eats (e.g., several small meals a day versus fasting approaches) is still not clear – some studies show at least three meals a day in children might result in better outcomes, but other recent work indicates restricting one's calorie intake to fewer hours of the day might be beneficial [14].

Box 2.1 Examples of Established Diets: Definitions and Specifics [46, 62, 63]

Mediterranean diet – high level of monounsaturated fat relative to saturated fat; moderate consumption of alcohol, mainly as wine; a high consumption of vegetables, fruits, legumes, and grains; a moderate consumption of milk and dairy products, mostly in the form of cheese; and a relatively low intake of meat and meat products.

Dietary Approaches to Stop Hypertension (DASH) diet – four to five servings of fruit, four to five servings of vegetables, two to three servings of low-fat dairy per day, and <25 percent dietary intake from fat.

Low-fat diets – if a food "melts" in your mouth, it probably has fat in it and it is best to avoid it, and individuals can be instructed in counting fat grams as an alternative to counting calories.

Low-carbohydrate diets – involves restricting all carbohydrates, not just high sucrose or fructose carbohydrates or processed or high glycemic index foods, making healthy choices for fat (mono- and polyunsaturated fats), and getting adequate protein intake.

Low-glycemic index diets – consuming foods with a lower glycemic index or glycemic load.

High-protein diets – eating most of ones calories from protein, ideally low fat.

Very low-calorie diets – consumed calorie levels are between 200 and 800 kcal/day; starvation diets involve consumption of less than 200 kcal/day and are not recommended.

Ketogenic diets – if carbohydrates are taken in at less than 50 g per day, then there is glycogen mobilization and ketosis with rapid weight loss primarily due to glycogen breakdown and fluid loss (rather than fat loss) and increase in energy expenditure from ketosis that wanes over time.

Commercial weight loss programs (e.g., Jenny Craig, Weight Watchers) – comprehensive lifestyle management programs using balanced nutritional recommendations.

Popular diets [e.g., Atkins (carbohydrate restriction to promote ketosis), Ornish (low-fat, vegetarian diet that focuses on plant-based ingredients like fruits, veggies, whole grains, and legumes), Zone (high low-fat protein, like skinless chicken, turkey, or fish; carbs as mostly fruits and veggies; and a small amount of "good" fat, like olive oil, almonds, and avocado)].

Fad diets – diets involving unusual combinations of foods or eating sequences; often not sustainable.

Intermittent fasting [e.g., time restricted feeding (limiting calorie intake to a certain window of time each day, ideally 8 hours or less), alternate day fasting (consuming 25% of energy needs on the "fast" day and adlib on alternate "feed" days)] – intermittent fasting for more than 20 hours promotes ketogenesis and is anti-inflammatory/antioxidant which might increase satiety.

Portion controlled meals – using individually packaged foods, such as formula diet drinks using powdered or liquid formula diets, nutrition bars, frozen food, and prepackaged meals, that can be stored at room temperature.

For example, in several large meta-analysis, all diet programs (e.g., low carbohydrate, low fat, DASH, Mediterranean, Atkins, Ornish, and/or Zone) resulted in significant weight loss (approximately 6–8 kg at 6 months) compared with no diet, and at 12-month follow-up, the average weight losses of all diet programs were 1–2 kg less than they had been at 6 month follow-up with minimal differences between diets [46, 59, 61]. That said, some interesting differences and subtleties still deserve mention.

For one, controlled trials and epidemiological analyses suggest a more adverse role for simple sugars than for fats in obesity [60]. Furthermore, highly processed and high-sugar foods may impact body weight beyond the effects of the calories they contain by their effects on hedonic eating pathways in the brain, systemic and brain inflammation, mood symptoms, and gut microbiome profiles, for example [46] (Chaps. 8 and 9). So it's not just about "calories in < calories out" when these and other mechanisms underlying obesity are taken into consideration.

Fasting approaches may have similar short- and long-term weight loss and adherence outcomes [46, 62, 64–68] to other approaches. However, these approaches may also outshine other dietary programs in their effects on overall health. In trials comparing fasting to a more standard weight loss diet, the group assigned to 5:2 intermittent fasting had a similar weight loss, but also a greater increase in insulin sensitivity, and a larger reduction in waist circumference [63]. Furthermore, fasting approaches have been shown to have numerous health benefits including on metabolic syndrome markers, brain function and neurodegenerative markers, cancer risk, and overall life span [63]. That said, caloric restriction alone also causes improvement in cognitive function [69].

In addition, the Mediterranean diet appears to be associated with several health benefits above and beyond the weight loss effects. These include cardiovascular risk reduction and diabetes prevention [46]. Similarly the DASH diet has been studied in both normo- and hypertensive populations and found to lower systolic and diastolic pressure more than a diet rich in fruits and vegetables alone [46].

In terms of low-carbohydrate versus low-fat diets, some interesting differences between these approaches have emerged and deserve mention. For one, low-fat diets seem to cause greater fat loss than balanced diets [46]. Furthermore a few studies show a low-fat diet outshines other diets like low-carbohydrate diets in terms of health benefits and weight loss [60], but most studies show that adherence and long-term weight loss is probably similar between the two diets, [46, 70]. On the other hand, low-carbohydrate (60–130 grams per day) and very-low-carbohydrate (0 to <60 grams) diets appear to be more effective for short-term weight loss than low-fat diets [46, 70]. This benefit of reduced carbohydrate intake earlier on in weight loss attempts makes sense since they can lead to ketosis, and diets that increase ketones (e.g., Atkins) may temporarily aid in weight management by reducing appetite, increasing satiety, and increasing fat breakdown while sparing lean muscle [71]; ketosis may also increase body fluid loss, which would produce a temporary advantage only [46]. That said, long-term success of low ketogenic diets may be similar to other diets, and adherence to a strict ketogenic diet long term is very difficult for most [46]. It is likely, also, that the sources of carbohydrate do not behave equally and that carbohydrates high in whole grains are healthier, promoting more weight loss and improved health, whereas highly processed foods or foods high in sugar are considered "toxic" by some [46, 70, 72, 73]. High-carbohydrate diets that emphasize foods containing whole grains (especially oats and barley), fruit, and high fiber (especially viscous fiber sources) decrease intermediate cardiometabolic risk factors and are associated with weight loss and decreased incidence of diabetes, cardiovascular disease, and cardiovascular mortality in cohort studies [70, 72]. Finally, choosing carbohydrates based on glycemic index is of uncertain benefit [46, 60], with studies showing varied results. Side effects of very-low-carbohydrate diets include constipation, headache, halitosis, muscle cramps, diarrhea, and general weakness which all occur at rates of 25% or higher [46].

Higher protein intake is also beneficial for obesity treatment, with higher levels of protein intake associated with improved weight maintenance [46, 74], although not all studies show any particular benefit of high protein intake on weight loss [46, 60]. For example, in one study, only individuals in a high-protein, low-glycemic index diet group continued to lose weight (mean change −0.38 kg) after 6 months compared to other diets [46, 74]. High-protein diets tend to be less palatable and more satiating, stimulate thermogenesis [46, 75], have beneficial effects on appetite-regulating hormones, and may increase ketogenesis contributing to increased satiety [74]. Protein intake also prevents a decrease in fat-free mass with weight loss, which helps maintain resting energy expenditure despite weight loss [74]. High-protein diets have also not been reported to have adverse effects on health in terms of bone density or renal function in healthy adults [74].

Very-low-calorie diets (VLCD) (calorie intake of 200–800 calories per day) have not been shown to be superior to conventional diets for long-term weight loss [76]. Furthermore, they come with side effects of hair loss, thinning of the skin, and coldness. There is increased cholesterol mobilization from peripheral fat stores, thus increasing the risk of gallstones too, although this occurs with all diets but at higher rates for VLCD: after 8 weeks of VLCD, 25% of patients developed gallstones and 6% required cholecystectomy [46, 76]. VLCD also may increase risk of binge eating disorder (BED) development and cause behavioral fatigue and poor compliance [76], although regarding BED results are mixed and some work shows that VLCD might be easier to follow than other diets with no increases of binge eating [76, 77]. Despite this, VLCD should be reserved for individuals who require rapid weight loss for a specific purpose, such as surgery [46]. A subcategory of a VLCD (a very-low-calorie ketogenic diet which provides less than 800 kcal/day, no more than 20–50 g/day of carbohydrates, and 0.8–1.5 g/kg ideal body weight of protein) leads to a rapid weight loss and reduces waist circumference and fat mass and improves satiety while preserving lean body mass and resting metabolic rate [78].

2.6.4 Physical Activity Component

Exercise is an essential component of all weight loss interventions. Increasing energy expenditure through physical activity is a strong predictor of weight loss maintenance, although it is not as strong of a predictor of weight loss, per se, as diet. Physical activity is helpful because it increases calorie expenditure, but more importantly it promotes adherence by causing positive shifts in many other ways which favor weight loss and maintenance. For example, exercise increases ghrelin and gastric inhibitory peptide while also decreasing leptin, peptide YY, and cholecystokinin (CCK) [46]. Physical activity should be performed for approximately 30 minutes or more, 5–7 days a week, to prevent weight gain and to improve cardiovascular health [44]. Endurance exercise prevents the loss of lean mass, increases high-density lipoprotein, and augments visceral fat loss [62]. It also improves mood and sleep and impulse control, all key factors for weight maintenance (Chap. 14). Some interesting recent work is exploring the effectiveness of wearable technologies and circuit training, and it shows beneficial effects on weight loss outcomes [79].

2.6.5 Behavioral Modification Component

Behavioral therapy is the third core aspect of comprehensive lifestyle interventions for obesity treatment. Integrating behavioral therapy with the other weight-loss-promoting methods have been shown to enhance the magnitude and duration of weight loss [80]. During behavior modification for obesity treatment, patients receive counselling around ways to modify food intake and physical activity, are taught how to self-monitor with food diaries, and are told to weigh themselves no more than once per day and no less than once per week [44]. Behavioral therapy for weight loss also usually includes a cognitive behavior therapy-like platform which involves skills training around stimulus control (e.g., identifying and dealing with cues and environmental stimuli that trigger overeating, since cues play an important role for many [26]), problem solving (e.g., teaching people how to go to restaurants or fit grocery shopping into a busy schedule), goal setting using the SMART (specific, manageable, realistic, time-limited) principle (e.g., typically having people aim to lose 0.5–1 kg per week, get their weight down by 5–10%), meal planning, and giving positive reinforcement for success [80, 81]. Other important components included in most programs include efforts to increase social support, assertiveness training, helping with stress reduction, teaching people about how to engage in cognitive restructuring (e.g., identifying and modifying or replacing maladaptive thoughts that contribute to overeating or physical inactivity such as "If I can't exercise for 45 minutes I might as well not do it at all" or "I deserve to eat whatever, I had a hard day" with more adaptive thoughts), and encouraging people to adopt positive rather than negative self-talk [14, 80, 81]. Relapse prevention components are also included, and patients are taught to anticipate problem situations and are helped to develop a coping plan, with emphasis placed on the fact that slips are to be expected and to avoid all-or-nothing thinking [14, 80, 81]. All of these behavioral concepts and components are usually delivered and conducted by psychologists, other trained personnel, and/or through self-help groups [44, 80]. Behavioral interventions help improve compliance [46], and commercial weight loss programs such as Jenny Craig qualify as "behavioral weight loss" approaches [80].

There are several features that may improve the likelihood of success with behavioral interventions. Guidance and personalized feedback from trained interventionists and treatment that lasts at least months with at least 14 sessions [80] increases successful outcomes. Success is proportional to the frequency of interactions and their longevity – even if some of the interactions are via telephone, the longer programs are more effective than the shorter length programs [80]. Regular patient education on healthy diet choices, physical activity, weight loss goals, and barriers to weight loss, as well as regular weight checks and peer support, help facilitate weight loss [80]. Follow-up phone calls may help prevent weight regain [80].

There's a growing literature on mindfulness-based therapeutic approaches to supplement standard behavioral weight loss programs, as well [82, 83]. A recent meta-analysis showed that mindful eating was as effective as common diet programs for weight loss [84], but other studies including another meta-analysis have demonstrated less robust effects, showing that mindfulness-based interventions have no significant effect on weight loss in obesity, despite improvements in physical activity, binge eating, and physical activity [85]. Also there has been limited evidence for the effectiveness of intuitive eating, so far [86]. Ultimately, mindfulness-based approaches, including mindfulness-based stress reduction (MBSR) appear most effective in addressing binge eating, emotional eating, and eating in response to external cues; via these mechanisms, MBSR might, if nothing else, prevent weight gain [82, 86–89].

Motivational interviewing (MI) has not been found to be highly effective so far for improving weight loss outcomes in obesity compared to standard treatment, but studies are ongoing and sorely needed. One study performed MI in a small sample of patients in primary care with obesity with or without BED over the internet and the MI found to be more resource intensive compared to nutritional psychoeducation, and MI trended towards being less effective [90]. However, it was not studied as an add-on to see if it would improve outcomes if added to nutritional psychoeducation in this study.

2.6.6 Pharmacotherapy

Pharmacotherapy can help improve weight loss outcomes for people with obesity. In most cases, anti-obesity medications act by reducing appetite and food intake, although pharmacotherapy can also work by reducing absorption, too [26, 47, 56, 91–93]. For weight loss, orlistat, naltrexone-bupropion, phentermine-topiramate, and liraglutide are FDA approved for the treatment of obesity [56], as are several other sympathomimetic agents (Table 2.1).

Drug therapy can be considered for those with a BMI greater than 30 kg/m or a BMI of 27–29.9 kg/m with comorbidities and who have not lost at least 5 percent of total body weight at 3–6 months with a comprehensive lifestyle intervention [44]. Like with diet, patients should be advised that the medication only takes people so far, and that when the maximal therapeutic effect is achieved, weight loss ceases, and that when

Table 2.1 Treatments for obesity, binge eating disorder, and bulimia nervosa. Included are FDA-approved treatments and most frequently used off-label treatments

Medication	Dose	Results	Mechanism	Side effects	Contraindications	Monitoring	FDA Approval
FDA approved for obesity							
Benzphetamine	25 mg to 50 mg once daily to TID, max dose of 50 mg TID [91]		Stimulant: Increased norepinephrine release [94]	Cardiovascular, CNS, dermatologic, endocrine, GI, neuromuscular side effects [95]	Hypersensitivity to benzphetamine, cardiovascular disease, moderate or severe hypertension, hyperthyroidism, glaucoma, drug abuse history, current/ recent MAO-I use, pregnancy [95]	Baseline cardiac evaluation, cardiac echo during treatment, weight, waist circumference, blood pressure and heart rate [95]	1960 [92] (infrequent use in the USA)
Diethylpropion	25 mg TID or 75 mg daily [91]		Stimulant: Increased norepinephrine release [94]	Cardiovascular, CNS, dermatologic, endocrine, GI, genitourinary, hematologic, neuromuscular, ophthalmic, renal and urinary side effects [96]	Hypersensitivity to diethylpropion, cardiovascular disease, pulmonary hypertension, hyperthyroidism, drug abuse history, current/ recent MAO-I [96]	Baseline cardiac evaluation; cardiac echo during treatment, weight, waist circumference, blood pressure and heart rate, renal function [96]	1959 [92] (infrequent use in the USA)
Liraglutide (semaglutide and exenatide too)	3.0 mg [97] (requires injection, high cost)	−5.5 kg maximal weight loss [98]	GLP-1 receptor agonist [91]	Nausea, vomiting, abdominal pain, gallbladder pathology, pancreatitis, renal impairment [97]	Hypersensitivity to liraglutide, history of medullary thyroid cancer, history of multiple endocrine neoplasia, pregnancy [99]	Serum glucose, Hgb A1c, renal function, triglycerides, gallbladder and pancreatic function [99]	2014 [92]
Naltrexone-bupropion	8 mg/90 mg tab, 2 tabs BID [92]	−6.15 kg maximal weight loss [98]	Opioid antagonist/ stimulant – naltrexone blocks inhibitory feedback circuit of bupropion [91]	Nausea, headache, constipation, dizziness, vomiting and dry mouth, heart rate and blood pressure elevation, psychiatric [91] Increased risk of suicide in patients under age 25 [101]	Hypersensitivity to medication, opioid use or withdrawal, hypertension, seizure disorder, anorexia or bulimia, sedative withdrawal [100]	Blood pressure, heart rate, serum glucose, kidney/liver function, mental status, suicidality [100]	2014 [92]

Orlistat	120 mg [98]	−2.94 kg maximal weight loss [98]	Inhibits gastrointestinal lipase, reduces fat absorption [91]	Fecal urgency, fecal incontinence, flatus with discharge, oily spotting, bloating, diarrhea, malabsorption (vitamin D), kidney stones [92]	Hypersensitivity to orlistat, chronic malabsorption, cholestasis, anorexia and bulimia [101]	BMI, waist circumference, lipid profile [101]	1999 [92]
Phendimetrazine	35 mg BID or TID prior to meals [91]		Stimulant: Increased norepinephrine release [94]	Cardiovascular, CNS, endocrine, GI, genitourinary, hematologic, neuromuscular, ophthalmic, respiratory side effects [102]	Hypersensitivity to phendimetrazine, glaucoma, pregnancy, drug abuse history, hyperthyroidism, current or recent MAO-I treatment [102]	Baseline cardiac evaluation, weight, waist circumference, blood pressure, pulse [102]	1959 [92] (infrequent use in USA)
Phentermine	8, 15, 30, 37.5 mg [91]	−7.39 kg (mean weight loss) [103]	Stimulant [91]	Increased blood pressure and pulse, dry mouth, insomnia [91]	Hypersensitivity to phentermine, cardiovascular disease, hyperthyroidism, drug abuse history, current or recent MAO-I use, pregnancy, breast feeding [104]	Weight/waist circumference, blood pressure and heart rate [104]	1959 [92]
Phentermine-topiramate	7.5/46 mg [98]	−7.45 kg maximal weight loss [98]	Stimulant, anticonvulsant, glutamate AMPA antagonist, GABA agonist, sodium channel blocker [91]	Dry mouth, paresthesia, constipation, insomnia, dizziness and dysgeusia [91]	Hypersensitivity to either medication, Hyperthyroidism, glaucoma, current or recent MAO-I use, pregnancy, caution with hypertension [105]	Weight, blood pressure and heart rate, mood, glaucoma, labs: bicarbonate, potassium, creatinine, glucose, acidosis [105]	2012 [92]
Setmelanotide	2–3 mg daily [106] (requires injection, high cost)		Melanocortin-4 receptor agonist [107]	Headache, arthralgia, nausea, spontaneous penile erections, female genital sensitivity [107]	None listed [106]	Weight, sexual adverse reactions symptoms, depression symptoms [106]	FDA approved for rare genetic disorders of obesity [107]

(continued)

Table 2.1 (continued)

Medication	Dose	Results	Mechanism	Side effects	Contraindications	Monitoring	FDA Approval
Obesity treatments: Off-label or under review							
Bupropion-zonisamide	360 mg/120 mg and 360 mg/260 mg [107]	−6.1% and 7.5% of body weight [107]	Dopamine and serotonin reuptake inhibitor/antiepileptic agent with sodium channel modulation [107]	Nausea, headache, insomnia, blood pressure and heart rate elevation, psychiatric [107]	Not available	Not available	[107]
Metformin	850 mg BID [108]	−2 kg weight loss [108]	Inhibits mitochondrial ATP production. Possibly decreased appetite versus increased metabolism [108]	Diarrhea, flatulence, nausea and vomiting [109]	Hypersensitivity to metformin, renal dysfunction, acute or chronic metabolic acidosis [109]	Urine glucose/ketones, HgbA1c, CBC, creatinine, B12, folate [109]	Off-label for obesity [108] current type 2 diabetes treatment [109]
Tesofensine	0.25 mg, 0.5 mg, or 1 mg daily (under review) [91]	−4.5%, 9.2% or 10.6% of body weight [91]	Stimulant: presynaptic reuptake inhibitor of dopamine, norepinephrine, and serotonin [91]	Elevations in blood pressure and pulse [91]	Not available	Not available	Phase III Review [91]
Topiramate	64 mg–384 mg for obesity [91]	−5–6.3% of body weight in obesity [91] −4.5–5.9 kg in BED [110]	Anticonvulsant, sodium channel blocker, glutamate AMPA antagonist, GABA agonist [91]	Paresthesia, somnolence and difficulty with memory, concentration and attention, kidney stones [91]	Metabolic acidosis with metformin treatment, glaucoma [111]	Symptoms of acidosis, symptoms of glaucoma, suicidality, labs: bicarbonate, potassium, creatinine, glucose, acidosis [111]	Off-label for obesity and BED
Semaglutide/exenatide	2.5 mg to 40 mg/5–10 mcg BID [91]	−6.7 kg for 40 mg dose (semaglutide) [91]	GLP-1 analog [91]	Abdominal pain, nausea, other endocrine, metabolic and gastrointestinal disturbances [112]	Hypersensitivity to semaglutide/exenatide, personal or family history of medullary thyroid carcinoma, multiple endocrine neoplasia type 2, pregnancy, breastfeeding [112]	Plasma glucose, HbA1c, renal function, pancreatic pathology, triglycerides, gallbladder pathology [112]	Phase III review for obesity [91]; current type 2 diabetes treatment [112]

Treatment for eating disorders

Fluoxetine	20 mg/ 60 mg [113]	Reduction in binge eating behavior [113]	SSRI: inhibit reuptake of serotonin [113]	Insomnia, drowsiness, headache, nausea, asthenia, anxiety, tremor, dizziness, yawning, and decreased libido, increased risk of suicide in patients under age 25 [115]	Hypersensitivity to fluoxetine, current/ recent use of MAOI, linezolid, methylene blue, pimozide, thioridazine [114]	Suicidality, signs/ symptoms of serotonin syndrome, akathisia [114]	FDA approved for BN [113]
Lisdexamfetamine	50 mg, 70 mg [113]	Reduction in binge eating behavior [113]	Stimulant: amphetamine pro-drug [113]	Dry mouth, decreased appetite, insomnia, headache, elevated blood pressure and heart rate [113]	Hypersensitivity to lisdexamfetamine, cardiovascular disease, moderate-to-severe hypertension, hyperthyroidism, glaucoma, drug abuse history [115]	Cardiac symptoms, blood pressure, heart rate, weight, signs of peripheral vasculopathy, sleep/ behavior changes [115]	FDA approved for BED [115]
SSRIs (other than fluoxetine)	Varies	Reduction in binge eating behavior, equivalent to fluoxetine (above) [116]	Inhibit reuptake of serotonin [116]	Sexual dysfunction, drowsiness, weight gain, insomnia, anxiety, dizziness, headache, increased risk of suicide in patients under age 25 [117]	Hypersensitivity to medication, current/ recent use of MAOI, caution with other serotonergic medication [117]	Varies with medication	Off-label use for BN and BED [116]
TCAs: Imipramine, amitriptyline, desipramine	Varies	Reduction in bulimic behavior/ reduction of binge behavior in BED [116]	Tricyclic antidepressant: inhibit reuptake of serotonin and norepinephrine [118]	Blurred vision, constipation, dry mouth, and urinary retention, elevated blood pressure and heart rate [118]	Prolonged QTC [118], other (varies with medication)	Blood pressure, heart rate, other (varies with medication)	Off-label use for BN and BED [116]
Topiramate	64–384 mg for obesity [91]	−5–6.3% body weight in obesity [91] -4.5–5.9 kg body weight in BED [110]	Anticonvulsant, sodium channel blocker, glutamate AMPA antagonist, GABA agonist [91]	Paresthesia, somnolence and difficulty with memory, concentration and attention, kidney stones [91]	Metabolic acidosis with metformin treatment, glaucoma [111]	Symptoms of acidosis, symptoms of glaucoma, suicidality, labs: bicarbonate, potassium, creatinine, glucose, acidosis [111]	Off-label for obesity and BED
Zonisamide	100–600 mg [119]	Reduction in binge eating and weight loss [119]	Anticonvulsant, sodium and calcium channels [119]	Dizziness, drowsiness [111]	Hypersensitivity to medication [111]	Labs: BUN, creatinine, bicarbonate, ammonia [111]	Off-label use for BED [119]

drug therapy is discontinued, weight may rise again [47]. Monitoring degree of weight loss is important of course, but it's also important to monitor whether or not health or mental health status has improved during determinations of how long to continue drug therapy given potential risks [47]. The fact that there is a lack of long-term safety (and efficacy), data should be made known to patients as well before initiating pharmacotherapy: the longest-term clinical trial to date examining the safety and efficacy of pharmacotherapy was done in orlistat and lasted 4 years [47]. Also, patients should be told that no approved weight loss medication appears to promote long-term thermogenesis, just reduction in appetite and calorie intake [26], and appetite may rebound after medication cessation.

Despite these caveats, weight loss promoting medications can be helpful for many patients and should be considered for those who fail standard treatment and are interested. Pharmacologic options for the treatment of obesity in the United States include orlistat, liraglutide (a daily injection), combination phentermine-extended release topiramate (in one capsule), combination bupropion-naltrexone (in one extended-release tablet), and the sympathomimetics including phentermine, benzphetamine, phendimetrazine, and diethylpropion [26, 47]. For patients who are candidates for pharmacologic therapy, the choice of anti-obesity drugs is usually governed by the comorbidities and relative contraindications present in the individual patient [47].

Orlistat may be the best first choice for most patients, given known benefits with glycemia, lipids and blood pressure, and the availability of long-term safety data [47]. Orlistat alters fat digestion by inhibiting pancreatic lipases, causing fat not to be completely hydrolyzed which results in increased fecal fat excretion. The use of this medicine is limited by unpleasant gastrointestinal side effects and malabsorption [47].

The glucagon-like peptide-1(GLP-1) receptor agonists, like liraglutide, exenatide, and semaglutide, are especially good options for patients with type 2 diabetes and cardiovascular disease since they have demonstrated benefits with regard to cardiometabolic risk factors, glycemia, and quality of life. These drugs are administered by injection at varying frequencies [47]. These peptides affect appetite (Chap. 1) but also stimulate glucose-dependent insulin release from pancreatic islet cells and so are also often used in combination with metformin in patients with type 2 diabetes mellitus who fail one or two of the oral agents and are obese [47]. However, unpleasant gastrointestinal side effects often also occur [47, 120].

Phentermine-topiramate (extended release) is a good option for people without hypertension or coronary heart disease who don't tolerate orlistat or liraglutide. They both suppress appetite via different mechanisms: phentermine has stimulant effects, and topiramate also reduces appetite but also improves impulse control and reduces the ability of food cues to trigger craving via its effects on the glutamate AMPA receptors. Because phentermine is a stimulant, it is associated with cardiovascular and addiction risks, and topiramate may cause cognitive dulling and renal stones. Clinicians who prescribe phentermine-topiramate are encouraged to enroll in a Risk Evaluation and Mitigation Strategy (REMS), which includes an online or print formal training module detailing safety information [47] and pharmacies that dispense the drug require certification, which involves identifying a representative to oversee the REMS program and providing patients with a medication guide and brochure each time the drug is dispensed, detailing the risks of birth defects.

Combination bupropion-naltrexone (sustained release) is another good option acting on appetite and food craving. Naltrexone is believed to block the feedback inhibitory circuit of bupropion to give greater weight loss [91]. Bupropion has some cardiovascular and psychiatric side effects especially in individuals less than 24 years of age, and experts recommend it not be first line, but reserved for smokers with obesity [47].

The currently available sympathomimetic drugs (phentermine, diethylpropion, benzphetamine, and phendimetrazine) are only approved for use for up to 12 weeks, because of their potential cardiovascular side effects and potential for abuse. Use requires regulatory surveillance. They are contraindicated in patients with coronary heart disease, hypertension, hyperthyroidism, or in patients with a history of drug abuse.

There are few head-to-head trials comparing the efficacy, safety, and tolerability of the approved medications to each other, and meta-analyses haven't demonstrated large differences between the medications [47]. Many of the trials have limitations including short duration of study, high attrition rates, heterogeneity, and inadequate reporting of important clinical outcomes [47]. One head-to-head trial deserves mention, however: in this trial, the efficacy of liraglutide was compared to orlistat. Patients on the two highest doses of liraglutide (2.4 and 3.0 mg) lost significantly more weight than those assigned to orlistat (6.3, 7.2, and 4.1 kg, respectively), and these results persisted in a 2-year extension [47].

2.6.7 Dietary Supplements and Procedures to Avoid

Due to safety concerns, several over-the-counter and dietary supplements are not recommended for use by experts, and these include Emagrece Sim (also known as the Brazilian diet pill), Herbathin dietary supplement (contains prescription drugs, including amphetamines, benzodiazepines, and fluoxetine), *Citrus aurantium* (contains synephrine and increases heart rate and blood pressure), *Garcinia cambogia* (causes hepatic failure), ephedrine (a sympathomimetic amine with a prolonged duration of action), and ephedra and ephedra alkaloids like Ma huang (ephedrine-like molecules with cardiac concerns) [47].

Several other supplements are not recommended as they have not demonstrated efficacy. These include but are not limited to green tea, conjugated linoleic acid, chitosan, chromium, gambisan, *Hoodia gordonii*, *Cynanchum auriculatum*, guar gum preparations, human chorionic gonadotropin,and calcium [47].

Liposuction should also be avoided as there is no evidence that it improves insulin sensitivity or coronary risk factors and is associated with increased risk of several adverse surgery-related outcomes [44].

2.6.8 Bariatric Surgery

There are several types of bariatric surgeries, all of which are associated with greater weight loss than comprehensive lifestyle interventions (15–30% as opposed to 4%) and much longer periods of successful weight-loss maintenance (years as opposed to months) [44]. The mean changes in body weight for 2, 10, 15, and 20 years after bariatric surgery are 23%, 17%, 16%, and 18%, respectively [56]. It is similarly much more effective in the short and long term compared to the available pharmacotherapeutic agents for obesity and morbid obesity. Candidates for bariatric surgery include adults with a BMI ≥40 kg/m or a BMI of 35 to 39.9 kg/m^2 with at least one serious comorbidity, who have not met weight loss goals with diet, exercise, and drug therapy [44]. In an important intervention study, after 10–20 years of follow-up after surgery (gastric banding, vertical banded gastroplasty, or gastric bypass), reductions in obesity-related morbidity (diabetes, hypertension, dyslipidemia) and overall mortality (hazard ratio 0.71) were observed in the bariatric surgery group compared with the conventionally treated group receiving a comprehensive lifestyle intervention [44]. Robust weight loss effects are reported in many other systematic reviews and meta-analyses of randomized trials [44]. Besides weight loss, other health benefits include normalization of other hormone imbalances (e.g., testosterone), reduced inflammation, and reduced incidences of diabetes, myocardial infarction, stroke, cancer, and improved overall mortality [56].

It is important for surgeons to collaborate with mental health providers. Neuropsychiatric complications, such as increased suicide risk, may also occur after surgeries [15]. Inadequate weight loss or weight regain after bariatric surgery can be found with several psychiatric conditions including BED, so higher monitoring and collaborative care should be utilized more in high-risk patients such as these pre- and post-surgery [121].

Bariatric surgical procedures affect weight loss through two fundamental mechanisms: by causing malabsorption and by reducing the stomach's reservoir capacity, the latter oftentimes referred to as a restrictive mechanism [122]. Malabsorptive procedures decrease the effectiveness of nutrient absorption by shortening the length of the functional small intestine, either through bypass of the small bowel absorptive surface area or diversion of the biliopancreatic secretions that facilitate absorption [122]. Restrictive procedures work by reducing the stomach's reservoir capacity by resection, bypass, or creation of a gastric outlet [122]. Malabsorptive procedures come with complications, such as protein calorie malnutrition and various micronutrient deficiencies [122]. There is also growing recognition that bariatric surgical procedures contribute to weight loss via several other important mechanisms; these mechanisms include beneficial effects on neurohormone function (ghrelin, GLP-1, CCK) [56, 122], normalization of hedonic brain circuitry (e.g., restoration of dopamine imbalances, reduction in attentional bias to food cues, and improved impulse control) [12, 15, 56, 93, 123] (Chap. 10), increased total energy expenditure [12], negative conditioning (when it causes "dumping syndrome," which is an unpleasant syndrome of nausea, diarrhea, diaphoresis, lightheadedness after eating high-sugar foods), and inflammation-reduction [56, 122]. Weight loss induced by the surgeries can also cause leptin, ghrelin, and insulin function to normalize, which might further promote weight loss [124].

The most commonly performed procedures are Roux-en-Y gastric bypass (RYGB), vertical sleeve gastrectomy (VSG), and adjustable gastric band (BAND). The RYGB procedure is both a restrictive and malabsorptive procedure and is the most commonly performed bariatric procedures, with expected weight loss of 70% by 2 years [56, 122]. VSG is a partial gastrectomy and is a primarily restrictive procedure [56, 122] with expected weight loss of 60% by 2 years. Adjustable gastric banding is the least likely to be performed of the three [56, 122].There are several other procedures which are even less likely performed and outside the scope of this book.

2.7 Conclusion

In conclusion, obesity is important to identify and address, and there are numerous available treatment options, although the mainstays of treatment are to (1) teach people how to adopt a healthy diet which they can adhere to long-term despite reduction in calorie intake, (2) encourage an increase in physical exercise, and (3) provide behavioral support for these major lifestyle changes and to help people cope with the barriers and pitfalls that arise along the way.

References

1. Perrault L. Obesity in adults: prevalence, screening and evaluation. 2018 Pi-Sunyer FX, Martin CA. Accessed Aug 2 2018. In: UpToDate. Wolters Kluwer. Available from: www.uptodate.com.
2. Ng M, Fleming T, Robinson M, Thomson B, Graetz N, Margono C, et al. Global, regional, and national prevalence of overweight and obesity in children and adults during 1980–2013: a systematic analysis for the Global Burden of Disease Study 2013. Lancet. 2014;384(9945):766–81.
3. Adams RC, Sedgmond J, Maizey L, Chambers CD, Lawrence NS. Food addiction: implications for the diagnosis and treatment of overeating. Nutrients. 2019;11(9)
4. Sinha R. Role of addiction and stress neurobiology on food intake and obesity. Biol Psychol. 2018;131:5–13.
5. De Lorenzo A, Romano L, Di Renzo L, Di Lorenzo N, Cenname G, Gualtieri P. Obesity: a preventable, treatable, but relapsing disease. Nutrition. 2020;71:110615.
6. Wiss D, Brewerton T. Separating the signal from the noise: how psychiatric diagnoses can help discern food addiction from dietary restraint. Nutrients. 2020;12(10)
7. Schulte EM, Wadden TA, Allison KC. An evaluation of food addiction as a distinct psychiatric disorder. Int J Eat Disord. 2020;53(10):1610–22.
8. Jia H, Lubetkin EI. Trends in quality-adjusted life-years lost contributed by smoking and obesity. Am J Prev Med. 2010;38(2):138–44.

9. Cherikh F, Frey S, Bel C, Attanasi G, Alifano M, Iannelli A. Behavioral food addiction during lockdown: time for awareness, time to prepare the aftermath. Obes Surg. 2020;30(9):3585–7.
10. Rolland B, Haesebaert F, Zante E, Benyamina A, Haesebaert J, Franck N. Global changes and factors of increase in caloric/salty food intake, screen use, and substance use during the early COVID-19 containment phase in the general population in France: survey study. JMIR Public Health Surveill. 2020;6(3):e19630.
11. Van de Graaf RC, Hofstra L. Obesity and covid-19: the role of the food industry. BMJ. 2020;370:m2813.
12. O'Rourke RW. The pathophysiology of obesity and obesity-related disease. In: Nguyen N, et al., editors. The ASMBS textbook of bariatric surgery. Cham: Springer; 2020.
13. Kauffman BY, Manning K, Rogers AH, Garey L, Gallagher MW, Viana AG, et al. The role of anxiety sensitivity in terms of weight-related impairment and fatigue severity among adulst with obesity and chronic low back pain. Cogn Ther Res. 2020;
14. Perrault L. Obesity in adults: etiology and risk factors. 2018. Pi-Sunyer FX, Martin KA. Accessed Aug 2 2018. In: UpToDate. Wolters Kluwer. Available from: www.uptodate.com.
15. Morin JP, Rodriguez-Duran LF, Guzman-Ramos K, Perez-Cruz C, Ferreira G, Diaz-Cintra S, et al. Palatable hyper-caloric foods impact on neuronal plasticity. Front Behav Neurosci. 2017;11:19.
16. Schiestl ET, Rios JM, Parnarouskis L, Cummings JR, Gearhardt AN. A narrative review of highly processed food addiction across the lifespan. Prog Neuro-Psychopharmacol Biol Psychiatry. 2021;106:110152.
17. Lohman BJ, Neppl TK, Lee Y, Diggs ON, Russell D. The association between household food insecurity and body mass index: a prospective growth curve analysis. J Pediatr. 2018;202:115–20 e1.
18. Palmisano GL, Innamorati M, Vanderlinden J. Life adverse experiences in relation with obesity and binge eating disorder: a systematic review. J Behav Addict. 2016;5(1):11–31.
19. Wiss DA, Brewerton TD. Adverse childhood experiences and adult obesity: a systematic review of plausible mechanisms and meta-analysis of cross-sectional studies. Physiol Behav. 2020;223:112964.
20. Tobore TO. Towards a comprehensive theory of obesity and a healthy diet: the causal role of oxidative stress in food addiction and obesity. Behav Brain Res. 2020;384:112560.
21. Nedeltcheva AV, Kilkus JM, Imperial J, Schoeller DA Penev PD. Insufficient sleep undermines dietary efforts to reduce adiposity. Ann Intern Med. 2010;153(7):435–41.
22. Greer SM, Goldstein AN, Walker MP. The impact of sleep deprivation on food desire in the human brain. Nat Commun. 2013;4:2259.
23. Spiegel K, Tasali E, Penev P, Van Cauter E. Brief communication: sleep curtailment in healthy young men is associated with decreased leptin levels, elevated ghrelin levels, and increased hunger and appetite. Ann Intern Med. 2004;141(11):846–50.
24. Katsunuma R, Oba K, Kitamura S, Motomura Y, Terasawa Y, Nakazaki K, et al. Unrecognized sleep loss accumulated in daily life can promote brain hyperreactivity to food cue. Sleep. 2017;40(10)
25. Jensen CD, Duraccio KM, Barnett KA, Carbine KA, Stevens KS, Muncy NM, et al. Sleep duration differentially affects brain activation in response to food images in adolescents with overweight/obesity compared to adolescents with normal weight. Sleep. 2019;42(4)
26. Apovian CM, Aronne LJ, Bessesen DH, McDonnell ME, Murad MH, Pagotto U, et al. Pharmacological management of obesity: an endocrine Society clinical practice guideline. J Clin Endocrinol Metab. 2015;100(2):342–62.
27. Cope RJ, Fischetti BS, Kavanagh RK, Lepa TM, Sorbera MA. Safety and efficacy of weight-loss pharmacotherapy in persons living with HIV: a review of the literature and potential drug-drug interactions with antiretroviral therapy. Pharmacotherapy. 2019;39(12):1204–15.
28. Abela AR, Ji XD, Li Z, Le AD, Fletcher PJ. Clozapine reliably increases the motivation for food: parsing the role of the 5-HT2c and H1 receptors. Psychopharmacology. 2020;237(4):957–66.
29. Kaisari P, Dourish CT, Higgs S. Attention Deficit Hyperactivity Disorder (ADHD) and disordered eating behaviour: a systematic review and a framework for future research. Clin Psychol Rev. 2017;53:109–21.
30. Faber A, Dube L, Knauper B. Attachment and eating: a meta-analytic review of the relevance of attachment for unhealthy and healthy eating behaviors in the general population. Appetite. 2018;123:410–38.
31. Ouwens MA, van Strien T, van Leeuwe JF. Possible pathways between depression, emotional and external eating. A structural equation model. Appetite. 2009;53(2):245–8.
32. Alblas MC, Mollen S, Fransen ML, van den Putte B. Food at first sight: visual attention to palatable food cues on TV and subsequent unhealthy food intake in unsuccessful restrained eaters. Appetite. 2020;147:104574.
33. Lescher M, Wegmann E, Muller SM, Laskowski NM, Wunder R, Jimenez-Murcia S, et al. A randomized study of food pictures-influenced decision-making under ambiguity in individuals with morbid obesity. Front Psych. 2020;11:822.
34. Weiss F, Barbuti M, Carignani G, Calderone A, Santini F, Maremmani I, et al. Psychiatric aspects of obesity: a narrative review of pathophysiology and psychopathology. J Clin Med. 2020;9(8)
35. Wardle J, Carnell S, Haworth CM, Plomin R. Evidence for a strong genetic influence on childhood adiposity despite the force of the obesogenic environment. Am J Clin Nutr. 2008;87(2):398–404.

36. Perrault L. Genetic contribution and pathophysiology of obesity. 2018. Pi-Sunyer FX, Martin KA. Accessed Aug 2 2018. In: UpToDate. Wolters Kluwer. Available from: www.uptodate.com.
37. Willyard C. Heritability: the family roots of obesity. Nature. 2014;508(7496):S58–60.
38. Locke AE, Kahali B, Berndt SI, Justice AE, Pers TH, Day FR, et al. Genetic studies of body mass index yield new insights for obesity biology. Nature. 2015;518(7538):197–206.
39. Li J, Song J, Zaytseva YY, Liu Y, Rychahou P, Jiang K, et al. An obligatory role for neurotensin in high-fat-diet-induced obesity. Nature. 2016;533(7603):411–5.
40. Heber D, Carpenter CL. Addictive genes and the relationship to obesity and inflammation. Mol Neurobiol. 2011;44(2):160–5.
41. Kinasz KR, Ross DA Cooper JJ. Eat to live or live to eat? The neurobiology of appetite regulation. Biol Psychiatry. 2017;81(9):e73–e5.
42. Milaneschi Y, Lamers F, Bot M, Drent ML, Penninx BW. Leptin dysregulation is specifically associated with major depression with atypical features: evidence for a mechanism connecting obesity and depression. Biol Psychiatry. 2017;81(9):807–14.
43. Espeso-Gil S, Halene T, Bendl J, Kassim B, Ben Hutta G, Iskhakova M, et al. A chromosomal connectome for psychiatric and metabolic risk variants in adult dopaminergic neurons. Genome Med. 2020;12(1):19.
44. Perrault L. Obesity in adults: Overview of management. 2018. Pi-Sunyer FX, Seres D, Martin KA. Accessed Aug 2 2018. In: UpToDate. Wolters Kluwer. Available from: www.uptodate.com.
45. Bray GA, Fruhbeck G, Ryan DH, Wilding JP. Management of obesity. Lancet. 2016;387(10031):1947–56.
46. Perrault L. Obesity in adults: dietary therapy. 2021. Kiunins L, Seres D, Pi-Sunyer FX. Accessed Jan 1 2021. In: UpToDate. Wolters Kluwer. Available from: www.updtodate.com.
47. Perrault L. Obesity in adults: drug therapy. 2018. Mulder J, Pi-Sunyer FX. Accessed Aug 2 2018. In: UpToDate. Wolters Kluwer. Available from: www.uptodate.com.
48. Buchanan RW. How much of an advance is the addition of samidorphan to olanzapine? Am J Psychiatry. 2020;177(12):1113–4.
49. Siskind DJ, Leung J, Russell AW, Wysoczanski D, Kisely S. Metformin for clozapine associated obesity: a systematic review and meta-analysis. PLoS One. 2016;11(6):e0156208.
50. Preuss H, Pinnow M, Schnicker K, Legenbauer T. Improving inhibitory control abilities (ImpulsE)-a promising approach to treat impulsive eating? Eur Eat Disord Rev. 2017;25(6):533–43.
51. Meule A. A critical examination of the practical implications derived from the food addiction concept. Curr Obes Rep. 2019;8(1):11–7.
52. Webber KH, Casey EM, Mayes L, Katsumata Y, Mellin L. A comparison of a behavioral weight loss program to a stress management program: a pilot randomized controlled trial. Nutrition. 2016;32(7–8):904–9.
53. Naumann E, Svaldi J, Wyschka T, Heinrichs M, von Dawans B. Stress-induced body dissatisfaction in women with binge eating disorder. J Abnorm Psychol. 2018;127(6):548–58.
54. Forman EM, Butryn ML. A new look at the science of weight control: how acceptance and commitment strategies can address the challenge of self-regulation. Appetite. 2015;84:171–80.
55. Forman EM, Shaw JA, Goldstein SP, Butryn ML, Martin LM, Meiran N, et al. Mindful decision making and inhibitory control training as complementary means to decrease snack consumption. Appetite. 2016;103:176–83.
56. Lin Z, Qu S. Legend of weight loss: a crosstalk between the bariatric surgery and the brain. Obes Surg. 2020;30(5):1988–2002.
57. Higgins GA, Zeeb FD, Fletcher PJ. Role of impulsivity and reward in the anti-obesity actions of 5-HT2C receptor agonists. J Psychopharmacol. 2017;31(11):1403–18.
58. Brownell KD. The Learn Program for Weight Management. 10th ed. American Health Publishing Company; 2004.
59. Dansinger ML, Gleason JA, Griffith JL, Selker HP, Schaefer EJ. Comparison of the Atkins, Ornish, Weight Watchers, and Zone diets for weight loss and heart disease risk reduction: a randomized trial. JAMA. 2005;293(1):43–53.
60. San-Cristobal R, Navas-Carretero S, Martinez-Gonzalez MA, Ordovas JM, Martinez JA. Contribution of macronutrients to obesity: implications for precision nutrition. Nat Rev Endocrinol. 2020;16(6):305–20.
61. Ge L, Sadeghirad B, Ball GDC, da Costa BR, Hitchcock CL, Svendrovski A, et al. Comparison of dietary macronutrient patterns of 14 popular named dietary programmes for weight and cardiovascular risk factor reduction in adults: systematic review and network meta-analysis of randomised trials. BMJ. 2020;369:m696.
62. Bhutani S, Klempel MC, Kroeger CM, Trepanowski JF, Varady KA. Alternate day fasting and endurance exercise combine to reduce body weight and favorably alter plasma lipids in obese humans. Obesity. 2013;21(7):1370–9.
63. de Cabo R, Mattson MP. Effects of intermittent fasting on health, aging, and disease. N Engl J Med. 2019;381(26):2541–51.

64. Hoddy KK, Kroeger CM, Trepanowski JF, Barnosky AR, Bhutani S, Varady KA. Safety of alternate day fasting and effect on disordered eating behaviors. Nutr J. 2015;14:44.
65. Barnosky A, Kroeger CM, Trepanowski JF, Klempel MC, Bhutani S, Hoddy KK, et al. Effect of alternate day fasting on markers of bone metabolism: an exploratory analysis of a 6-month randomized controlled trial. Nutr Healthy Aging. 2017;4(3):255–63.
66. Trepanowski JF, Kroeger CM, Barnosky A, Klempel M, Bhutani S, Hoddy KK, et al. Effects of alternate-day fasting or daily calorie restriction on body composition, fat distribution, and circulating adipokines: secondary analysis of a randomized controlled trial. Clin Nutr, 6 Pt A. 2018;37:1871–8.
67. Trepanowski JF, Kroeger CM, Barnosky A, Klempel MC, Bhutani S, Hoddy KK, et al. Effect of alternate-day fasting on weight loss, weight maintenance, and cardioprotection among metabolically healthy obese adults: a randomized clinical trial. JAMA Intern Med. 2017;177(7):930–8.
68. Catenacci VA, Pan Z, Ostendorf D, Brannon S, Gozansky WS, Mattson MP, et al. A randomized pilot study comparing zero-calorie alternate-day fasting to daily caloric restriction in adults with obesity. Obesity. 2016;24(9):1874–83.
69. Grigolon RB, Brietzke E, Trevizol AP, McIntyre RS, Mansur RB. Caloric restriction, resting metabolic rate and cognitive performance in non-obese adults: a post-hoc analysis from CALERIE study. J Psychiatr Res. 2020;128:16–22.
70. Sievenpiper JL. Low-carbohydrate diets and cardiometabolic health: the importance of carbohydrate quality over quantity. Nutr Rev. 2020;78(Suppl 1):69–77.
71. Gershuni VM, Yan SL, Medici V. Nutritional ketosis for weight management and reversal of metabolic syndrome. Curr Nutr Rep. 2018;7(3):97–106.
72. Wang W, Li J, Chen X, Yu M, Pan Q, Guo L. Whole grain food diet slightly reduces cardiovascular risks in obese/overweight adults: a systematic review and meta-analysis. BMC Cardiovasc Disord. 2020;20(1):82.
73. Lustig RH, Schmidt LA Brindis CD. Public health: the toxic truth about sugar. Nature. 2012;482(7383):27–9.
74. Moon J, Koh G. Clinical evidence and mechanisms of high-protein diet-induced weight loss. J Obes Metab Syndr. 2020;29(3):166–73.
75. Onaolapo AY, Onaolapo OJ. Food additives, food and the concept of 'food addiction': is stimulation of the brain reward circuit by food sufficient to trigger addiction? Pathophysiology. 2018;25(4):263–76.
76. Alhamdan BA, Garcia-Alvarez A, Alzahrnai AH, Karanxha J, Stretchberry DR, Contrera KJ, et al. Alternate-day versus daily energy restriction diets: which is more effective for weight loss? A systematic review and meta-analysis. Obes Sci Pract. 2016;2(3):293–302.
77. Sethi Dalai S, Sinha A, Gearhardt AN. Low carbohydrate ketogenic therapy as a metabolic treatment for binge eating and ultraprocessed food addiction. Curr Opin Endocrinol Diabetes Obes. 2020;27(5):275–82.
78. Di Rosa C, Lattanzi G, Taylor SF, Manfrini S, Khazrai YM. Very low calorie ketogenic diets in overweight and obesity treatment: effects on anthropometric parameters, body composition, satiety, lipid profile and microbiota. Obes Res Clin Pract. 2020;14(6):491–503.
79. Yen HY, Chiu HL. The effectiveness of wearable technologies as physical activity interventions in weight control: a systematic review and meta-analysis of randomized controlled trials. Obes Rev. 2019;20(10):1485–93.
80. Perrault L. Obesity in adults: behavioral therapy. 2018. Pi-Sunyer FX, Kunins L. Accessed Dec 8 2018. In: UpToDate. Wolters Kluwer. Available from: www.uptodate.com.
81. Gokee-LaRose J. Adult behavioral weight loss treatment. Med Health R I. 2009;92(2):50–2.
82. Levoy E, Lazaridou A, Brewer J, Fulwiler C. An exploratory study of Mindfulness Based Stress Reduction for emotional eating. Appetite. 2017;109:124–30.
83. Tapper K. Can mindfulness influence weight management related eating behaviors? If so, how? Clin Psychol Rev. 2017;53:122–34.
84. Fuentes Artiles R, Staub K, Aldakak L, Eppenberger P, Ruhli F, Bender N. Mindful eating and common diet programs lower body weight similarly: systematic review and meta-analysis. Obes Rev. 2019;20(11):1619–27.
85. Ruffault A, Czernichow S, Hagger MS, Ferrand M, Erichot N, Carette C, et al. The effects of mindfulness training on weight-loss and health-related behaviours in adults with overweight and obesity: a systematic review and meta-analysis. Obes Res Clin Pract. 2017;11(5 Suppl 1):90–111.
86. Warren JM, Smith N, Ashwell M. A structured literature review on the role of mindfulness, mindful eating and intuitive eating in changing eating behaviours: effectiveness and associated potential mechanisms. Nutr Res Rev. 2017;30(2):272–83.
87. Wangen KE. Mindful eating. In: Zerbo E, Schlechter A, Desai S, Levounis P, editors. Becoming mindful integrating mindfulness into your psychiatric practice. Virginia: American Psychiatric Association Publishing; 2017.
88. Palmeira L, Pinto-Gouveia J, Cunha M. Exploring the efficacy of an acceptance, mindfulness & compassionate-based group intervention for women struggling with their weight (Kg-Free): a randomized controlled trial. Appetite. 2017;112:107–16.

89. O'Reilly GA, Cook L, Spruijt-Metz D, Black DS. Mindfulness-based interventions for obesity-related eating behaviours: a literature review. Obes Rev. 2014;15(6):453–61.
90. Barnes RD, Ivezaj V, Martino S, Pittman BP, Grilo CM. Back to basics? No weight loss from motivational interviewing compared to nutrition psychoeducation at one-year follow-up. Obesity. 2017;25(12):2074–8.
91. Coulter AA, Rebello CJ, Greenway FL. Centrally acting agents for obesity: past, present, and future. Drugs. 2018;78(11):1113–32.
92. Gadde KM, Atkins KD. The limits and challenges of antiobesity pharmacotherapy. Expert Opin Pharmacother. 2020;21(11):1319–28.
93. Ben-Porat T, Weiss R, Sherf-Dagan S, Rottenstreich A, Kaluti D, Khalaileh A, et al. Food addiction and binge eating during one year following sleeve gastrectomy: prevalence and implications for postoperative outcomes. Obes Surg. 2021;31(2):603–11.
94. Bray GA. Drug treatment of obesity. Bailliere Clin Endocrinol Metab. 1999;13(1):131–48.
95. Lexicomp. Benzphetamine. Available from: http://online.lexi.com/lco/action/doc/retrieve/docid/patch_f/6438.
96. Lexicomp. Diethylpropion. Available from: http://online.lexi.com/lco/action/doc/retrieve/docid/patch_f/6740.
97. Pi-Sunyer X, Astrup A, Fujioka K, Greenway F, Halpern A, Krempf M, et al. A randomized, controlled trial of 3.0 mg of liraglutide in weight management. N Engl J Med. 2015;373(1):11–22.
98. Dong Z, Xu L, Liu H, Lv Y, Zheng Q, Li L. Comparative efficacy of five long-term weight loss drugs: quantitative information for medication guidelines. Obes Rev. 2017;18(12):1377–85.
99. Lexicomp. Liraglutide. Available from: http://online.lexi.com/lco/action/doc/retrieve/docid/patch_f/2144379.
100. Lexicomp. Naltrexone and Bupropion. Available from: http://online.lexi.com/lco/action/doc/retrieve/docid/patch_f/5338462.
101. Bansal AB, Al Khalili Y. Orlistat Treasure Island (FL): StatPearls Publishing; 2020. [updated 2020/11/22. Available from: https://www.statpearls.com/articlelibrary/viewarticle/26335/.
102. Lexicomp. Phendimetrazine. Available from: http://online.lexi.com/lco/action/doc/retrieve/docid/patch_f/7475.
103. Garcia Ramirez AV, Filho DR Zotarelli Filho IJ (2020) Meta-analysis and approach of the real impact of anorexigenic drugs in the obesity in humans: the last five years of the randomized studies. Curr Diabetes Rev 16(7):750–758.
104. Lexicomp. Phentermine. Available from: http://online.lexi.com/lco/action/doc/retrieve/docid/patch_f/7481.
105. Lexicomp. Phentermine Topiramate. Available from: http://online.lexi.com/lco/action/doc/retrieve/docid/patch_f/3832942.
106. Lexicomp. Setmelanotide. Available from: http://online.lexi.com/lco/action/doc/retrieve/docid/patch_f/7037631.
107. Srivastava G, Apovian C. Future pharmacotherapy for obesity: new anti-obesity drugs on the horizon. Curr Obes Rep. 2018;7(2):147–61.
108. Yerevanian A, Soukas AA. Metformin: mechanisms in human obesity and weight loss. Curr Obes Rep. 2019;8(2):156–64.
109. Lexicomp. Metformin. Available from: http://online.lexi.com/lco/action/doc/retrieve/docid/patch_f/7260.
110. Reas DL, Grilo CM. Pharmacological treatment of binge eating disorder: update review and synthesis. Expert Opin Pharmacother. 2015;16(10):1463–78.
111. Lexicomp. Topiramate. Available from: http://online.lexi.com/lco/action/doc/retrieve/docid/patch_f/7789.
112. Lexicomp. Semaglutide. Available from: http://online.lexi.com/lco/action/doc/retrieve/docid/patch_f/6577162.
113. Bello NT, Yeomans BL. Safety of pharmacotherapy options for bulimia nervosa and binge eating disorder. Expert Opin Drug Saf. 2018;17(1):17–23.
114. Lexicomp. Fluoxetine. Available from: http://online.lexi.com/lco/action/doc/retrieve/docid/patch_f/6931.
115. Lexicomp. Lisdexamfetamine. Available from: http://online.lexi.com/lco/action/doc/retrieve/docid/patch_f/810062.
116. Aigner M, Treasure J, Kaye W, Kasper S, Disorders WTFOE. World Federation of Societies of Biological Psychiatry (WFSBP) guidelines for the pharmacological treatment of eating disorders. World J Biol Psychiatry. 2011;12(6):400–43.
117. Hirsch M. Selective serotonin reuptake inhibitors: pharmacology, administration, and side effects. Waltham, MA: UpToDate; 2020. [updated 2020/3/16. Available from: https://www.uptodate.com/contents/selective-serotonin-reuptake-inhibitors-pharmacology-administration-and-side-effects.
118. Hirsch M. Tricyclic and tetracyclic drugs: pharmacology, administration, and side effects. Waltham, MA: UpToDate; 2020. [updated 2020/12/3. Available from: https://www.uptodate.com/contents/tricyclic-and-tetracyclic-drugs-pharmacology-administration-and-side-effects.
119. McElroy SL, Kotwal R, Guerdjikova AI, Welge JA, Nelson EB, Lake KA, et al. Zonisamide in the treatment of binge eating disorder with obesity: a randomized controlled trial. J Clin Psychiatry. 2006;67(12):1897–906.
120. Wilding JPH, Batterham RL, Calanna S, Davies M, Van Gaal LF, Lingvay I, et al. Once-weekly semaglutide in adults with overweight or obesity. N Engl J Med. 2021;
121. Mechanick JI, Youdim A, Jones DB, Garvey WT, Hurley DL, McMahon MM, et al. Clinical practice guidelines for the perioperative nutritional, metabolic, and nonsurgical support of the bariatric sur-

gery patient–2013 update: cosponsored by American Association of Clinical Endocrinologists, The Obesity Society, and American Society for Metabolic & Bariatric Surgery. Obesity. 2013;21 Suppl 1:S1–27.
122. Lim RB. Bariatric operations for management of obesity: indications and perioperative preparation. 2018. Jones D, Chen W. Accessed Aug 2 2018. In: UpToDate. Wolters Kluwer. Available from: www.uptodate.com.
123. Schafer L, Schmidt R, Muller SM, Dietrich A, Hilbert A. Changes in visual attention towards food cues after obesity surgery: an eye-tracking study. J Psychiatr Res. 2020;129:214–21.
124. Jimenez-Murcia S, Aguera Z, Paslakis G, Munguia L, Granero R, Sanchez-Gonzalez J, et al. Food addiction in eating disorders and obesity: analysis of clusters and implications for treatment. Nutrients. 2019;11(11)

3 Binge-Related Eating Disorders (Binge Eating Disorder and Bulimia Nervosa)

3.1 Epidemiology

Binge eating, characterized as uncontrollably consuming objectively large quantities of food in a discrete period of time, was recognized as a clinical condition as early as 1959; was a provisional diagnosis in the fourth edition of the DSM-IV needing more study; [1] and was first recognized as a distinct diagnosis in 2013 with the advent of the DSM-V [2, 3]. BED is a heterogeneous and complex disorder [1, 4] with several levels of severity and varied pictures. Furthermore, subthreshold BED does not differ significantly from full-syndrome BED regarding outcomes such as body weight, eating disorder (ED) symptoms, and associated psychiatric symptoms.

The prevalence of BED among American women is 3.5%, among men it is 2.0% [5], and it is 2.6% across genders [1]. BED is more prevalent than either anorexia nervosa or BN, is more common across both sexes than the other eating disorders [6, 7], and is the most common eating disorder in the world [1]. It typically emerges in adolescence or early adulthood and may persist well beyond midlife [3]. BED is more common in obese individuals and can be present in up to 5–30% of those seeking obesity treatment [3].

3.2 Diagnosis and Assessment of BED

To meet criteria for a BED diagnosis, individuals have to report a lack of control over eating and related emotional distress, binge eating at least once per week. Furthermore, they need to not demonstrate compensatory (e.g., vomiting, excessive exercising) behavior. (Box 3.1).

Box 3.1 DSM-V Criteria for BED [2, 8, 9]

1. Recurrent episodes of binge eating
   - (i) Eating, in a discrete period of time (e.g., within any 2-hour period), an amount of food that is definitely larger than what most people would eat in a similar period of time under similar circumstances.
   - (ii) A sense of lack of control over eating during the episode (e.g., a feeling that one cannot stop eating or control what or how much one is eating).
2. The binge eating episodes are associated with three (or more) of the following:
   - (i) Eating much more rapidly than normal.

C. E. Wilcox, *Food Addiction, Obesity, and Disorders of Overeating*,
https://doi.org/10.1007/978-3-030-83078-6_3

(ii) Eating until feeling uncomfortably full.
(iii) Eating large amounts of food when not feeling physically hungry.
(iv) Eating alone because of feeling embarrassed by how much one is eating.
(v) Feeling disgusted with oneself, depressed, or very guilty afterward.
(vi) Marked distress regarding binge eating is present.

3. The binge eating occurs, on average, at least once a week for 3 months.
4. The binge eating is not associated with the recurrent use of inappropriate compensatory behavior as in bulimia nervosa and does not occur exclusively during the course of bulimia nervosa or anorexia nervosa.

BED is associated with numerous psychiatric and nonpsychiatric disorders [3, 6, 7]. A diagnosis of BED is often accompanied by impairment in psychosocial functioning, which can be severe in up to 20% of individuals [6]. BED is associated with poorer psychological well-being, including major depressive disorders, anxiety disorders, and substance use disorders, relationship distress and impaired social role functioning, as well as physical problems, including chronic pain, obesity, diabetes, metabolic syndrome and cardiovascular disease, gastrointestinal problems such as gastroesophageal reflux disease (GERD) or hepatobiliary disease, obstructive sleep apnea, and urinary incontinence [3, 6, 10]. Diabetes and metabolic syndrome can develop independent of weight [3, 10]. Therefore, the evaluation of the patient with BED should involve an in-depth psychological/psychiatric and physical evaluation, including measurement of body mass index (BMI), waist circumference, and blood pressure, and laboratory screens for diabetes, hyperlipidemia, and hepatobiliary disease [6].

For the development of a treatment plan, a comprehensive nutritional assessment is needed, and the treating clinician should ask about weight and dieting history, current eating pattern and food choices, types of overeating (at meals, snacking and grazing, night eating), frequency and intensity of binge eating episodes, physical activity, and exercise patterns [6]. Patients should also be asked about self-concept and attitudes towards body weight and shape and self-esteem [6]. Finally, the clinician should ask about compensatory behavior to assess for BN. If obese, treatment recommendations may be different (see below section for special considerations in individuals with BED and obesity) because treatment goals may also include reduction of body weight [6].

3.3 Epidemiology of BN

BN is more common in females than males (3:1), and the median age of onset is age 20 years [11]. Lifetime prevalence has been estimated to be approximately 2.3% [12]. Mild psychosocial impairment (home, work, personal life, or social life) was observed in 78% of patients and severe impairment in 16% [11]. Clinical features of BN share significant overlap with anorexia nervosa; however, unlike in anorexia, body weight in those with BN is usually at or above the normal range [11].

3.4 Diagnosis and Assessment of BN

Like with BED, a diagnosis of BN requires binge eating and loss of control but also includes a requirement for compensatory measures and excessive concern about body weight and shape (Box 3.2).

Box 3.2 DSM-V Criteria for BN [2, 13]

1. Recurrent episodes of binge eating. An episode of binge eating is characterized by both of the following:
   (i) Eating, in a discrete period of time (e.g., within any 2-hour period), an amount of food that is definitely larger than what most individuals would eat in a similar period of time under similar circumstances.
   (ii) A sense of lack of control over eating during the episode (e.g., a feeling that one cannot stop eating or control what or how much one is eating).
2. Recurrent inappropriate compensatory behaviors in order to prevent weight gain, such as self-induced vomiting; misuse of laxatives, diuretics, or other medications; fasting; or excessive exercise.
3. The binge eating and inappropriate compensatory behaviors both occur, on average, at least once a week for 3 months.
4. Self-evaluation is unduly influenced by body shape and weight.
5. The disturbance does not occur exclusively during episodes of anorexia nervosa.

The sequence of symptom behaviors is typically calorie restriction (due to desires for weight loss, usually), followed by bingeing, and finally engagement in compensatory measures to counteract the weight gain from bingeing [11]. Typical triggers for binges, other than hunger from restriction, include emotional dysregulation, dysphoria, and interpersonal stressors [11]. Binge eating and inappropriate compensatory behaviors occur at least once a week.

BN is associated with many psychiatric comorbidities. The lifetime prevalences of common comorbidities are unipolar major depression, 50%; specific phobia, 50%; posttraumatic stress disorder (PTSD), 45; social anxiety disorder, 41%; attention-deficit/hyperactivity disorder, 35%; alcohol use disorder, 34%; oppositional defiant disorder, 27%; conduct disorder, 27%; and illicit drug use disorder, 26% [11]. Suicide attempts (SA) are a common experience with a study of more than 3000 subjects diagnosed with BN which indicated 17% of participants having a history of SA [11, 14].

The medical comorbidities of BN are numerous and can include gastrointestinal complications of BN which include but are not limited to gastroesophageal reflux disease (GERD), gastric dilation, malabsorption syndromes, dysmotility syndromes, Mallory-Weiss syndrome (characterized by esophageal tears), diarrhea and constipation, and salivary gland hypertrophy (for which signs on physical exam may include puffy or swollen cheeks). In the medical assessment of individuals with BN, it is common to see type 2 diabetes mellitus (DM), dental enamel erosion, and B12 deficiency. Addison's disease and osteoporosis can develop due to low weight, sex steroid suppression, and malabsorption [10, 13, 15, 16]. Electrolyte imbalances (e.g., hypokalemia, hypochloremia, hyponatremia, metabolic alkalosis, hypomagnesemia, hypophosphatemia) and dehydration are possible complications from compensatory behaviors, and thus patients should be asked about palpitations and dizziness. Blood pressure for hypotension, electrocardiograms (ECG), serum amylase (which can be elevated in recurrent vomiting), and serum electrolytes should be checked [10, 13, 15, 16].

3.5 Etiology and Mechanisms of BED and BN

BED and BN are believed to result from a variety of biopsychosocial factors, which individually vary in degree of contribution. Both disorders are believed to involve placing excessive attention on body image and overvaluing societal messages that "thin is best," engaging in restrictive behaviors (e.g., dysfunctional dieting) leading to compensatory bingeing in an effort to restore caloric balance and maladaptive thought patterns including cognitive distortions [5, 6]. The pattern of restriction and compensatory bingeing typically involves cycles of learning to favor the highly palatable foods which have more rapid calorie restoration effects, leading to cycles of bingeing on these calorie-dense foods.

BED and BN are both characterized by increased impulsivity including general rash-spontaneous behavior in general and specifically towards food [17–21]. Underlying psychiatric conditions including depression, anxiety, and difficulties regulating emotions can also contribute to binge-eating and relate to a tendency to eat emotionally as can attachment security [17]. The emotion regulation model of binge eating posits that individuals with BED binge as a means of regulating emotions. This is supported by the "escape theory," which when applied to binge eating posits that bingeing allows an individual to focus on their immediate environment, the binge, and distract from and avoid their emotional overwhelm and negative affect [22]. Individuals with BED have been shown to have greater difficultly with emotion regulation [23], and individuals with BN report bingeing more in response to negative emotion [24]. Further, the escape theory of binge eating posits that binge eating functions as a method of avoidance of negative emotions, and therefore the cycle of binge eating is maintained by this mechanism.

Biopsychosocial factors such as childhood trauma [25], epigenetics [26], genetics (such as the D4 receptor) [27], and food insecurity can cause and contribute to binge eating behavior and worsening of the disorders [28]. Hormone imbalances (e.g., leptin, ghrelin; see Chap. 1) are observed in BED and BN. For example, ghrelin, an appetite stimulant, is at lower levels in BED than in controls. In a study of individuals with obesity, those with BED had significantly lower concentrations of acyl ghrelin (AG) compared to those without BED. Fasting and post-meal hunger rates in those with BED were also higher than the non-BED group, and so the lower AG concentrations were thought to be related to downregulation secondary to the overeating behavior [29].

3.6 Treatment of BED: General Considerations

Depending on comorbidities, treatment goals may vary from patient to patient, so establishing these goals during treatment plan development is important [6]. Treatment goals will almost always include reducing binge eating episodes [6]. If the patient is overweight (BMI 25–30) or obese (BMI > 30), another treatment goal may be to reduce excess weight [6]. Enhancing self-acceptance of body image may be another goal if the patient is excessively concerned about body image [6, 30]. Further, treatments for body image are an important element of CBT and should be considered for all eating disorder patients with binge eating [30, 31]. However, whether they reduce binge eating or promote weight loss is not entirely clear from the research [31].

Finally, the treatment of psychiatric comorbidities such as anxiety, depression, and substance use disorder and related medical problems are an essential part of the recovery plan [6]. BED treatment nearly always takes place on an outpatient basis unless the patient has other acute psychiatric or medical needs that require a more intense level of care [6].

Regarding psychotherapy, treatments are recommended based on patient preference and disorder severity. This may include several forms of psychotherapy such as CBT, interpersonal psychotherapy (IPT), dialectical behavior therapy (DBT), psychodynamic psychotherapy, self-help treatment and behavioral weight loss treatment (discussed more in Chap. 2), and pharmacotherapy [6].

3.7 Psychotherapies for BED

The first-line treatment for BED is CBT. CBT for BED was originally adapted from CBT for BN [5] (see Table 3.1 for key elements of treatment). CBT for all eating disorders is based on the prin-

Table 3.1 Elements of psychotherapies for BED [5, 6, 9]

Cognitive behavior therapy	Interpersonal therapy	Dialectical behavior therapy
1. Education about binge eating and its causes 2. Improving recognition of high-risk situations to trigger bingeing 3. Teaching coping skills (e.g., stimulus control, problem-solving, restructuring feelings) 4. Relapse prevention	1. Identifying the interpersonal problem area or areas that are most closely linked to binge eating (e.g., grief, interpersonal role dispute, role transition, interpersonal deficit) 2. Use of discussion, problem solving, and experimentation to correct problems (do not frame BED as the problem) 3. When combined with CBT can help address common underlying contributors such as low self-esteem, perfectionism and interpersonal challenges	1. Improve emotion regulation through psychoeducation and skills 2. Increased mindfulness (present moment awareness) 3. Teach distress tolerance skills to manage feelings related to binge eating 3. Improve interpersonal effectiveness skills to manage interpersonal distress

ciple that one of the core pathologies is an overvaluation of shape and weight in determining self-worth, which is in part fueled by either societal or familial pressures to eat less or lose weight [5, 8]. As a general rule however, CBT doesn't result in weight loss [5, 6, 32]. Another guiding principle of CBT for BED is that individuals with BED are especially sensitive to cues in the environment such as particular settings or food availability that can trigger cravings, which can then override proper satiety mechanisms, and lead to subsequent binge eating. Individuals in treatment will complete food diaries where they monitor food intake as well as the circumstances and emotional reactions surrounding the binge episode in order to identify and modify maladaptive patterns [32–34]. The vicious cycle of bingeing starts because an individual's overweight causes distress and low self-esteem which leads to dietary restraint which leads to more binge eating and weight gain [5, 32]. CBT is usually delivered in 20 weekly sessions for both BN and BED and is focused on providing education, generating insight into the pattern of binge eating, facilitating behavioral change, and altering maladaptive thinking patterns that maintain this cycle [13, 15]. Self-help CBT is based on the same principles as therapist-led CBT and utilizes many of the same techniques with favorable results [5]. "Overcoming binge eating" has been the most studied and longest-used version of self-help CBT for BED [32]. Clinicians can also serve as guides for self-help treatment, meeting with the patient a total of 10 times with each session lasting about 25 minutes [5].

There are several other psychotherapies often used instead of or in addition to CBT [6]. IPT shows similar efficacy to CBT and is also often utilized in the treatment of BED, based on theories that interpersonal struggles play an important role in BED [6]. In practice, IPT is sometimes combined with CBT and is useful for patients with more complex psychopathology that may include perfectionism, low self-esteem, and interpersonal difficulties [6]. Psychodynamic psychotherapy may also help reduce binge eating in some patients [6], and mindfulness-based interventions are used to help individuals with BED [6, 35].

DBT targets emotion regulation, and as a part of regulating difficult feeling and urges, impulse control is also often utilized as an effective part of the treatment protocol [6, 33]. The rationale for the effectiveness of DBT is based on theories that BED primarily stems from high-stress vulnerability and that stress and negative effect may be important triggers for binge eating [31] either by way of body dissatisfaction or directly due to emotional distress. Acute socio-evaluative stress during a commonly utilized task (Trier Social Stress Test) led to greater body dissatisfaction in subjects with BED but not in controls [31] which supports the potential validity of this stress-based theory. Inspiration for studying DBT for the treatment of BED has also come from theories positing that impulse control is impaired in individuals who overeat and who develop BED. For example, negative urgency (as defined as the tendency to act rashly when distressed) predicts later development of BED (sixth grade to tenth grade, respectively) [18, 19]. Another third-wave CBT treatment, ACT, has also been found to be effective in improving self-regulation [35–37]. Both DBT and ACT utilize mindfulness skills, and mindfulness training and mindfulness-based therapies have been found to be helpful too in reducing binge eating [35, 37, 38]. Additional work shows that mindfulness-based stress reduction (MBSR) reduces emotional eating scores [39]. A recent literature review [40, 41] also concluded that mindfulness-based interventions can be effective in reducing binge eating, reducing both emotional and external eating, food cravings, and body image concerns. Mindfulness skills also, helpfully, increase awareness of internal cues to overeat [38]. Whether intuitive eating-based approaches are helpful for binge-eating is unknown [38].

Summary of key elements of three psychotherapies for treatment of BED.

3.8 Pharmacotherapy for BED

SSRIs, imipramine, lisdexamfetamine, zonisamide, and topiramate are the primary medications utilized for BED treatment [6, 7, 18, 19] (Table 3.2). That said, although often utilized clinically, SSRIs have not received FDA approval for treatment of BED due to underwhelming evidence for efficacy [42, 43]. Most clinical trials that established efficacy for these medications have lasted 12 weeks or less, with the exception of one study of topiramate which lasted 21 weeks [44]. Thus, little is known regarding longer-term effects of medication on binge eating and what happens when medications are discontinued [4, 6].

In patients with BED, it is generally suggested that clinicians use SSRIs first-line because of efficacy, safety, and tolerability [6, 18]. SSRIs (e.g., citalopram, escitalopram, fluoxetine, fluvoxamine, and sertraline) are the most well-studied class of medications for BED [7], in part because fluoxetine is FDA approved for use in the treatment of BN [18]. Doses are comparable or greater than those usually used for major depressive disorder, and titration intervals are comparable [6, 18]. SSRIs are considered first-line treatment for BED, lisdexamfetamine or topiramate are second-line, and there is growing evidence for zonisamide and orlistat to be utilized in obese patients with BED [6, 18]. Imipramine also can be considered as an effective medication choice based on 2012 guidelines regarding pharmacotherapy for BED [68]. Serotonin and norepinephrine reuptake inhibitors (SNRI) are also likely also efficacious, but there is less study and insufficient research on the use of these medications [6]. For patients with BED who do not respond to one to two courses of an SSRI, imipramine, topiramate, or lisdexamfetamine can be tried [6, 71]. Both topiramate and lisdexamfetamine have advantages over SSRIs in that they are associated with weight reduction [6]. When choosing medications, it is important to consider that no head-to-head trials have compared an SSRI with either topiramate or lisdexamfetamine [6]. Further, adding an SSRI to CBT has not been found to improve outcomes, but adding topiramate might confer additional benefit [6].

Lisdexamfetamine is the first medication to be FDA approved for moderate-to-severe BED, and it was approved in 2015, and lisdexamfetamine use may be limited by adverse events such as cardiac effects (tachycardia and elevated BP) and an abuse risk (it is a stimulant) [6, 18]. Lisdexamfetamine has also been found to improve disability on the Sheehan Disability Scale [72]. Lisdexamfetamine is also FDA approved for the treatment of ADHD and likely reduces impulsivity [73].

Topiramate has been associated with adverse effects including cognitive dulling, paresthesia, and somnolence. There is a significant amount of concern about the negative cognitive effects of topiramate, but cognitive effects are usually associated with higher doses, and anecdotally low doses, as low as 25 or 50 mg, might improve symptoms. There is no clear relationship between

Table 3.2 Treatments for obesity, binge eating disorder, and bulimia nervosa. Included are FDA-approved treatments and most frequently used off-label treatments

Medication	Dose	Results	Mechanism	Side effects	Contraindications	Monitoring	FDA Approval
FDA approved for obesity							
Benzphetamine	25–50 mg once daily to TID, max dose of 50 mg TID [45]		Stimulant: increased norepinephrine release [46]	(Frequencies not defined) Cardiovascular, CNS, dermatologic, endocrine, GI, neuromuscular side effects [47]	Hypersensitivity to benzphetamine, cardiovascular disease, mod or severe hypertension, hyperthyroidism, glaucoma, drug abuse history, current/recent MAO-I use, pregnancy [47]	Baseline cardiac evaluation, cardiac echo during treatment, weight, waist circumference, blood pressure and heart rate [47]	1960 [48] (infrequent use in the USA)
Diethylpropion	25 mg TID or 75 mg daily [45]		Stimulant: increased norepinephrine release [46]	Cardiovascular, CNS, dermatologic, endocrine, GI, genitourinary, hematologic, neuromuscular, ophthalmic, renal and urinary side effects [49]	Hypersensitivity to diethylpropion, cardiovascular disease, pulmonary hypertension, hyperthyroidism, drug abuse history, current/recent MAO-I [49]	Baseline cardiac evaluation; cardiac echo during treatment, weight, waist circumference, blood pressure and heart rate, renal function [49]	1959 [48] (infrequent use in the USA)
Liraglutide (semaglutide and exenatide too)	3.0 mg [50] (requires injection, high cost)	−5.5 maximal weight loss [51]	GLP-1 receptor agonist [45]	Nausea, vomiting, abdominal pain, gallbladder pathology, pancreatitis, renal impairment; [50]	Hypersensitivity to liraglutide, history of medullary thyroid cancer, history of multiple endocrine neoplasia, pregnancy [52]	Serum glucose, Hgb A1c, renal function, triglycerides, gallbladder and pancreatic function [52]	2014 [48]

(continued)

Table 3.2 (continued)

Medication	Dose	Results	Mechanism	Side effects	Contraindications	Monitoring	FDA Approval
Naltrexone-bupropion	8 mg/90 mg tab, 2 tabs BID [48]	−6.15 kg maximal weight loss [51]	Opioid antagonist/ stimulant – naltrexone blocks inhibitory feedback circuit of bupropion [45]	Nausea, headache, constipation, dizziness, vomiting and dry mouth, heart rate and blood pressure elevation, psychiatric [45] Increased risk of suicide in patients under age 25 [53]	Hypersensitivity to medication, opioid use or withdrawal, hypertension, seizure disorder, anorexia or bulimia, sedative withdrawal [53]	Blood pressure, heart rate, serum glucose, kidney/ liver function, mental status, suicidality [53]	2014 [48]
Orlistat	120 mg [51]	−2.94 kg maximal weight loss [51]	Inhibits gastrointestinal lipase, reduces fat absorption [45]	Fecal urgency, fecal incontinence, flatus with discharge, oily spotting, bloating, diarrhea, malabsorption (vitamin D), kidney stones [48]	Hypersensitivity to orlistat, chronic malabsorption, cholestasis, anorexia and bulimia [54]	BMI, waist circumference, lipid profile [54]	1999 [48]
Phendimetrazine	35 mg 2–3 times daily prior to meals [45]		Stimulant: increased norepinephrine release [46]	(Frequencies not defined) Cardiovascular, CNS, endocrine, GI, genitourinary, hematologic, neuromuscular, ophthalmic, respiratory side effects [55]	Hypersensitivity to phendimetrazine, glaucoma, pregnancy, hx of drug abuse, hyperthyroidism, current or recent MAOI treatment [55]	Baseline cardiac evaluation, weight, waist circumference, blood pressure, pulse [55]	1959 [48] (infrequent use in the USA)
Phentermine	8, 15, 30, 37.5 mg [45]	−7.39 kg (mean weight loss) [56]	Stimulant [45]	Increased blood pressure and pulse, dry mouth, insomnia [45]	Hypersensitivity to phentermine, cardiovascular disease, hyperthyroidism, hx of drug abuse, current or recent MAOI use, pregnancy, breast feeding [57]	Weight/waist circumference, blood pressure and heart rate [57]	1959 [48]

Phentermine-topiramate	7.5/46 mg [51]	−7.45 kg maximal weight loss [51]	Stimulant; anticonvulsant, glutamate AMPA antagonist, GABA agonist, sodium channel blocker [45]	Dry mouth, paresthesia, constipation, insomnia, dizziness and dysgeusia [45]	Hypersensitivity to either medication, hyperthyroidism, glaucoma, current or recent MAOI use, pregnancy, caution with hypertension [58]	Weight, blood pressure and heart rate, mood, glaucoma, labs: bicarb, potassium, creatinine, glucose, acidosis [58]	2012 [48]
Setmelanotide	2–3 mg daily [59] (requires injection, high cost)		Melanocortin-4 receptor agonist [60]	Headache, arthralgia, nausea, spontaneous penile erections, female genital sensitivity [60]	None listed [59]	Weight, sexual adverse reactions symptoms, depression symptoms [59]	FDA approved for rare genetic disorders of obesity [60]
Obesity treatments: Off-label or under review							
Bupropion-zonisamide	360 mg/120 mg and 360 mg/260 mg [60]	−6.1% and 7.5% of body weight [60]	Dopamine and serotonin reuptake inhibitor/ antiepileptic agent with sodium channel modulation [60]	Nausea, headache, insomnia, blood pressure and heart rate elevation, psychiatric [60]	Not available	Not available	[60]
Metformin	850 mg BID [61]	−2 kg [61]	Inhibits mitochondrial ATP production. Possibly decreased appetite versus increased metabolism [61]	Diarrhea, flatulence, nausea and vomiting [62]	Hypersensitivity to metformin, renal dysfunction, acute or chronic metabolic acidosis [62]	Urine glucose/ ketones, HgbA1c, CBC, creatinine, B12, folate [62]	Off-label for obesity [61] Current type 2 diabetes treatment [62]
Tesofensine	0.25 mg, 0.5 mg, or 1 mg daily (under review) [45]	−4.5%, 9.2% or 10.6% of body weight [45]	Stimulant: Presynaptic reuptake inhibitor of dopamine, norepinephrine, and serotonin [45]	Elevations in blood pressure and pulse [45]	Not available	Not available	Phase III review [45]

(continued)

Table 3.2 (continued)

Medication	Dose	Results	Mechanism	Side effects	Contraindications	Monitoring	FDA Approval
Topiramate	64–384 mg for obesity [45]	–5–6.3% body weight in obesity [45] –4.5–5.9 kg body weight in BED [7]	Anticonvulsant, sodium channel blocker, glutamate AMPA antagonist, GABA agonist [45]	Paresthesias, somnolence and difficulty with memory, concentration and attention, kidney stones [45]	Metabolic acidosis with metformin treatment, glaucoma [63]	Symptoms of acidosis, symptoms of glaucoma, suicidality, labs: bicarbonate, potassium, creatinine, glucose, acidosis [63]	Off-label for obesity and BED
Semaglutide/ exenatide	2.5–40 mg/5–10 mcg BID [45]	–6.7 kg for 40 mg dose (semaglutide) [45]	GLP-1 analog [45]	Abdominal pain, nausea, other endocrine, metabolic and gastrointestinal disturbances [64]	Hypersensitivity to semaglutide/exenatide, personal or family history of medullary thyroid carcinoma, multiple endocrine neoplasia type 2, pregnancy, breastfeeding [64]	Labs: plasma glucose, HbA1c, renal function, pancreatic pathology, triglycerides, gallbladder pathology [64]	Phase III review for obesity [45]; current type 2 diabetes treatment [64]
Treatment for eating disorders							
Fluoxetine	20 mg/60 mg [65]	Reduction in binge eating behavior [65]	SSRI: inhibit reuptake of serotonin [65]	Insomnia, drowsiness, headache, nausea, asthenia, anxiety, tremor, dizziness, yawning, and decreased libido, increased risk of suicide in patients under age 25 [66]	Hypersensitivity to fluoxetine, current/recent use of MAOI, linezolid, methylene blue, pimozide, thioridazine [66]	Suicidality, signs/ symptoms of serotonin syndrome, akathisia [66]	FDA approved for BN [65]
Lisdexamfetamine	50 mg, 70 mg [65]	Reduction in binge eating behavior [65]	Stimulant: amphetamine pro-drug [65]	Dry mouth, decreased appetite, insomnia, headache, elevated blood pressure and heart rate [65]	Hypersensitivity to lisdexamfetamine, cardiovascular disease, moderate-to-severe hypertension, hyperthyroidism, glaucoma, history of drug abuse [67]	Cardiac symptoms, blood pressure, heart rate, weight, signs of peripheral vasculopathy, sleep/ behavior changes [67]	FDA approved for BED [67]

SSRIs (other than fluoxetine)	Varies	Reduction in binge eating behavior, equivalent to fluoxetine (above) [68]	Inhibit reuptake of serotonin [68]	Sexual dysfunction, drowsiness, weight gain, insomnia, anxiety, dizziness, headache, increased risk of suicide in patients under age 25 [69]	Hypersensitivity to medication, current/recent use of MAOI, caution with other serotonergic medication [69]	Varies with medication	Off-label use for BN and BED [68]
TCAs: imipramine, amitriptyline, desipramine	Varies	Reduction in bulimic behavior/reduction of binge behavior in BED [68]	Tricyclic antidepressant: inhibit reuptake of serotonin and norepinephrine [69]	Blurred vision, constipation, dry mouth, and urinary retention, elevated blood pressure and heart rate [69]	Prolonged QTC [69], other (varies with medication)	Blood pressure, heart rate, other (varies with medication)	Off-label use for BN and BED [68]
Topiramate	64–384 mg for obesity [45]	–5–6.3% body weight in obesity [45] –4.5–5.9 kg in BED [7]	Anticonvulsant, sodium channel blocker, glutamate AMPA antagonist, GABA agonist [45]	Paresthesia, somnolence and difficulty with memory, concentration and attention, kidney stones [45]	Metabolic acidosis with metformin treatment, glaucoma [63]	Symptoms of acidosis, symptoms of glaucoma, suicidality, labs: bicarb, potassium, creatinine, glucose, acidosis [63]	Off-label for obesity and BED
Zonisamide	100–600 mg [70]	Reduction in binge eating and weight loss [70]	Anticonvulsant, sodium and calcium channels [70]	Dizziness, drowsiness [63]	Hypersensitivity to mediation [63]	BUN, creatinine, bicarb, ammonia [63]	Off-label use for BED [70]

topiramate dose and efficacy, but no trial of dose-dependent efficacy has been published, and target dose ranges of 100–400 mg have been utilized in previous studies [44].

Imipramine is not FDA approved for the treatment of BED, but the World Federation of Societies of Biological Psychiatry guidelines listed it as having Grade A evidence, meaning there are two or more randomized control trials showing superiority to placebo, based on positive results from several studies (along with topiramate and SSRIs) [68].

One study of zonisamide deserves mention, as it is a medication similar to topiramate in its mechanism, but has a more tolerable side effect profile. Preliminary work shows binge eating behavior reduction and weight loss, however, more studies of this medication are in order [6, 7].

Further, preliminary work suggests obesity medicines may also prove to be effective in BED management. Although liraglutide (a glucagon-like peptide-1 receptor agonist) has not been tested in EDs, it has been shown in obese patients to cause short-term (up to 6 months) reductions in weight. A randomized control trial compared the use of intensive behavioral therapy (IBT), a behavioral intervention designed to target obesity, alone to IBT with liraglutide. The IBT with liraglutide was associated with greater short-term improvements in dietary disinhibition, global eating disorder psychopathology, and shape concern than IBT alone [74]. The IBT and liraglutide condition also showed reductions in food cravings, and therefore this medication may be more generally applicable to individuals with BED.

Another medication that is beneficial when combined with psychotherapy is orlistat, an anti-obesity drug that inhibits the absorption of dietary fat. When compared with self-help CBT, the medication led to no direct changes in binge eating (6–7) but was shown to promote weight loss.

An open-label trial on the efficacy and tolerability of naltrexone/bupropion SR for treating altered eating behaviors and weight loss in BED showed a significant and similar weight loss (approx. 8%) for both a group of obese and non-obese patients with BED. The trial showed improvement in pathological eating behavior including binge eating, grazing, emotional eating, craving for carbohydrates, and post-dinner eating as well as reduction of scores on the binge eating scale (BES) score, and a reduction in food addiction (FA) severity. Patients with BED fared particularly well, and dropout rates were low with good medication tolerability [75]. However, bupropion is contraindicated in BN due to increased risk of seizure associated with electrolyte imbalances [76]; therefore, it shouldn't be used as first-line treatment until safety and efficacy data are available. In a couple of cases, phentermine/topiramate extended-release showed cessation of binge eating and weight loss in obese women with BED, and no adverse events were reported. However, the use of any medication with phentermine, a psychostimulant, should be cautiously monitored because of possible cardiovascular effects [77]. Results from a completed crossover trial to assess the efficacy and safety of phentermine/topiramate for treatment of BED and BN are not yet available (https://clinicaltrials.gov/ct2/show/NCT02553824?term=02553824&rank=1).

3.9 Nutritional Recommendations for BED

Current dietary recommendations for BED are mainly based on nutritional approaches that have been utilized for decades in other eating disorders [32, 78–80], but whether they are the best interventions for BED still needs further study. That said, nutritional psychoeducation and meal-plan development should be a component of all BED treatments. Patients are asked to develop a regular pattern of eating and also monitor their eating behavior every day and for every meal, looking for patterns and antecedents to bingeing. Further, patients are asked to modify dieting behavior and minimize food avoidance, such as avoidance of particular macronutrients or excessive calorie restriction [6]. A typical food plan might involve three meals a day and two or three snacks, without skipping or snacking, no more than four hours between meals, and at least (usually significantly more) 1500 kcal/day [32].

3.10 Best Practices and Guidelines for BED Treatment

In terms of best practices and guidelines about what should be recommended for whom, there is still some controversy in the literature by experts about how medication use in BED should fit into treatment protocols. The American Psychiatric Association (APA) guidelines and the National Institute for Health and Care Excellence (NICE) both support the use of cognitive behavior therapy (CBT) and SSRIs, although APA endorses CBT as the cornerstone of treatment and medications as adjunctive therapy, whereas NICE endorses either as reasonable treatment [3, 6].

Based on existing evidence and guidelines, psychotherapy is generally considered first-line treatment for BED. Medications are also efficacious for the treatment of BED and are recommended as either a first-line or add-on to psychotherapy treatment [6]. Pharmacotherapy may be preferred over psychotherapy by some patients even though there is less evidence for long-term efficacy, because pharmacotherapy may require less time or be less expensive [6]. It is therefore reasonable to use pharmacotherapy as first-line treatment for patients who prefer medication and decline psychotherapy, as well as patients who do not have access to psychotherapy [6] .

A clinical effect for psychotherapy (CBT and DBT) was reported by one meta-analysis in reducing binge eating [6]. Another recent comprehensive meta-analysis demonstrated the medium-term (1 year) effectiveness for BED outcomes (including binge eating episodes and abstinence, eating disorder, and general psychopathology) following psychotherapy, structured self-help treatment, and combined treatment for patients with BED. Results supported the long-term (greater than 1 year) effectiveness of psychotherapy, particularly CBT with strong evidence for IPT as well; however, there was little effect of psychotherapy on weight [81]. Although CBT usually outshines behavioral weight loss therapy and other psychotherapeutic modalities for binge eating, some studies show they are comparable [6].

It is also important to compare psychotherapy and psychiatric interventions and understand the differences in efficacy. Randomized pharmacotherapy trials, mostly of antidepressants such as SSRIs, found only a medium-sized clinical effect [6]. Another review and meta-analysis found CBT, lisdexamfetamine, or SSRIs as treatment options with similar efficacy [3], whereas a subsequent editorial expressed concern about this conclusion, highlighting that most medication studies have only lasted 12 weeks, unlike psychotherapy studies which have long-term (months to years) outcomes. In those medication studies (primarily studies of SSRIs) that have followed patients over a longer period of time, the significant posttreatment reductions of binge eating episodes and BMI were no longer significant at 6–12 months in the few studies providing data [82] indicating more efficacy of psychotherapy. Finally, another recent systematic review and network meta-analysis measured the comparative effectiveness of second-generation antidepressants (mostly SSRIs), lisdexamfetamine, CBT, IPT, behavioral weight loss, and several other psychotherapeutic interventions and concluded that lisdexamfetamine was better at increasing binge abstinence than second-generation antidepressants, therapist-led CBT was better at reducing binge eating frequency than behavioral weight loss, and behavioral weight loss was better at reducing weight [82, 83]. Another meta-analysis of many different treatments including pharmacotherapy found only three statistically significant differences emerged: lisdexamfetamine was better at increasing binge abstinence than second-generation antidepressants; therapist-led cognitive behavioral therapy was better at reducing binge eating frequency than behavioral weight loss, but behavioral weight loss was better at reducing weight [83]. That said, other meta-analyses have found that remission from binge eating occurred in more patients who received pharmacotherapy in general (usually with antidepressants or topiramate) compared to those who did not [6].

In summary, regarding psychotherapy, CBT is the best practice for the management of BED. Given the emotional distress underpinning the disorder, integration of DBT has also been shown to be effective, as is guided self-help. From a medications perspective, SSRIs and lisdexamfetamine have been shown to improve bingeing behavior and reduce symptoms of BED.

3.11 Obesity and BED Treatment

CBT is generally not helpful for weight loss in individuals with BED who are overweight or obese; however, patients who stop binge eating with CBT may show a clinically modest weight advantage compared with patients who continue to experience binge eating episodes [6]. Similarly, treatments such as IPT and DBT also do not produce weight loss [4, 6]. It remains to be seen whether mindfulness is helpful, as weight loss is indicated in some but not all studies and more needs to be seen [35]. Behavioral weight loss therapy has been found to work better than CBT for weight loss in patients with BED [4]. Best practices for weight management in obese individuals in BED are unclear [3], however may include behavioral weight loss therapy [6] and medications that promote weight loss as well as reduce binge eating, such as topiramate, zonisamide, or lisdexamfetamine [6, 42, 43].

Bariatric surgery, including gastric bypass, gastric banding, or sleeve gastrectomy, has been used to help obese patients with BED lose weight [6, 84]. This is not surprising since bariatric surgery procedures anatomically restrict the capacity to binge eat or overeat [84], although growing evidence indicates it also has brain-level beneficial effects (Chap. 10). Binge eating post-surgery predicts worse weight loss outcomes [84]. Vomiting may result from overeating or attempts to binge eat, although vomiting often occurs postoperatively, both acutely and involuntarily, or in response to dysphagia [84]. Self-induced vomiting related to concerns of body weight and shape tends to appear more rarely following bariatric surgery [84, 85]. In summary, there is not any strong clinical basis for excluding people with BED from bypass surgery.

An intervention program, titled BE*free*, developed to integrate psychoeducation, mindfulness, and self-compassion, demonstrated efficacy over weight-list control in a study of obese or overweight women with BED. This program was shown to address the underlying mechanism of BED including reducing binge eating and shame, reducing impulsivity and negative internal experiences, and improving body acceptance in BED and obesity. While the program was deemed effective across these domains, it did not result in weight loss within the small sample included in the study [86].

3.12 Treatment of BN

Treatments for BED are adapted from the known treatments of BN, and therefore there are many similarities. Both treatments target binge-eating and the underlying causes of binge eating, and here we will focus on highlighting the differences in treatment modalities below. As with BED, CBT is the mainstay of treatment using principles similar to BED [32, 78, 79], and DBT, ACT, and mindfulness approaches may also be attempted and have some evidence of utility [87]. Treatment for BN is often more structured, sometimes in a partial hospitalization program (PHP) or inpatient setting given medical comorbidities [16]. Nutritional approaches are also similar involving psychoeducation, modification of eating habits, and the cessation of bingeing and purging behaviors [88].

When treating BN, pharmacotherapy alone appears to be less efficacious than psychotherapy alone, and combining the two appears to be the best approach. Nevertheless, pharmacotherapy is efficacious for BN and may be included in the initial treatment regimen, along with nutritional rehabilitation and psychotherapy, primarily first-line treatment using SSRIs [76] (Table 3.2). Using pharmacotherapy alone is reasonable if specialized nutritional services or psychotherapy is not available [76]. Fluoxetine is first-line treatment with a target dose of 60 mg per day. Second-line treatment involves other SSRIs, often sertraline, but escitalopram or fluvoxamine are other alternatives often used. In the treatment of BN, these SSRIs are often prescribed at higher doses than when are used to treat major depression [89].

Third-line medication options for BN include other antidepressants or topiramate (Table 3.2). In order of recommendation, for individuals with anxiety, these include tricyclic antidepressants, trazodone, monoamine oxidase inhibitors, or topiramate for those with comorbid anxiety. Prescriptions for those without comorbid anxiety-related disorders include topiramate, tricyclics, trazodone, or monoamine oxidase inhibitors. Medications that are contraindicated for individuals with BN include bupropion and lisdexamfetamine, due to their stimulant effects [76].

In a meta-analysis, it was determined that the treatments that are most likely to achieve full remission for BN are individual CBT and guided cognitive behavioral self-help, although there continues to be a limited evidence base for the treatment on BN [90].

What distinguishes BN from BED is the presence of purging, which is medically dangerous. Treatments for that element are CBT, including rapid response CBT (CBT-RR) [91], and for more information, we refer readers to other sources for guidance on this [16]. These patients are more likely than BED to require PHP and residential or inpatient care due to the heightened medical dangers (cardiac, dehydration, cognitive, seizure) related to electrolyte imbalances and medical consequences of vomiting such as tooth damage or esophageal tears.

In comorbid BN and obesity, an addition of behavioral weight loss management to other ED treatments might be useful for patients with BN and obesity. Structured and professionally run obesity treatment is associated with reduced ED prevalence, ED risk, and symptoms [92]. Individuals with BN are typically excluded from bariatric surgery until symptoms are managed, as the binge-purge cycle makes them poor candidates for surgery and reduces the efficacy of the medical procedure [93].

3.13 Treatments for both BED and BN

Given the similar mechanisms and clinical presentations of BN and BED, there is significant overlap in treatment for both disorders. A systematic review and meta-analysis aimed to examine the empirical status of various newer psychotherapies in disordered eating patients. Only 13 randomized controlled trials (RCT) were identified that studied these newer therapies, most focusing on BED. Large pre-post symptom improvements were observed for all treatments examined, including dialectical behavior therapy (DBT), schema therapy (ST), acceptance and commitment therapy (ACT), mindfulness-based interventions (MBI), and compassion-focused therapy (CFT), but none were better than CBT in active comparison studies. The article concluded that CBT should retain its status as the recommended treatment approach for BN and BED in adults, with IPT considered a strong empirically supported alternative [94].

Several app-based studies targeting binge eating in general (therefore applying to people with either BED or BN) have been published recently. One examined the effects of an intervention using health coaches via telemedicine combined with smartphone cognitive-behavioral-guided self-help therapy for BED and BN which showed that at 1-year follow-up, individuals who received the treatment were reported to have remission rates of 57%, compared with 30% for the treatment as usual group [95, 96]. Another study published a free (and soon-to-be-available) smartphone app and found the app was associate with reductions in attitudinal and behavioral eating disorder symptoms, including binge eating, in a randomized, controlled trial [97]. In a systematic review of 50-manualized self-help interventions for BED and BN, including 34 RCTs, rates of remission varied from 9% to 64%. Individuals with BED were less likely to drop out of the studies and more likely to benefit from other guided and unguided self-help, whereas patients with BN benefited primarily from guided self-help [98].

3.14 Conclusion

In summary, both BED and BN share many commonalities in their etiology, maintenance mechanisms, and behavioral characteristics. There is a strong body of empirical evidence in support of the psychological and psychiatric treatment of these disorders. An approach combining behavioral and cognitive approaches as well as medications is most likely to be effective in the treatment of BN and BED. However, more solutions are needed, especially for individuals with comorbid EDs and obesity.

References

1. Bogusz K, Kopera M, Jakubczyk A, Trucco EM, Kucharska K, Walenda A, et al. Prevalence of alcohol use disorder among individuals who binge eat: a systematic review and meta-analysis. Addiction. 2021;116(1):18–31.
2. Diagnostic and statistical manual of mental disorders (5th ed.). (DSM-V). Washington, DC: American Psychiatric Association; 2013.
3. Brownley KA, Berkman ND, Peat CM, Lohr KN, Cullen KE, Bann CM, et al. Binge-eating disorder in adults: a systematic review and meta-analysis. Ann Intern Med. 2016;165(6):409–20.
4. Wilfey DE, Fitzsimmons-Craft EE, Eichen DM. Binge eating disorder in adults (letter to editor). Ann Intern Med. 2017;166(3):230–1.
5. Sysko R, Devlin M. Binge eating disorder: cognitive-behavior therapy (CBT). 2018. Yager J, Solomon D. Accessed 2018. In: UpToDate. Wolters Kluwer. Available from: www.uptodate.com.
6. Sysko R, Delvin M. Binge eating disorder in adults: overview of treatment. 2018. Yager J, Solomon D. Accessed 2018. In: UpToDate. Wolters Kluwer. Available from: www.uptodate.com.
7. Reas DL, Grilo CM. Pharmacological treatment of binge eating disorder: update review and synthesis. Expert Opin Pharmacother. 2015;16(10):1463–78.
8. Karasu SR. Gravity of weight: the daunting science of weight control. Washington, D.C.: American Psychiatric Publishing Incorporated; 2010.
9. Wilcox CE. Binge eating disorder. Accessed. CMEtoGo.com: American Physician Institute; 2019. Available.
10. Mitchell JE, Zunker C. Bulimia nervosa and binge eating disorder in adults: medical complications and their management. 2018. Yager J, Solomon D. Accessed Aug 2 2018. In: UpToDate. Wolters Kluwer. Available from: www.uptodate.com.
11. Engel S, Steffen K, Mitchell JE. Bulimia nervosa in adults: clinical features, course of illness, assessment, and diagnosis. 2018. Yager J, Solomon D. Accessed Aug 2 2018. In: UpToDate. Wolters Kluwer. Available from: www.uptodate.com.
12. Castillo M, Weiselberg E. Bulimia Nervosa/Purging Disorder. Curr Probl Pediatr Adolesc Health Care. 2017;47(4):85–94.
13. Hay PJ, Claudino AM. Bulimia nervosa. BMJ Clin Evidnce. 2010;2010
14. Yao S, Kuja-Halkola R, Thornton LM, Runfola CD, D'Onofrio BM, Almqvist C, et al. Familial liability for eating disorders and suicide attempts: evidence from a population registry in Sweden. JAMA Psychiat. 2016;73(3):284–91.
15. Hay P. Current approach to eating disorders: a clinical update. Intern Med J. 2020;50(1):24–9.
16. Mehler PS, Andersen AE. Eating disorders: a guide to medical care and complications. Baltimore, MD: John's Hopkins University Press; 2017.
17. Faber A, Dube L, Knauper B. Attachment and eating: a meta-analytic review of the relevance of attachment for unhealthy and healthy eating behaviors in the general population. Appetite. 2018;123:410–38.
18. Davis H, Attia E. Pharmacotherapy of eating disorders. Curr Opin Psychiatry. 2017;30(6):452–7.
19. Davis HA, Smith GT. An integrative model of risk for high school disordered eating. J Abnorm Psychol. 2018;127(6):559–70.
20. Giel KE, Teufel M, Junne F, Zipfel S, Schag K. Food-related impulsivity in obesity and binge eating disorder-a systematic update of the evidence. Nutrients. 2017;9(11)
21. Hutson PH, Balodis IM, Potenza MN. Binge-eating disorder: clinical and therapeutic advances. Pharmacol Ther. 2018;182:15–27.
22. Blackburn SJL, Blampied N, Popp D, Kallen R. An application of escape theory to binge-eating. Eur Eat Disord Rev. 2006;14(1):23–31.
23. Kenny TE, Singleton C, Carter JC. Testing predictions of the emotion regulation model of binge-eating disorder. Int J Eat Disord. 2017;50(11):1297–305.
24. Meule A, Richard A, Schnepper R, Reichenberger J, Georgii C, Naab S, et al. Emotion regulation and emotional eating in anorexia nervosa and bulimia nervosa. Eat Disord. 2019:1–17.
25. Wiss DA, Brewerton TD. Adverse childhood experiences and adult obesity: a systematic review of plausible mechanisms and meta-analysis of cross-sectional studies. Physiol Behav. 2020;223:112964.
26. Thaler L, Steiger H. Eating disorders and epigenetics. Adv Exp Med Biol. 2017;978:93–103.
27. Botticelli L, Micioni Di Bonaventura E, Del Bello F, Giorgioni G, Piergentili A, Romano A, et al. Underlying susceptibility to eating disorders and drug abuse: genetic and pharmacological aspects of dopamine D4 receptors. Nutrients. 2020;12(8)
28. Lohman BJ, Neppl TK, Lee Y, Diggs ON, Russell D. The association between household food insecu-

rity and body mass index: a prospective growth curve analysis. J Pediatr. 2018;202(115–20):e1.
29. Hernandez D, Mehta N, Geliebter A. Meal-related acyl and des-acyl ghrelin and other appetite-related hormones in people with obesity and binge eating. Obesity. 2019;27(4):629–35.
30. Thompson KJ. Body image, eating disorders and obesity: an integrative guide for assessment and treatment. Washington, DC: American Psychological Association; 2000.
31. Naumann E, Svaldi J, Wyschka T, Heinrichs M, von Dawans B. Stress-induced body dissatisfaction in women with binge eating disorder. J Abnorm Psychol. 2018;127(6):548–58.
32. Fairburn CG. Overcoming binge eating, second edition: the proven program to learn why you binge and how you can stop. New York, NY: The Guilford Press; 2013.
33. Kinasz KR, Ross DA Cooper JJ. Eat to live or live to eat? The neurobiology of appetite regulation. Biol Psychiatry. 2017;81(9):e73–e5.
34. Boutelle KN, Knatz S, Carlson J, Bergmann K, Peterson CB. An open trial targeting food cue reactivity and satiety sensitivity in overweight and obese binge eaters. Cogn Behav Pract. 2017;24(3):363–73.
35. Wangen KE. Mindful eating. In: Zerbo E, Schlechter A, Desai S, Levounis P, editors. Becoming mindful integrating mindfulness into your psychiatric practice. Virginia: American Psychiatric Association Publishing; 2017.
36. Forman EM, Butryn ML. A new look at the science of weight control: how acceptance and commitment strategies can address the challenge of self-regulation. Appetite. 2015;84:171–80.
37. Forman EM, Shaw JA, Goldstein SP, Butryn ML, Martin LM, Meiran N, et al. Mindful decision making and inhibitory control training as complementary means to decrease snack consumption. Appetite. 2016;103:176–83.
38. Warren JM, Smith N, Ashwell M. A structured literature review on the role of mindfulness, mindful eating and intuitive eating in changing eating behaviours: effectiveness and associated potential mechanisms. Nutr Res Rev. 2017;30(2):272–83.
39. Levoy E, Lazaridou A, Brewer J, Fulwiler C. An exploratory study of Mindfulness Based Stress Reduction for emotional eating. Appetite. 2017;109:124–30.
40. O'Reilly GA, Cook L, Spruijt-Metz D, Black DS. Mindfulness-based interventions for obesity-related eating behaviours: a literature review. Obes Rev. 2014;15(6):453–61.
41. Palmeira L, Pinto-Gouveia J, Cunha M. Exploring the efficacy of an acceptance, mindfulness & compassionate-based group intervention for women struggling with their weight (Kg-Free): a randomized controlled trial. Appetite. 2017;112:107–16.
42. Higgins GA, Sellers EM, Fletcher PJ. From obesity to substance abuse: therapeutic opportunities for 5-HT2C receptor agonists. Trends Pharmacol Sci. 2013;34(10):560–70.
43. Higgins GA, Zeeb FD, Fletcher PJ. Role of impulsivity and reward in the anti-obesity actions of 5-HT2C receptor agonists. J Psychopharmacol. 2017;31(11):1403–18.
44. Arbaizar B, Gomez-Acebo I, Llorca J. Efficacy of topiramate in bulimia nervosa and binge-eating disorder: a systematic review. Gen Hosp Psychiatry. 2008;30(5):471–5.
45. Coulter AA, Rebello CJ, Greenway FL. Centrally acting agents for obesity: past, present, and future. Drugs. 2018;78(11):1113–32.
46. Bray GA. Drug treatment of obesity. Bailliere Clin Endocrinol Metab. 1999;13(1):131–48.
47. Lexicomp. Benzphetamine. Available from: http://online.lexi.com/lco/action/doc/retrieve/docid/patch_f/6438.
48. Gadde KM, Atkins KD. The limits and challenges of antiobesity pharmacotherapy. Expert Opin Pharmacother. 2020;21(11):1319–28.
49. Lexicomp. Diethylpropion. Available from: http://online.lexi.com/lco/action/doc/retrieve/docid/patch_f/6740.
50. Pi-Sunyer X, Astrup A, Fujioka K, Greenway F, Halpern A, Krempf M, et al. A randomized, controlled trial of 3.0 mg of liraglutide in weight management. N Engl J Med. 2015;373(1):11–22.
51. Dong Z, Xu L, Liu H, Lv Y, Zheng Q, Li L. Comparative efficacy of five long-term weight loss drugs: quantitative information for medication guidelines. Obes Rev. 2017;18(12):1377–85.
52. Lexicomp. Liraglutide. Available from: http://online.lexi.com/lco/action/doc/retrieve/docid/patch_f/2144379.
53. Lexicomp. Naltrexone and Bupropion. Available from: http://online.lexi.com/lco/action/doc/retrieve/docid/patch_f/5338462.
54. Bansal AB, Al Khalili Y. Orlistat Treasure Island (FL): StatPearls Publishing; 2020. [updated 2020/11/22. Available from: https://www.statpearls.com/articlelibrary/viewarticle/26335/.
55. Lexicomp. Phendimetrazine. Available from: http://online.lexi.com/lco/action/doc/retrieve/docid/patch_f/7475.
56. Garcia Ramirez AV, Filho DR, Zotarelli Filho IJ. Meta-analysis and approach of the real impact of anorexigenic drugs in the obesity in humans: the last five years of the randomized studies. Curr Diabetes Rev. 2020;16(7):750–8.
57. Lexicomp. Phentermine. Available from: http://online.lexi.com/lco/action/doc/retrieve/docid/patch_f/7481.
58. Lexicomp. Phentermine Topiramate. Available from: http://online.lexi.com/lco/action/doc/retrieve/docid/patch_f/3832942.
59. Lexicomp. Setmelanotide. Available from: http://online.lexi.com/lco/action/doc/retrieve/docid/patch_f/7037631.
60. Srivastava G, Apovian C. Future pharmacotherapy for obesity: new anti-obesity drugs on the horizon. Curr Obes Rep. 2018;7(2):147–61.

61. Yerevanian A, Soukas AA. Metformin: mechanisms in human obesity and weight loss. Curr Obes Rep. 2019;8(2):156–64.
62. Lexicomp. Metformin. Available from: http://online.lexi.com/lco/action/doc/retrieve/docid/patch_f/7260.
63. Lexicomp. Topiramate. Available from: http://online.lexi.com/lco/action/doc/retrieve/docid/patch_f/7789.
64. Lexicomp. Semaglutide. Available from: http://online.lexi.com/lco/action/doc/retrieve/docid/patch_f/6577162.
65. Bello NT, Yeomans BL. Safety of pharmacotherapy options for bulimia nervosa and binge eating disorder. Expert Opin Drug Saf. 2018;17(1):17–23.
66. Lexicomp. Fluoxetine. Available from: http://online.lexi.com/lco/action/doc/retrieve/docid/patch_f/6931.
67. Lexicomp. Lisdexamfetamine. Available from: http://online.lexi.com/lco/action/doc/retrieve/docid/patch_f/810062.
68. Aigner M, Treasure J, Kaye W, Kasper S, Disorders WTFOE. World Federation of Societies of Biological Psychiatry (WFSBP) guidelines for the pharmacological treatment of eating disorders. World J Biol Psychiatry. 2011;12(6):400–43.
69. Hirsch M. Selective serotonin reuptake inhibitors: pharmacology, administration, and side effects Waltham, MA: UpToDate; 2020. updated 2020/3/16. Available from: https://www.uptodate.com/contents/selective-serotonin-reuptake-inhibitors-pharmacology-administration-and-side-effects.
70. McElroy SL, Kotwal R, Guerdjikova AI, Welge JA, Nelson EB, Lake KA, et al. Zonisamide in the treatment of binge eating disorder with obesity: a randomized controlled trial. J Clin Psychiatry. 2006;67(12):1897–906.
71. Hudson JI, McElroy SL, Ferreira-Cornwell MC, Radewonuk J, Gasior M. Efficacy of lisdexamfetamine in adults with moderate to severe binge-eating disorder: a randomized clinical trial. JAMA Psychiat. 2017;74(9):903–10.
72. Sheehan DV, Gasior M, McElroy SL, Radewonuk J, Herman BK, Hudson J. Effects of lisdexamfetamine dimesylate on functional impairment measured on the Sheehan disability scale in adults with moderate-to-severe binge eating disorder: results from two randomized, placebo-controlled trials. Innov Clin Neurosci. 2018;15(5–6):22–9.
73. Najib J, Didenko E, Meleshkina D, Yusupov K, Maw K, Ramnarain J, et al. Review of lisdexamfetamine dimesylate in children and adolescents with attention deficit/hyperactivity disorder. Curr Med Res Opin. 2020;36(10):1717–35.
74. Chao AM, Wadden TA, Walsh OA, Gruber KA, Alamuddin N, Berkowitz RI, et al. Effects of liraglutide and behavioral weight loss on food cravings, eating behaviors, and eating disorder psychopathology. Obesity. 2019;27(12):2005–10.
75. Carbone EA, Caroleo M, Rania M, Calabro G, Staltari FA, de Filippis R, et al. An open-label trial on the efficacy and tolerability of naltrexone/bupropion SR for treating altered eating behaviours and weight loss in binge eating disorder. Eat Weight Disord. 2020;
76. Crow SJ. (Downloaded 12/8/2018) Bulemia nervosa in adults: Pharmacotherapy. Yager J, Solomon D. Accessed. In: UpToDate. www.uptodate.com. Available.
77. Sethi Dalai S, Sinha A, Gearhardt AN. Low carbohydrate ketogenic therapy as a metabolic treatment for binge eating and ultraprocessed food addiction. Curr Opin Endocrinol Diabetes Obes. 2020;27(5):275–82.
78. Fairburn CG. Cognitive behavior therapy and eating disorders. New York: The Guilford Press; 2018.
79. Fairburn CG, Cooper Z, Shafran R. Cognitive behaviour therapy for eating disorders: a "transdiagnostic" theory and treatment. Behav Res Ther. 2003;41(5):509–28.
80. Wiss D, Brewerton T. Separating the signal from the noise: how psychiatric diagnoses can help discern food addiction from dietary restraint. Nutrients. 2020;12(10)
81. Hilbert A, Bishop ME, Stein RI, Tanofsky-Kraff M, Swenson AK, Welch RR, et al. Long-term efficacy of psychological treatments for binge eating disorder. Br J Psychiatry. 2012;200(3):232–7.
82. Hilbert A, Petroff D, Herpertz S, Pietrowsky R, Tuschen-Caffier B, Vocks S, et al. Meta-analysis of the efficacy of psychological and medical treatments for binge-eating disorder. J Consult Clin Psychol. 2019;87(1):91–105.
83. Peat CM, Berkman ND, Lohr KN, Brownley KA, Bann CM, Cullen K, et al. Comparative effectiveness of treatments for binge-eating disorder: systematic review and network meta-analysis. Eur Eat Disord Rev. 2017;25(5):317–28.
84. Ben-Porat T, Weiss R, Sherf-Dagan S, Rottenstreich A, Kaluti D, Khalaileh A, et al. Food addiction and binge eating during one year following sleeve gastrectomy: prevalence and implications for postoperative outcomes. Obes Surg. 2021;31(2):603–11.
85. Williams-Kerver GA, Steffen KJ, Mitchell JE. Eating pathology after bariatric surgery: an updated review of the recent literature. Curr Psychiatry Rep. 2019;21(9):86.
86. Pinto-Gouveia J, Carvalho SA, Palmeira L, Castilho P, Duarte C, Ferreira C, et al. BEfree: a new psychological program for binge eating that integrates psychoeducation, mindfulness, and compassion. Clin Psychol Psychother. 2017;24(5):1090–8.
87. Kristeller JL BR, Quillian-Wolever R. Mindfulness-based approaches to eating disorders. Mindfulness-based treatment approaches: Clinician's guide to evidence base and applications 75; 2006.
88. Gómez CCPM, Miján-de-la-Torre A, Rodríguez OP, Matía MP, Loria CV, Campos DP, Virgili CM, Martínez OM, Mories ÁM, Castro AM. Consensus document about the nutritional evaluation and management of eating disorders: bulimia nervosa, binge-eating disorder, and others. Nutr Hosp. 2018;35(49)

89. Group FBNCS. Fluoxetine in the treatment of bulimia nervosa. A multicenter, placebo controlled, double-blind trial. Arch Gen Psychiatry. 1992;49:139–47.
90. Slade E, Keeney E, Mavranezouli I, Dias S, Fou L, Stockton S, et al. Treatments for bulimia nervosa: a network meta-analysis. Psychol Med. 2018;48(16):2629–36.
91. MacDonald DE, McFarlane TL, Dionne MM, David L, Olmsted MP. Rapid response to intensive treatment for bulimia nervosa and purging disorder: a randomized controlled trial of a CBT intervention to facilitate early behavior change. J Consult Clin Psychol. 2017;85(9):896–908.
92. Jebeile H, Gow ML, Baur LA, Garnett SP, Paxton SJ, Lister NB. Treatment of obesity, with a dietary component, and eating disorder risk in children and adolescents: a systematic review with meta-analysis. Obes Rev. 2019;20(9):1287–98.
93. Sekula M, Boniecka I, Pasnik K. Bulimia nervosa in obese patients qualified for bariatric surgery – clinical picture, background and treatment. Wideochir Inne Tech Maloinwazyjne. 2019;14(3):408–14.
94. Linardon J, Fairburn CG, Fitzsimmons-Craft EE, Wilfley DE Brennan L. The empirical status of the third-wave behaviour therapies for the treatment of eating disorders: a systematic review. Clin Psychol Rev. 2017;58:125–40.
95. Hildebrandt T, Michaeledes A, Mayhew M, Greif R, Sysko R, Toro-Ramos T, et al. Randomized controlled trial comparing health coach-delivered smartphone-guided self-help with standard care for adults with binge eating. Am J Psychiatry. 2020;177(2):134–42.
96. Kalin NH. Treating substance use disorders, binge eating, and depression, and identifying factors underlying psychosis risk. Am J Psychiatry. 2020;177(2):101–3.
97. Linardon J, Shatte A, Rosato J, Fuller-Tyszkiewicz M. Efficacy of a transdiagnostic cognitive-behavioral intervention for eating disorder psychopathology delivered through a smartphone app: a randomized controlled trial. Psychol Med. 2020:1–12.
98. Beintner I, Jacobi C, Schmidt UH. Participation and outcome in manualized self-help for bulimia nervosa and binge eating disorder – a systematic review and metaregression analysis. Clin Psychol Rev. 2014;34(2):158–76.

Part II

Can the Food Addiction Concept Improve Treatment?

4 Problems with Current Approaches to Treating Disorders of Overeating

4.1 Weight Loss with Available Treatments Is Modest

On the whole, behavioral, nutritional, and pharmacotherapeutic interventions lead to only modest weight loss, with questionable clinical significance. Adopting a healthier diet, caloric restriction, physical activity, behavioral weight loss, CBT-based interventions, and/or medications typically results in no more than a 5–10% reduction in body weight [1–5]. Adherence to dietary recommendations is a challenge for most people, likely due to innate counterregulatory mechanisms and primed brain hedonic eating pathways [3, 6, 7].

A meta-analysis comparing dietary interventions and resulting weight loss found that in 21,942 individuals and 212 trials undergoing low carb diets, low fat diets, or several popular named diets (Atkins, Zone, DASH) as opposed to usual diet, mean weight loss was about 4.5 kg. Of the popular named diets, Atkins had the largest effect on weight (5.5 kg loss) [8]. Although a number of commercially available weight loss programs boast >10% weight loss, meta-analyses show that attrition is greater than one third, with weight loss of less than 5% of initial body weight and effects diminishing further after 6 months [9–11]. Finally, a recent meta-analysis focused on primary care settings showed an average weight loss of about 5% of body weight [12, 13]. In the primary care setting, the optimal approach is not yet clear, with nutritional counseling alone actually outshining combined interventions (including a behavioral, exercise and nutritional component) in some studies [13]. Fasting strategies, such as alternate day fasting (ADF), don't appear to be any better for short-term weight loss, either [14–16].

Medications for weight loss may slightly augment degree of weight loss from nutritional and/or behavioral interventions [17]. In randomized controlled trials, currently approved anti-obesity drugs have yielded an average weight loss ranging from approximately 3% to 9% relative to placebo at 1 year [17]. In a meta-analysis of 43,443 obese individuals undergoing pharmacotherapy from 50 publications, the maximal mean weight loss relative to placebo for orlistat (120 mg), lorcaserin, naltrexone-bupropion, phentermine-topiramate (7.5/46 mg), and liraglutide was −2.94, − 3.06, − 6.15, − 7.45, and − 5.5 kg, at weeks 60, 54, 67, 59, and 65, respectively (Chap. 2, Table 2.1) [18]. Phentermine-topiramate has yielded the highest degree of loss and orlistat the lowest in most studies [17, 19].

However, the drug therapy has been questioned because typically body weight loss slows and then plateaus with continued treatment, degree of additional weight loss over behavioral and nutritional support is modest, and most patients regain weight when their weight loss drugs are stopped [19]. Most medication studies are rarely longer than several months except in

C. E. Wilcox, *Food Addiction, Obesity, and Disorders of Overeating*,
https://doi.org/10.1007/978-3-030-83078-6_4

the case of orlistat for which several long term studies are available [19]. Furthermore, medications act primarily on appetite, or in one case (orlistat) on absorption [19], but no approved weight loss medication appears to promote long-term thermogenesis, which also limits their efficacy potential [20]. The majority of participants in phase 3 trials of anti-obesity drugs have been white women; therefore, the efficacy and safety of these medicines in men and other ethic/racial groups is unknown [17, 19]. High attrition in weight loss medication clinical trials introduces serious bias to clinical trial results, making it difficult to trust favorable results and to know if they can be generalized to clinical practice [17, 19].

Bariatric surgery is the most effective weight loss intervention [1]. The most commonly performed procedures are Roux-en-Y gastric bypass (RYGB), vertical sleeve gastrectomy (VSG), and adjustable gastric band (BAND) [1]. The mean changes in body weight for 2, 10, 15, and 20 years after surgery are 23%, 17%, 16%, and 18%, respectively [1]. However, many patients still plateau earlier than desired [17] and a substantial proportion of individuals achieve inadequate weight loss post-surgery [21].

4.2 Maintenance of Weight Loss Is Difficult

Over time, most people gain back much if not all of the weight they lost after behavioral, lifestyle-based, and nutritional interventions [1, 10, 11], and relapse rates are quite high within a few months or years [2, 5]. In the aforementioned meta-analysis of 21,942 individuals, weight loss diminished at 12 months among all macronutrient patterns and popular named diets [8]. Even in studies that show promise for a particular diet in the short term (e.g., one found that VLCD works better than LCD), long-term (1–5 years) outcomes tend to be similar from diet to diet, and significant differences for an intervention demonstrated early on tend to disappear after 6 months to a year [5, 8, 22]. A study based on a large prospective cohort from the UK suggests that over a 9-year period, the probability of going from obese to normal was 1 in 210 for men and 1 in 124 for women [23, 24].

Pharmacotherapy is also associated with weight plateauing and then relapse or weight regain [19]. In the aforementioned meta-analysis of 43,443 obese individuals undergoing pharmacotherapy with orlistat, lorcaserin, naltrexone-bupropion, phentermine-topiramate, and liraglutide, mean rates of weight regain were 0.51 kg, 0.48 kg, 0.91 kg, 1.27 kg, and 0.43 kg per year, respectively [18]. Unfortunately, given poor adherence to these medications, and the fact that few trials continue treatment long term, it's difficult to accurately determine long-term outcomes with medication treatment [17]. One study showed that at 2 years, only 27% of patients in a trial were still taking naltrexone/bupropion, and weight loss was only 2.5% above placebo [17]. Similar rates of medication continuation (27%) were seen for phentermine-topiramate during the second year of another longer-term study [17]. There is limited evidence for sustained weight loss from medication treatment beyond 1 year in children and adolescents and in post-bariatric surgery patients [17].

Bariatric surgery is the most effective long-lasting weight loss intervention [1], but plateauing and rebound even occur following bariatric surgery [17, 25]. For example, nearly one in three patients undergoing BAND regained all their lost weight (to within 5% of baseline) by 4 years after surgery, and 15% of patients undergoing VSG regained to within 5% [26]. Furthermore, 24–28% of patients do not maintain a 20% or greater weight loss at 10 years following RYGB [26–28]. However, only around 3% regain weight back within 5% of their original baseline weight, indicating that possible long-term failure of weight loss of this particular surgery is low [26–28]. In another study of female surgical patients after RYGB surgery, half of whom met BED criteria according to the binge eating scale, binge eating was lowest at month six and was still only 1/5 of baseline at 1 year [21]. At follow-up years later, binge eating symptoms may revert and even return to pre-surgery levels [21, 29]. Medications post-surgery to minimize weight regain and plateauing are under study, with several open-label studies and chart reviews, but no published randomized controlled studies as of yet [17].

4.3 The Biology Behind the Difficulty of Weight Loss and Maintenance

The fact that minimal weight loss and high relapse rates occur with available treatments [1, 3, 4] suggests that weight loss involves more than just simple choice: "motivation to lose weight is necessary but often not sufficient" [30]. Some claim that this is because interventions address the outcomes of the disorder and not the underlying cause, e.g., altered biology [3]. Indeed, appetite increases with weight loss and dieting in large part due to our ingrained biology and homeostatic compensatory homeostatic mechanisms (Chaps. 1 and 2) [30]. These compensatory mechanisms include increases in circulating levels of the orexigenic (feeding-promoting) hormone ghrelin and reductions in the levels of the anorexigenic (satiety-promoting) hormones peptide YY (PYY), cholecystokinin (CCK), leptin, and insulin with dieting [20]. These changes may persist for at least 1 year after weight reduction and may remain that way indefinitely, promoting increased energy intake and ultimately weight regain years later [20, 31–33]. Metabolic rate also slows with weight loss, and the body decreases energy expenditure to match the reduced calorie intake [30, 34].

Furthermore, the obese state itself can cause the body to cease to respond to hunger and satiety signals properly [30]. Leptin resistance occurs over time, with chronically high circulating leptin levels due to excess adipose tissue. The response from the brain to leptin becomes blunted, and leptin no longer produces the same degree of satiety after a meal [30].

Hedonically mediated eating, or eating for pleasure [also the basis for the food addiction (FA) concept], is also not adequately addressed with standard treatment: for people with FA, reward, cognitive and emotional factors play a key role in food craving and food intake. Homeostatic mechanisms such as hunger and fullness are not the only cause of overeating [20]. Food deprivation during dieting also increases hedonically mediated eating and activation of associated brain pathways, which could cause food craving. Studies show that sensory cues associated with palatable food elicit greater activation in the brain with food restriction short term (hours) and following weight loss (2 weeks of dieting) [1, 35] and that regional cerebral blood flow is increased in key attention, motivation, and reward circuits during fasting states [36].

Interestingly, the brain pathways mediating hedonic eating are generally altered in the obese state with hyperresponsivity to food cues in reward and attentional circuits and reduced activation to a meal in brain areas responsible for self-control like the prefrontal cortex (Chap. 8); these changes have been found to predict greater future weight gain [1, 37, 38].

4.4 Eating Disorder (ED) Treatment Success Rates

Treatments [CBT and interpersonal psychotherapy (IPT)] for BED show long-lasting effects for some people, with full recovery seen in 2/3 of patients after 4 years, but 20% still have either no response or relapse [24, 39, 40]. BN is more difficult to treat, with relapse rates up to 43% over 60 months [24, 40]. Relapse might be mitigated if more attention were paid to biological factors driving binge eating, such as effects of cues on the brain, craving, and impulse control [24, 41].

Furthermore, these treatments do not generally lead to weight loss, which is a significant concern for obese patients with comorbid health problems [42, 43]. Studies show that reduction in binge episodes during treatment is not associated with weight loss initially (although, in one study, reduction in binging during treatment did predict modest weight loss at longer-term follow-up months later, indicating binging might be a slightly helpful treatment target for weight loss) [42, 43]. In a meta-analysis and systemic review of 114 studies totaling 8862 individuals with BED including many treatments (behavioral and pharmacotherapy, self-help and therapist-mediated), only behavioral weight loss therapy and inpatient treatment were associated with modest weight loss [44]. Most studies did not include long-term (greater than 1 year) follow-up data, but for behavioral weight loss therapy, the effect on BMI loss at posttreatment was reduced by about 80% at follow-ups longer than 12 months, and weight loss for inpatient treatment didn't remain significant beyond 1 year [44].

The addition of SSRIs can be helpful for binge eating but these medications generally have only modest benefits, and they do not reduce weight [45]. For patients with BED who have marked weight problems, some clinicians use drugs that may promote weight loss, such as lisdexamfetamine, topiramate, or zonisamide, although as reviewed above, weight loss is still modest, and their utility for long-term weight control and binge reduction is currently mostly unknown (Chap. 2, Table 2.1) [42]. Most medication trials have been short term (12 weeks) and exclude comorbid psychopathology (from which 43% of patients with BED suffer), making it difficult to know real-world efficacy [46].

4.5 ED and Obesity Treatments Give Conflicting Messages

Patients who are overweight or obese and suffer from BED or bulimia may receive conflicting treatment recommendations. Standard obesity treatment involves calorie restriction, combined with a behavioral approach to support weight loss. By contrast, a core assumption in ED treatment models is that dieting precipitates bingeing and that the pursuit of weight loss is counterproductive [24]. Standard CBT-based approaches to ED treatment discourage dieting [24, 47] and instead encourage eating all types of food, and eating frequent healthy meals, under the assumption that it's the restriction of food intake that triggers the binge eating. Instead of focusing on weight loss, mindful eating and body acceptance are encouraged [24]. But some overweight or obese patients with BED or bulimia wish to lose weight in addition to reducing binge eating and bulimic compensatory measures [42]. This is of particular clinical importance if a patient is obese or even overweight, or if they have health consequences from their overweight state. Although discouraging caloric restriction in patients with anorexia nervosa and some people with significant binge eating is best, it is not clear that all patients with binge eating benefit from approaches that discourage dieting and weight loss.

Where did this belief in the ED treatment world come from that BED treatment should turn focus away from weight loss or an abstinence-based approach to nutritional recommendations? Is it rooted in evidence or is it cultural? Probably both are true. In 2003, Fairburn introduced a transdiagnostic theory of EDs proposing that the actual ED diagnosis is not relevant to the treatment [24, 48], and his CBT-based model of ED treatment was adopted as the standard of care. This occurred when BED was in the Diagnostic and Statistical Manual of Mental Disorders (DSM-IV) appendix but not yet an official diagnosis [24]. In fact, because this is such a strongly ingrained part of ED treatment, many eating disorder treatment clinicians have abandoned trying to help patients lose weight in order to avoid being shamed by colleagues [24, 47]. The fact that most diets fail also supports this cultural belief [24, 47]. Some argue that this transdiagnostic model will not be useful for certain people, especially those who have FA [41].

Indeed, the data is mixed regarding whether dieting is a root cause for later development of BED or further weight gain. Some studies indicate that typical dieting behavior predicts higher risk of later weight gain. An animal study showed that bingeing occurs in animals from whom food has been restricted and that food-restricted animals end up having more weight gain overall [49]. In humans, fasting predicts binge eating and bulimic pathology 5 years later [1, 50, 51], and dieting predicts weight gain during the freshman year of college [52]. A twin study suggested that frequent intentional weight loss attempts increased the risk of future weight gain [53]. Other studies show mixed results. In one study of almost 100 BED outpatients, 65% reported an onset of dieting prior to their first binge, and 35% reported that binge eating preceded their first diet [24, 54]. In women with body image concerns, weight suppression correlated with future onset of eating disorders characterized by dietary restriction or compensatory weight control behaviors, but not with BED [24, 55]. In some cases, restraint is related to a lower body weight, better weight regulation, and a better diet quality, while in others, restraint predicts poor diet, overeating, and obesity [24, 56]. In terms of whether a rapid weight loss is more dangerous long term than slow or no weight loss, one study showed that a larger initial weight loss in obesity may predict better clinical outcomes including maintenance although cause and effect in this case is not entirely clear [57, 58].

The data is also mixed regarding whether weight loss interventions are safe and efficacious for individuals who binge eat. On the one hand, low and very low calorie diets (VLCD) are similarly effective for weight loss in obese patients who binge eat compared to obese patients who do not binge eat and can be equally effective for reducing binge eating in patients with and without BED [42, 59, 60]. In another study, although binge eating behavior developed among 62% of obese subjects undergoing a VLCD regimen, binge eating decreased among 39% [42, 60, 61]. Structured and professionally run obesity treatment programs utilizing caloric restriction and behavioral weight loss techniques in pediatric and adolescent populations have been found to reduce ED prevalence, ED risk, and ED symptoms [24, 62] and lead to weight loss. ADF, which involves pretty significant restriction of calorie intake several days a week, was not found to trigger an increase in binge eating in obese individuals [24, 63]. Interestingly, shape and weight concern appear to respond most effectively to weight loss rather than to psychotherapeutic intervention [43]. On the other hand, individuals with BED are at higher risk of not responding to weight control interventions [24, 64].

Clearly more treatments are needed to address concurrent eating disorders and obesity as well as studies to identify who would be more likely to benefit or worsen from a more restrictive approach and what kind of approach would work best in which individuals [24]. For example, individuals with higher impulsivity and lower inhibitory control have worse outcomes to eating disorder and weight loss interventions, with minimal weight loss and high relapse as well as binge eating and bulimic symptoms [1, 50, 51, 65], and medications and other interventions to target this impulsivity trait might be particularly useful in this subgroup, for example, as well [24]. Considering the possibility of FA may be key to improving outcomes as well, as we will discuss throughout the rest of this book.

4.6 Side Effects of Diets

There are several possible negative medical consequences from adopting some of the more extreme forms of dietary restriction. For example, a VLCD is associated with increased risk of developing gallstones: one study showed that after 8 weeks of VLCD, 25% of patients developed gallstones, and 6% required cholecystectomy [60]. There is also growing concern about the potential adverse effects of ultra-processed VLCD on gut microbiota, which can in turn adversely affect mood and food craving [66]. Furthermore, high protein, high fat, and ketogenic diets, including the Atkins diet and the ketogenic diets, have been found to be associated with development of nonalcoholic fatty liver disease (NAFLD) and insulin resistance and may have negative effects on lipid profiles per animal studies, but in humans, there appear to be generally positive cardiometabolic effects, with mixed results regarding insulin resistance [67]. Finally, as mentioned above, restrictive dieting of any kind, especially in those with eating disorder vulnerabilities, can lead to binge eating, other disordered eating behavior, and ED diagnoses in some individuals.

4.7 Limitations and Side Effects of Medications

Although medications can help promote weight loss and improve binge eating, poor tolerability limits the use of medications for obesity and ED [1, 17]. Indeed, clinical trials show high dropout rates for weight loss medications, with 1-year dropout rates for orlistat, lorcaserin, naltrexone-bupropion, phentermine-topiramate, and liraglutide as high as 29.0, 40.9, 49.1, 34.9, and 24.3%, respectively, mainly due to adverse effects [1, 68]. Dropout rates in phase 3 trials of approved anti-obesity drugs were in the range of 40–50% over 1 year [17]. In the real world, adherence to these medicines seems to significantly drop after a month of treatment [17, 69]. Furthermore, among the approximate 71.6 million US adults with obesity, anti-obesity drug utilization is only at an estimated 660,000 people per year, and only about 3% of people trying to lose weight between 2013 and 2016 reported using prescription medication for weight loss [17]. Another similar study in the same time period at the Veterans Health Administration's MOVE! Weight Management Program from 2013 through 2016 found that only 1% of veterans enrolled in the program were prescribed an anti-obesity drug [17]. Physicians and other providers cite ineffectiveness and safety as concerns that limit their prescribing, often referring to the removal of fenfluramine and dexfenfluramine from the market in 1997 [17].

Several medications which have come (or were almost FDA approved for marketing) but since gone, have dampened enthusiasm for obesity and ED medications in general. For example, lorcaserin was recently taken off the market for increased risk of cancer [70]. Rimonabant, a CB-1 antagonist which had initially shown efficacy, was found to be associated with a variety of psychiatric concerns (increased suicidal thinking and depression in persons who are already suffering from mental disorders). Sibutramine, a stimulant-like medication was withdrawn from the market due to cardiovascular concerns. Fenfluramine/phentermine was withdrawn for cardiac valvular abnormalities [71]. In addition, lack of insurance coverage, high out-of-pocket costs, and patients' inability to afford anti-obesity drugs contribute to the reluctance of healthcare providers to prescribe these drugs [17].

Nausea is the most common side effect of weight loss medications [1] as are insomnia, paresthesia, dry mouth, depression, anxiety, and constipation (Chap. 2, Table 2.1) [17]. In one review, the percentage of patients discontinuing drug due to AEs was found to be highest for naltrexone-bupropion (24.0%) [17]. In a trial of naltrexone-bupropion or placebo in combination with intensive lifestyle intervention, 42% dropped out in the lifestyle intervention plus placebo group, with 12% citing their early withdrawal to an adverse event [17, 72]. Combination medications such as naltrexone-bupropion and phentermine-topiramate may have worse tolerability and higher risk of drug-drug interactions by nature of the fact that they have two components, and indeed some studies indicate bupropion alone may work just as well for weight loss as the combination medication [17].

There are also expressed concerns about the safety of some of these medicines, especially the stimulant-based ones: phentermine-topiramate, naltrexone-bupropion, and lisdexamfetamine [1, 19]. Amphetamines can cause addiction, myocardial infarction, stroke, and death [73], and these risks might not be adequately emphasized in marketing. For example, a study of bias in continuing medical education (CME) modules concluded that lisdexamfetamine was over-marketed and the risks downplayed. Specifically, all of 27 online CME activities on BED in 2015 were found by this study to be funded by Shire, which manufactures lisdexamfetamine, 7 of 16 presenters disclosed financial ties with Shire, and none mentioned the cardiac (stroke, blood pressure, tachycardia) or addiction risks [73]. That said, experts argue that lisdexamfetamine is less addictive and abusable than the other stimulants due to its slow onset of action, since it's a "pro-drug" [74, 75]. Furthermore, naltrexone-bupropion has a black box warning for suicidality and suicide attempts [17]. Thankfully, tesofensine, which is a medicine under study with stimulant mechanisms, bupropion, and atomoxetine were found to have limited psychoactive and euphoric effects compared to d-amphetamine in a head-to-head study [18]. Phentermine also has a lower abuse potential [18, 71].

Finally, in terms of safety for other medications for BED and weight loss, SSRIs also have a black-box warning for suicide in individuals under the age of 25; topiramate is associated with fetal malformations, renal stones and gastrointestinal distress and causes cognitive dulling as well as paresthesias [18]. Orlistat, which blocks dietary fat absorption, can also cause fecal urgency and fecal incontinence [17]. Zonisamide, which has a similar mechanism to topiramate but a more favorable side effect profile, especially in attention and cognition, is understudied [76].

There is limited evidence for safety and efficacy of anti-obesity drugs in children and adolescents and in post-bariatric surgery patients [17]. At this point, only orlistat is approved for adolescent use [17, 77].

4.8 Side Effects of Bariatric Surgery

Bariatric surgery (BS) is clearly the most effective weight loss tool available which results in 15 to 30% total weight loss that can be sustained for years, but bariatric surgery is invasive with a relatively high potential for adverse effects [1, 78]. Risks of the BAND include port problems, slippage, reflux disease, and vomiting or dysphagia as well as infection [79]. Post-op risks of the RYGB and VSG include anesthesia-related risks, infection, obstruction, reflux, and esophageal dilation [80]. Sometimes people are not able to eat certain foods and lose weight too rapidly [80]. Others fail to lose weight [80]. Long-term risks include dumping syndrome, with nausea and dizziness and diarrhea, low blood sugar, malnutrition (protein and vitamin deficiencies, especially vitamin D and B and iron), chronic vomiting, ulcers, bowel obstruction and hernias, stomach perforation, and gallstones [81]. Vomiting may result from overeating or attempts to binge eat [21, 29]. Vomiting commonly occurs postoperatively, both acutely and involuntarily, or in response to dysphagia [21]. Self-induced vomiting related to concerns of body weight and shape appear much more rarely following BS [21]. Chronic pain is also a frequent complaint after gastric bypass surgery [1]. Rates of serious complications were 1% for VSG, 1.25% for RYGB and 0.25% for BAND [82]. Risks of minor complications for these surgeries were high; reflux went from 13% before surgery to 39% after BAND and 23% after VSG. Iron deficiency rates after RYGB are as high as 51%, and rates of gallstones after the surgeries range from 22% to 71% [80].

4.9 Difficulty of Exercising When Obese

Although physical activity plays a key role in health, mental well-being and successful weight loss, and a sedentary lifestyle promotes obesity, it is difficult for obese individuals to engage in significant amounts of exercise due to limitations of large body habitus. Once overweight or obesity develops, there is a vicious cycle of physical inactivity, low energy expenditure, and obesity [5]. Furthermore, exercise by obese people has been found to cause a decrease in leptin and an increase in ghrelin, both of which are hormone changes that tend to increase appetite [5].

4.10 Conclusion

In summary, there are numerous limitations, problems, and potential negative consequences associated with our currently available treatments for overweight, obesity, and clinically significant binge eating. New and improved approaches to treatment are needed.

References

1. Lin Z, Qu S. Legend of weight loss: a crosstalk between the bariatric surgery and the brain. Obes Surg. 2020;30:1988–2002.

2. Franz MJ, VanWormer JJ, Crain AL, Boucher JL, Histon T, Caplan W, et al. Weight-loss outcomes: a systematic review and meta-analysis of weight-loss clinical trials with a minimum 1-year follow-up. J Am Diet Assoc. 2007;107:1755–67.
3. Adams RC, Sedgmond J, Maizey L, Chambers CD, Lawrence NS. Food addiction: implications for the diagnosis and treatment of overeating. Nutrients. 2019;11
4. Guise S. Mini habits for weight loss: stop dieting. Form new habits. Change your lifestyle without suffering. Selective Entertainment LLC; 2016.
5. Tobore TO. Towards a comprehensive theory of obesity and a healthy diet: the causal role of oxidative stress in food addiction and obesity. Behav Brain Res. 2020;384:112560.
6. Bacon L, Aphramor L. Weight science: evaluating the evidence for a paradigm shift. Nutr J. 2011;10:9.
7. Mann T, Tomiyama AJ, Westling E, Lew A-M, Samuels B, Chatman J. Medicare's search for effective obesity treatments: diets are not the answer. Am Psychol. 2007;62:220–33.
8. Ge L, Sadeghirad B, Ball GDC, da Costa BR, Hitchcock CL, Svendrovski A, et al. Comparison of dietary macronutrient patterns of 14 popular named dietary programmes for weight and cardiovascular risk factor reduction in adults: systematic review and network meta-analysis of randomised trials. BMJ. 2020;369:m696.
9. McEvedy SM, Sullivan-Mort G, McLean SA, Pascoe MC, Paxton SJ. Ineffectiveness of commercial weight-loss programs for achieving modest but meaningful weight loss: systematic review and meta-analysis. J Health Psychol. 2017;22:1614–27.
10. Jensen MD, Ryan DH, Apovian CM, Ard JD, Comuzzie AG, Donato KA, et al. 2013 AHA/ACC/TOS guideline for the management of overweight and obesity in adults: a report of the American College of Cardiology/American Heart Association Task Force on Practice Guidelines and the Obesity Society. J Am Coll Cardiol. 2014;63:2985–3023.
11. Perreault L, Apovian C, Seres D. Obesity in adults: Overview of management. UpTo-Date Apr [Internet]. www.uptodate.com: uptodate.com; 2019 [cited 2018 Aug 2.]; Available from: https://www.uptodate.com/contents/obesity-in-adults-overview-of-management.
12. de Menezes MC, Duarte CK, Costa DV de P, Lopes MS, Freitas PP de, Campos SF, et al. A systematic review of effects, potentialities, and limitations of nutritional interventions aimed at managing obesity in primary and secondary health care. Nutrition. 2020;75–76:110784.
13. Canuto R, Garcez A, de Souza RV, Kac G, Olinto MTA. Nutritional intervention strategies for the management of overweight and obesity in primary health care: a systematic review with meta-analysis. Obes Rev. 2021;22:e13143.
14. Trepanowski JF, Kroeger CM, Barnosky A, Klempel M, Bhutani S, Hoddy KK, et al. Effects of alternate-day fasting or daily calorie restriction on body composition, fat distribution, and circulating adipokines: secondary analysis of a randomized controlled trial. Clin Nutr. 2018;37:1871–8.
15. Trepanowski JF, Kroeger CM, Barnosky A, Klempel MC, Bhutani S, Hoddy KK, et al. Effect of alternate-day fasting on weight loss, weight maintenance, and Cardioprotection among metabolically healthy obese adults: a randomized clinical trial. JAMA Intern Med. 2017;177:930–8.
16. Catenacci VA, Pan Z, Ostendorf D, Brannon S, Gozansky WS, Mattson MP, et al. A randomized pilot study comparing zero-calorie alternate-day fasting to daily caloric restriction in adults with obesity. Obesity. 2016;24:1874–83.
17. Gadde KM, Atkins KD. The limits and challenges of antiobesity pharmacotherapy. Expert Opin Pharmacother. 2020;21:1319–28.
18. Coulter AA, Rebello CJ, Greenway FL. Centrally acting agents for obesity: past, present, and future. Drugs. 2018;78:1113–32.
19. Perreault L. Obesity in adults: Drug therapy [Internet]. UpToDate. www.uptodate.com: UpToDate; 2018 [cited 2018 Aug 2]. Available from: https://www.uptodate.com/contents/obesity-in-adults-drug-therapy.
20. Apovian CM, Aronne LJ, Bessesen DH, McDonnell ME, Murad MH, Pagotto U. Pharmacological management of obesity: an Endocrine Society Clinical Practice Guideline. J Clin Endocrinol Metab. 2015;100:342–62.
21. Ben-Porat T, Weiss R, Sherf-Dagan S, Rottenstreich A, Kaluti D, Khalaileh A, et al. Food addiction and binge eating during one year following sleeve gastrectomy: prevalence and implications for postoperative outcomes. Obes Surg. 2021;31:603–11.
22. Perreault L. UpToDate [Internet]. UpToDate. 2018 [cited 2021 Apr 12]. Available from: https://www.uptodate.com/contents/obesity-in-adults-etiology-and-risk-factors.
23. Fildes A, Charlton J, Rudisill C, Littlejohns P, Prevost AT, Gulliford MC. Probability of an obese person attaining normal body weight: cohort study using electronic health records. Am J Public Health. 2015;105:e54–9.
24. Wiss D, Brewerton T. Separating the signal from the noise: how psychiatric diagnoses can help discern food addiction from dietary restraint. Nutrients. 2020;12:2937.
25. Schwartz J, Chaudhry UI, Suzo A, Durkin N, Wehr AM, Foreman KS, et al. Erratum to: pharmacotherapy in conjunction with a diet and exercise program for the treatment of weight recidivism or weight-loss plateau post-bariatric surgery: a retrospective review. Obes Surg. 2016;26:706.
26. Maciejewski ML, Arterburn DE, Van Scoyoc L, Smith VA, Yancy WS Jr, Weidenbacher HJ, et al. Bariatric

surgery and long-term durability of weight loss. JAMA Surg. 2016;151:1046–55.
27. Sjöström L. Review of the key results from the Swedish Obese Subjects (SOS) trial – a prospective controlled intervention study of bariatric surgery. J Intern Med. 2013;273:219–34.
28. Adams TD, Davidson LE, Litwin SE, Kolotkin RL, LaMonte MJ, Pendleton RC, et al. Health benefits of gastric bypass surgery after 6 years. JAMA. 2012;308:1122–31.
29. Spirou D, Raman J, Smith E. Psychological outcomes following surgical and endoscopic bariatric procedures: a systematic review. Obes Rev. 2020;21(6):e12998.
30. Kinasz KR, Ross DA, Cooper JJ. Eat to live or live to eat? The neurobiology of appetite regulation. Biol Psychiatry. 2017;81(9):e73–5.
31. Lutter M, Nestler EJ. Homeostatic and hedonic signals interact in the regulation of food intake. J Nutr. 2009;139:629–32.
32. Volkow ND, Wang G-J, Tomasi D, Baler RD. Obesity and addiction: neurobiological overlaps. Obes Rev. 2013;14:2–18.
33. Sumithran P, Prendergast LA, Delbridge E, Purcell K, Shulkes A, Kriketos A, et al. Long-term persistence of hormonal adaptations to weight loss. N Engl J Med. 2011;365:1597–604.
34. Fothergill E, Guo J, Howard L, Kerns JC, Knuth ND, Brychta R, et al. Persistent metabolic adaptation 6 years after "the biggest loser" competition. Obesity. 2016;24:1612–9.
35. Stice E, Burger K, Yokum S. Caloric deprivation increases responsivity of attention and reward brain regions to intake, anticipated intake, and images of palatable foods. NeuroImage. 2013;67:322–30.
36. DelParigi A, Chen K, Salbe AD, Hill JO, Wing RR, Reiman EM, et al. Persistence of abnormal neural responses to a meal in postobese individuals. Int J Obes Relat Metab Disord. 2004;28:370–7.
37. Val-Laillet D, Aarts E, Weber B, Ferrari M, Quaresima V, Stoeckel LE, et al. Neuroimaging and neuromodulation approaches to study eating behavior and prevent and treat eating disorders and obesity. Neuroimage Clin. 2015;8:1–31.
38. DelParigi A, Chen K, Salbe AD, Hill JO, Wing RR, Reiman EM, et al. Successful dieters have increased neural activity in cortical areas involved in the control of behavior. Int J Obes. 2007;31:440–8.
39. Hilbert A, Bishop ME, Stein RI, Tanofsky-Kraff M, Swenson AK, Welch RR, et al. Long-term efficacy of psychological treatments for binge eating disorder. Br J Psychiatry. 2012;200:232–7.
40. Grilo CM, Pagano ME, Stout RL, Markowitz JC, Ansell EB, Pinto A, et al. Stressful life events predict eating disorder relapse following remission: six-year prospective outcomes. Int J Eat Disord. 2012;45:185–92.
41. Treasure J, Leslie M, Chami R, Fernández-Aranda F. Are trans diagnostic models of eating disorders fit for purpose? A consideration of the evidence for food addiction. Eur Eat Disord Rev. 2018;26:83–91.
42. Sysko R, Delvin M. Binge eating disorder in adults: overview of treatment [Internet]. UpToDate. 2018 [cited 2018]. Available from: https://www.uptodate.com/contents/binge-eating-disorder-in-adults-overview-of-treatment.
43. Pacanowski CR, Mason TB, Crosby RD, Mitchell JE, Crow SJ, Wonderlich SA, et al. Weight change over the course of binge eating disorder treatment: relationship to binge episodes and psychological factors. Obesity. 2018;26:838–44.
44. Hilbert A, Petroff D, Herpertz S, Pietrowsky R, Tuschen-Caffier B, Vocks S, et al. Meta-analysis on the long-term effectiveness of psychological and medical treatments for binge-eating disorder. Int J Eat Disord. 2020;53:1353–76.
45. Wilcox CE. Binge eating disorder. CMEtoGo.com: American Physician Institute; 2019.
46. Wilfley DE, Fitzsimmons-Craft EE, Eichen DM. Binge-eating disorder in adults. Ann Intern Med. 2017:230–1.
47. Hunger JM, Dodd DR, Smith AR. Weight discrimination, anticipated weight stigma, and disordered eating. Eat Behav. 2020;37:101383.
48. Fairburn CG, Cooper Z, Shafran R. Cognitive behaviour therapy for eating disorders: a "transdiagnostic" theory and treatment. Behav Res Ther. 2003;41:509–28.
49. Berner LA, Avena NM, Hoebel BG. Bingeing, self-restriction, and increased body weight in rats with limited access to a sweet-fat diet. Obesity. 2008;16:1998–2002.
50. Stice E, Davis K, Miller NP, Marti CN. Fasting increases risk for onset of binge eating and bulimic pathology: a 5-year prospective study. J Abnorm Psychol. 2008;117:941–6.
51. Neumark-Sztainer D, Wall M, Guo J, Story M, Haines J, Eisenberg M. Obesity, disordered eating, and eating disorders in a longitudinal study of adolescents. J Am Diet Assoc. 2006;106(4):559–68.
52. Lowe MR, Annunziato RA, Markowitz JT, Didie E, Bellace DL, Riddell L, et al. Multiple types of dieting prospectively predict weight gain during the freshman year of college. Appetite. 2006;47:83–90.
53. Pietiläinen KH, Saarni SE, Kaprio J, Rissanen A. Does dieting make you fat? A twin study. Int J Obes (Springer Nature). 2012;36:456–64.
54. Grilo CM, Masheb RM. Onset of dieting vs binge eating in outpatients with binge eating disorder. Int J Obes Relat Metab Disord. 2000;24:404–9.
55. Stice E, Rohde P, Shaw H, Desjardins C. Weight suppression increases odds for future onset of anorexia nervosa, bulimia nervosa, and purging dis-

order, but not binge eating disorder. Am J Clin Nutr. 2020;112:941–7.

56. Bryant EJ, Rehman J, Pepper LB, Walters ER. Obesity and eating disturbance: the role of TFEQ restraint and disinhibition. Curr Obes Rep. 2019;8:363–72.
57. Casazza K, Brown A, Astrup A, Bertz F, Baum C, Brown MB, et al. Weighing the evidence of common beliefs in obesity research. Crit Rev Food Sci Nutr. 2015;55:2014–53.
58. Meule A. A critical examination of the practical implications derived from the food addiction concept. Curr Obes Rep. 2019;8:11–7.
59. Wadden TA, Foster GD, Letizia KA. One-year behavioral treatment of obesity: comparison of moderate and severe caloric restriction and the effects of weight maintenance therapy. J Consult Clin Psychol. 1994;62:165–71.
60. Alhamdan BA, Garcia-Alvarez A, Alzahrnai AH, Karanxha J, Stretchberry DR, Contrera KJ, et al. Alternate-day versus daily energy restriction diets: which is more effective for weight loss? A systematic review and meta-analysis. Obes Sci Pract. 2016;2:293–302.
61. Telch CF, Agras WS. The effects of short-term food deprivation on caloric intake in eating-disordered subjects. Appetite. 1996;26:221–33.
62. Jebeile H, Gow ML, Baur LA, Garnett SP, Paxton SJ, Lister NB. Treatment of obesity, with a dietary component, and eating disorder risk in children and adolescents: a systematic review with meta-analysis. Obes Rev. 2019;20:1287–98.
63. Hoddy KK, Kroeger CM, Trepanowski JF, Barnosky AR, Bhutani S, Varady KA. Safety of alternate day fasting and effect on disordered eating behaviors. Nutr J. 2015;14:44.
64. Dakanalis A, Clerici M. Tackling excess body weight in people with binge eating disorder. Aust N Z J Psychiatry. 2019;53(10):1027.
65. Nederkoorn C, Braet C, Van Eijs Y, Tanghe A, Jansen A. Why obese children cannot resist food: the role of impulsivity. Eat Behav. 2006;7:315–22.
66. Lane M, Howland G, West M, Hockey M, Marx W, Loughman A, et al. The effect of ultra-processed very low-energy diets on gut microbiota and metabolic outcomes in individuals with obesity: a systematic literature review. Obes Res Clin Pract. 2020;14:197–204.
67. Kosinski C, Jornayvaz FR. Effects of ketogenic diets on cardiovascular risk factors: evidence from animal and human studies. Nutrients [Internet]. 2017;9. Available from: https://doi.org/10.3390/nu9050517.
68. Dong Z, Xu L, Liu H, Lv Y, Zheng Q, Li L. Comparative efficacy of five long-term weight loss drugs: quantitative information for medication guidelines. Obes Rev. 2017;18:1377–85.
69. Ganguly R, Tian Y, Kong SX, Hersloev M, Hobbs T, Smolarz BG, et al. Persistence of newer anti-obesity medications in a real-world setting. Diabetes Res Clin Pract. 2018;143:348–56.
70. FDA requests the withdrawal of the weight-loss drug Belviq, Belviq XR (lorcaserin) from the market [Internet]. U.S. Food & Drug Administration. 2020 [cited 2021 Apr 23]. Available from: https://www.fda.gov/drugs/drug-safety-and-availability/fda-requests-withdrawal-weight-loss-drug-belviq-belviq-xr-lorcaserin-market.
71. Vardanyan GS, Harutyunyan HS, Aghajanov MI, Vardanyan RS. Neurochemical regulators of food behavior for pharmacological treatment of obesity: current status and future prospects. Future Med Chem. 2020;12:1865–84.
72. Wadden TA, Faulconbridge LF, Jones-Corneille LR, Sarwer DB, Fabricatore AN, Thomas JG, et al. Binge eating disorder and the outcome of bariatric surgery at one year: a prospective, observational study. Obesity. 2011;19:1220–8.
73. Jung J, Fugh-Berman A. Marketing messages in Continuing Medical Education (CME) modules on Binge-Eating Disorder (BED). J Am Board Fam Med. 2020;33:240–51.
74. Hudson JI, McElroy SL, Ferreira-Cornwell MC, Radewonuk J, Gasior M. Efficacy of Lisdexamfetamine in adults with moderate to severe binge-eating disorder: a randomized clinical trial. JAMA Psychiat. 2017;74:903–10.
75. McElroy SL, Hudson JI, Mitchell JE, Wilfley D, Ferreira-Cornwell MC, Gao J. Efficacy and safety of lisdexamfetamine for treatment of adults with moderate to severe binge-eating disorder: a randomized clinical trial. JAMA Psychiat. 2015;72:235–46.
76. McElroy SL, Kotwal R, Guerdjikova AI, Welge JA, Nelson EB, Lake KA, et al. Zonisamide in the treatment of binge eating disorder with obesity: a randomized controlled trial. J Clin Psychiatry. 2006;67:1897–906.
77. O'Connor EA, Evans CV, Burda BU, Walsh ES, Eder M, Lozano P. Screening for obesity and intervention for weight management in children and adolescents: evidence report and systematic review for the US Preventive Services Task Force. JAMA. 2017;317:2427–44.
78. Telem D, Greenstein AJ, Wolfe B. Outcomes of bariatric surgery [Internet]. UpToDate. Waltham, MA: UpToDate; 2021 [cited 2021 Apr 26]. Available from: https://www.uptodate.com/contents/outcomes-of-bariatric-surgery.

79. Kodner C, Hartman D. Complications of adjustable gastric banding surgery for obesity. Am Fam Physician. 2014;89:813–8.
80. Ma IT, Madura JA 2nd. Gastrointestinal complications after bariatric surgery. Gastroenterol Hepatol. 2015;11:526–35.
81. Bariatric Surgery Risks, Complications & Side Effects [Internet]. UPMC. [cited 2018]. Available from: https://www.upmc.com/services/bariatrics/candidate/risks-and-complications.
82. American Society for Metabolic and Bariatric Surgery. Studies weigh in on safety and effectiveness of newer bariatric and metabolic surgery procedure [Internet]. ASMBS. 2012 [cited 2018]. Available from: https://asmbs.org/resources/studies-weigh-in-on-safety-and-effectiveness-of-newer-bariatric-and-metabolic-surgery-procedure.

5 The Food Addiction Concept: History, Controversy, Potential Pitfalls, and Promises

5.1 History

The FA term suggests that individuals may experience addictive-like responses to food similar to those seen with substances of abuse [1], and the construct was first brought up in a research article in 1956 [2]. In 1960, Overeaters Anonymous (OA) was founded, in which the 12-step-based model of addiction was applied to food overconsumption, in the hopes the model might also support recovery from overeating and obesity [2]. In parallel, the world experienced a surge in availability of highly palatable (HP) and processed foods, and the obesity epidemic was born and grew [3–5].

Preclinical research, and human neuroimaging research into the addictive effects of certain foods, has provided growing support for the existence of a food addiction (FA) syndrome over the last several decades (Chaps. 7, 8, 9, and 10). In upcoming chapters, we will review research that excess palatable food can affect the brain in a similar manner as drugs of abuse, that animal models overfed with certain foods can develop craving, loss of control, and withdrawal symptoms, and that there are many similarities in the opioidergic and dopaminergic systems in the brain between overfed, bingeing animals, and animal models of stimulant or opioid dependence.

Clinical research in this area has also ballooned recently (Chap. 6), making it increasingly clear that some people experience addictive-like responses to certain food, particularly processed foods high in fat and/or sugar [6, 7]. To facilitate study of the construct in humans, in 2009, a scale designed after the Diagnostic and Statistical Manual of Mental Disorders (DSM), called the Yale Food Addiction Scale (YFAS), was developed and validated [2, 6–9]. Other FA scales have also been developed but are less widely used [6, 10]. Since the YFAS has been made available, the number of studies on FA has increased exponentially, with over 1000 peer-reviewed papers published in the past 5 years, in diverse populations, utilizing various methodologies with behavioral and biological measures [7]. With growing awareness of the parallels in the biological, psychological, and behavioral factors implicated in addiction and problematic eating, increasing numbers of investigators hypothesize that addictive processes may contribute to eating disorders (ED) associated with binge eating and obesity [3, 11, 12].

5.2 Is the FA Concept Valid?

5.2.1 Can Obesity Be Explained by FA?

Some assert that attributing all obesity and overeating behavior solely to FA and changes in addiction-based reward brain circuitry would be erroneous [3, 8, 13–15]. Indeed, it is true that the

C. E. Wilcox, *Food Addiction, Obesity, and Disorders of Overeating*,
https://doi.org/10.1007/978-3-030-83078-6_5

majority of obesity is, in fact, not associated with an FA diagnosis (Chap. 12) and that the causes of weight gain and obesity are diverse and complex [16]. However, many cases of obesity are likely caused or made worse by FA (Chap. 12), and just because most obesity is not due to FA does not invalidate the construct.

5.2.2 Is FA Distinct from BED and Bulimia?

Rates of FA are much higher in BED and bulimia nervosa (BN) populations (up to 100% in some smaller studies; Chaps. 6 and 12) compared to controls. For this reason, some question whether FA represents a distinct phenomenon separate from BED or BN or whether it is actually just a new name applied to an old construct, since these two groups of disorders are both characterized by loss of control around eating [1, 17, 18]. We will address this question in Chap. 6 when we discuss the discriminant validity of the YFAS, but the short answer is yes, research supports that it does represent a new entity [12]. There are also several important theoretical differences between EDs and FA. For example, FA diagnostic criteria include withdrawal, tolerance, and craving [2], whereas EDs emphasize the importance of shape and weight concern [12, 19]. Over-restriction is seen to be a primary cause and treatment target in the treatment of ED and "no forbidden foods" food plans are often utilized [20, 21], whereas FA treatment models will likely incorporate suggestions to abstain from certain foods [2, 22].

5.2.3 Do DSM Criteria for SUD Present in Relation to Food in Humans and Do Symptoms Cluster Together?

Some claim that despite the robust animal literature, there is not yet enough evidence to support the existence of FA in clinical populations. However, initial work done to validate the YFAS and YFAS 2.0 indicates the FA construct is valid and that the symptoms cluster together [8, 12]. Furthermore, a growing body of literature supports higher rates of SUD in BED and BN populations and higher rates of binge eating, sweet preference, and transfer of addictive behavior from drugs to food during abstinence in substance-using populations (Chap. 6).

5.2.4 Is It Valid to Claim Certain Foods Are "Addictive," and Might It Be More Accurate to Consider FA a Behavioral Disorder?

An underlying principal of FA is that there is something in the food, itself, which is toxic, and "addictive." But some question whether food can be considered addictive if it is necessary to our survival [6, 23]. Furthermore, one single or several single food items have not been identified as being consistently the culprits underlying addictive behavior [14, 24]. Indeed, whereas classic substances of abuse contain a clear addictive agent (e.g., ethanol in alcoholic beverages, nicotine in tobacco, delta-9-tetrahydrocannabinol in marijuana), a specific, addictive substance has not been identified in foods [2, 24–28]. Relatedly, people assert that cyclical addiction models, where substance use causes brain changes that lead to loss of control of use (Chaps. 7 and 8) don't apply to food and eating behaviors [29].

Questions such as these lead people to wonder about semantics and whether the addictive eating phenomenon would better be considered through the lens of other behavioral disorders, like gambling addiction [1, 14, 20, 24, 30, 31]. A behavioral addiction is characterized by compulsive behaviors and actions that have been reinforced over time, and that are associated with changes in many of the same brain circuits as is seen in SUD [6, 9, 32], but focus more on the reinforcing nature of the behaviors rather than the toxic substance itself. Supporters of a more behavioral addiction model suggest that the terms "eating addiction" or "food use disorder" might more accurately capture the construct. Indeed, "compulsive overeating" was recently considered for inclusion in the DSM-V [6, 33].

That said, there is a growing body of evidence that certain categories of food, such as many of the highly processed, high-carbohydrate, high caloric density, high-fat, and high-sugar foods, act on the brain in similar manner as substances of abuse [2, 6, 12, 20, 24, 28, 30, 31] (Chaps. 11 and 13) in ways that prime the reward system and lead to the downward spiral of addiction.

5.3 Is the FA Model Useful, and Do Benefits Outweigh Harms?

5.3.1 Abstinence-Based Food Plans

During treatment of an SUD, often (but not always) providers recommend patients to become abstinent from a problem substance, at least for a period of time [24]. That said, harm reduction models of SUD treatment are getting increasing attention [20, 34]. But, for most people with SUD, abstinence is often the easiest solution. As more and more FA-based treatments for obesity and binge eating are developed, we will likely see as part of these treatments nutritional recommendations that suggest abstention, or partial abstention, from certain foods, such as those that are highly processed or high in sugar and/or fat.

Abstinence models have been considered and proposed for the treatment of BN and obesity for decades, and such approaches are currently advocated by self-help groups such as OA [24, 35, 36]. However, many experts, and especially ED treatment professionals, raise red flags about the idea of labeling certain foods as addictive, out of concerns that this might cause more harm than good and might even being dangerous in some cases [24], worsening ED symptoms by encouraging restrictive behavior [20, 24]. Recall that food avoidance, calorie restriction, dieting, and the pursuit of weight loss are seen as major causes of bingeing behavior, and ED treatments discourage this (Chap. 3) [20] out of concern that both calorie restriction and avoidance of particular foods increase the risk for severe caloric restriction, purging, and resultant dangerous medical consequences. The Disordered Eating and Food Addiction Nutrition Guide (DEFANG) rejects the concept of food having addictive qualities and favors an "all foods fit" ("no bad foods") approach [20, 37]. The "Health at any size" movement is growing in popularity among ED treatment providers as well. However, whether this approach is appropriate for all ED patients is still unclear (Chap. 3). Further work is needed to determine whether all EDs should be treated with non-restrictive approaches or whether a subgroup might do better with FA-based models involving trigger food or HP food avoidance strategies, and if there were such a subgroup, how best to identify them (e.g., based on higher weight status, the absence of a restriction history, and/or an FA diagnosis) (Chap. 14).

5.3.2 Self-Efficacy

It is not clear what effects the application of the "disease model of addiction" (e.g., describing addition as a brain disease) [38] to overeating will have on eating behavior, and some have expressed concerns that such models might reduce self-efficacy, by increasing perceptions that one's weight and eating are out of one's control, which could undermine motivation for dietary and behavioral change [24, 39, 40]. On the other hand, the belief that there is a medical cause for one's condition may increase willingness to seek treatment and to try a medication or an abstinence-based approach to recovery [39]. Furthermore, the FA model might reduce perceptions of personal failure: in BN studies, using addiction as a treatment metaphor can be helpful to motivate change [24, 41]. Ultimately though, we do not know what impact telling people that they have FA will have on their adherence to recommendations, eating behavior, ED severity, and weight and more studies are needed [39].

5.3.3 Public Health

Whether applying the FA concepts to our understanding of disordered eating will help or harm obesity prevention efforts is unknown and also still a subject of debate [24, 42]. The food industry enhances the rewarding properties of food by manipulating salt, sugar, fat, flavors, and additives [24, 39, 43], and the spike in obesity rates has paralleled the rise in availability of cheap, highly refined, calorie-dense foods [39, 44]. Many conceptualize obesity more as a product of environmental exposure rather than due to personal choice [24, 39, 44–49]. Increased regulation, such as taxation of HP foods and warnings on labels has been touted by some as the only way to deal with the obesity epidemic successfully, especially the case in children and adolescents [15, 22, 39, 44]. However, like with tobacco, the food industry has actively resisted any restricting policies [39, 44], and governmental regulation of the food industry is minimal [24]. Interestingly, food regulation policies are not as popular with the general public as they are with tobacco [24, 39, 44], which makes it even harder to progress with prevention efforts.

Increased recognition of FA could theoretically undermine efforts to increase governmental regulation. For one, the food industry could use FA as an argument to sidestep regulations: if FA is perceived as a rare disorder not usually seen in the general public, then it could be pushed off as the individual's concern, not a corporate one. This argument has been made time and again by the alcohol industry [9, 24, 26, 39, 44, 50, 51]. That said, rates of food addiction are quite high [up to 20% in the general population (Chap. 12)] which are higher than current point prevalence rates for alcohol use disorder.

On the flip side, acceptance of the FA construct might also help boost regulatory efforts. For example, when nicotine was recognized as an addictive substance, there was increased public and political support for expanding governmental regulation, which was followed by a rapid decline in smoking rates [39]. Furthermore, if certain foods are seen by the general public as "addictive," people who are trying to abstain from certain foods might get more support around their efforts, especially, say, in social settings, where common messages like "just have one bite" can currently undermine weight loss attempts. A major challenge, though, is the absence of a process to define which foods are "addictive" and for whom [39, 44, 52, 53] and where and how to draw the line. More research will need to be done to clarify these questions.

5.3.4 Stigma

Obese individuals are subject to prejudicial messages from society that their struggles with food are due to laziness, an inherent character flaw, or a lack of self-control, motivation, and intelligence [39, 44, 52, 53]. Individuals who are not seen as responsible for their condition (e.g., Alzheimer's) receive more sympathy than obese individuals [39, 44]. Stigma gets in the way of policy changes that could reduce access to less health-promoting foods and harness support for better treatments and prevention for overweight and obesity [39, 44]. Stigma can be internalized (individual) or externalized (society). Externalized stigma can lead to weight-based discrimination which adversely affects employment outcomes, interpersonal friendships, and dating [9, 44] or result in victimization and teasing in children [9]. Internalized stigma causes shame, low self-esteem, poor mood, and self-loathing, all of which are important contributors to emotional eating and weight gain, and to restricting and subsequent binge eating [9, 20, 39, 44, 54, 55].

There is a concern that the FA concept, if embraced, could increase stigma associated with obesity [9, 20] by invoking stereotypes of someone untrustworthy or "on the outs" of society. In support of this, one study showed that the "obese food addict" label evoked more stigmatizing positions (e.g., study participants saw the use as a personal choice more) than the "food addict" or "obese" terms used alone [9, 44, 52, 53]. On the other hand, the disease model of addiction reduces stigma and negative attitudes towards people with SUDs [38], supporting arguments that the FA model will reduce stigma associated with obesity [9, 20, 39, 40, 44, 56–58]. The same may be true for FA: a study investigating the effect of an addiction model on public perceptions found that a FA-based explanatory model actually reduced stigma, blame, and perceived psychopathology, and the "addicted" individual was viewed as being less at fault for their weight compared to when obesity was attributed to personal control and personal choice around diet and exercise [9, 39, 44, 52, 53, 58]. It's also possible that the FA construct will not impact stigma much at all, as supported by a recent survey of people from the United States and Australia which found that viewpoints attributing obesity to FA did not reduce weight-based stigma [39, 44, 59].

5.4 Potential Promises for the Future

There are several other possible ways that increased adoption of the FA concept will help individuals who suffer from obesity and binge eating. For one, it will likely increase our range of treatment options for FA, both currently, and in the future. Researchers will be better informed, increasing the number of repurposing studies of medications and interventions that work for SUDs in obesity and BED or BN populations. Furthermore, even before such studies are undertaken, providers may start to help more people by utilizing treatments "off-label" in patients who are refractory to traditional approaches (Chap. 14). Some argue that the FA construct is not necessary for providers to offer treatments that target craving and loss of control, but ultimately there will be more recognition of the overlap between some forms of overeating and SUDs if there is more widespread use of the FA term in the fields. Second, because obesity, BED, and BN are heterogeneous conditions [15, 60, 61], progress in clinical and research settings may occur if it is used as a "treatment matching variable" within obese populations – e.g., people with FA might be more likely to respond than others to treatments that act directly on reward, conditioning, negative affect, and impulsivity circuitry and behavior or to nutritional interventions that encourage some degree of abstinence from problem foods. If true, this would be an invaluable tool for providers. Indeed, "precision medicine" is an important initiative dating back to the Obama administration [62], and the FA scale is already being explored as a tool to predict outcome after bariatric surgery and several other treatments (Chap. 14).

5.5 Increasing Community Acceptance

Regardless of whether FA is a true or useful entity, the reality is that the FA concept is increasingly accepted by popular culture, suggesting that it may be here to stay [20, 31, 52, 53]. A survey of over 600 American and Australian adults reported that 86% believed certain foods may be addictive, and 72% believed addictive eating is linked with an increased risk of obesity [17, 63]. Moreover, rates of a YFAS-based FA diagnosis are high in the general population, ranging from 11% to 20% in the United States (Chap. 12), those of self-perceived addictive eating are even higher among community samples, ranging from 27% to 50% [17, 31], and people with FA symptoms express a desire to have their perceived condition formally recognized in order to receive more appropriate treatment [20]. To reflect this, increased discussion and publication on the topic is seen in media reports, health blogs, and scientific literature [14] over the last several years.

For this reason alone, providers shouldn't ignore the concept and should be equipped to deal with it knowledgeably. In a study of health professionals, although half reported that they consider the term food addiction to be stigmatizing for individuals, 60% reported they were interested in addictive eating training [17].

5.6 Conclusion

In summary, the FA concept is growing in popularity, and there is growing evidence that it is a valid and useful construct. There are many who are not comfortable with widespread use of the term in clinical realms, but an initial review indicates that these concerns may not be warranted or at least addressable with some additional attention during clinical interactions and with more research.

References

1. Hauck C, Cook B, Ellrott T. Food addiction, eating addiction and eating disorders. Proc Nutr Soc. 2020;79(1):103–12.
2. Schulte EM, Wadden TA, Allison KC. An evaluation of food addiction as a distinct psychiatric disorder. Int J Eat Disord. 2020;53(10):1610–22.
3. Volkow ND, Wang GJ, Tomasi D, Baler RD. Obesity and addiction: neurobiological overlaps. Obes Rev. 2013;14(1):2–18.
4. Blanco-Gandia MC, Minarro J, Rodriguez-Arias M. Common neural mechanisms of palatable food intake and drug abuse: knowledge obtained with animal models. Curr Pharm Des. 2020;26(20):2372–84.
5. Baladi MG, Daws LC, France CP. You are what you eat: influence of type and amount of food consumed on central dopamine systems and the behavioral effects of direct- and indirect-acting dopamine receptor agonists. Neuropharmacology. 2012;63(1):76–86.
6. Gordon EL, Ariel-Donges AH, Bauman V, Merlo LJ. What is the evidence for "food addiction?" A systematic review. Nutrients. 2018;10(4):477.
7. Gordon EL, Lent MR, Merlo LJ. The effect of food composition and behavior on neurobiological response to food: a review of recent research. Curr Nutr Rep. 2020;9(2):75–82.
8. Gearhardt AN, Corbin WR, Brownell KD. Preliminary validation of the Yale Food Addiction Scale. Appetite. 2009;52(2):430–6.
9. Adams RC, Sedgmond J, Maizey L, Chambers CD, Lawrence NS. Food addiction: implications for the diagnosis and treatment of overeating. Nutrients. 2019;11(9):2086.
10. Ifland JR, Preuss HG, Marcus MT, Rourke KM, Taylor WC, Burau K, et al. Refined food addiction: a classic substance use disorder. Med Hypotheses. 2009;72(5):518–26.
11. Avena NM, Rada P, Hoebel BG. Evidence for sugar addiction: behavioral and neurochemical effects of intermittent, excessive sugar intake. Neurosci Biobehav Rev. 2008;32(1):20–39.
12. Gearhardt AN, Corbin WR, Brownell KD. Development of the Yale Food Addiction Scale Version 2.0. Psychol Addict Behav. 2016;30(1):113–21.
13. Davis C, Carter JC. Compulsive overeating as an addiction disorder. A review of theory and evidence. Appetite. 2009;53(1):1–8.
14. Onaolapo AY, Onaolapo OJ. Food additives, food and the concept of 'food addiction': is stimulation of the brain reward circuit by food sufficient to trigger addiction? Pathophysiology. 2018;25(4):263–76.
15. Ziauddeen H, Fletcher PC. Is food addiction a valid and useful concept? Obes Rev. 2013;14(1):19–28.
16. Vainik U, Misic B, Zeighami Y, Michaud A, Mottus R, Dagher A. Obesity has limited behavioural overlap with addiction and psychiatric phenotypes. Nat Hum Behav. 2020;4(1):27–35.
17. Burrows T, Verdejo-Garcia A, Carter A, Brown RM, Andrews ZB, Dayas CV, et al. Health professionals' and health professional trainees' views on addictive eating behaviours: a cross-sectional survey. Nutrients. 2020;12(9):2860.
18. Fletcher PC, Kenny PJ. Food addiction: a valid concept? Neuropsychopharmacology. 2018;43(13):2506–13.
19. Gearhardt AN, White MA, Potenza MN. Binge eating disorder and food addiction. Curr Drug Abuse Rev. 2011;4(3):201–7.
20. Wiss D, Brewerton T. Separating the signal from the noise: how psychiatric diagnoses can help discern food addiction from dietary restraint. Nutrients. 2020;12(10):2937.
21. Fairburn CG, Cooper Z, Shafran R. Cognitive behaviour therapy for eating disorders: a "transdiagnostic" theory and treatment. Behav Res Ther. 2003;41(5):509–28.
22. Gearhardt AN, Davis C, Kuschner R, Brownell KD. The addiction potential of hyperpalatable foods. Curr Drug Abuse Rev. 2011;4(3):140–5.
23. Ziauddeen H, Farooqi IS, Fletcher PC. Obesity and the brain: how convincing is the addiction model? Nat Rev Neurosci. 2012;13(4):279–86.
24. Meule A. A critical examination of the practical implications derived from the food addiction concept. Curr Obes Rep. 2019;8(1):11–7.
25. Ifland J, Preuss HG, Marcus MT, Rourke KM, Taylor W, Wright HT. Clearing the confusion around processed food addiction. J Am Coll Nutr. 2015;34(3):240–3.
26. Schulte EM, Avena NM, Gearhardt AN. Which foods may be addictive? The roles of processing, fat content, and glycemic load. PLoS One. 2015;10(2):e0117959.
27. Schulte EM, Potenza MN, Gearhardt AN. A commentary on the "eating addiction" versus "food addiction" perspectives on addictive-like food consumption. Appetite. 2017;115:9–15.
28. Schulte EM, Potenza MN, Gearhardt AN. Specific theoretical considerations and future research directions for evaluating addictive-like eating as a substance-based, food addiction: comment on Lacroix et al. (2018). Appetite. 2018;130:293–5.
29. Leigh SJ, Morris MJ. The role of reward circuitry and food addiction in the obesity epidemic: an update. Biol Psychol. 2016;131:31–42.
30. Hebebrand J, Albayrak O, Adan R, Antel J, Dieguez C, de Jong J, et al. "Eating addiction", rather than "food addiction", better captures addictive-like eating behavior. Neurosci Biobehav Rev. 2014;47:295–306.
31. Ruddock HK, Christiansen P, Halford JCG, Hardman CA. The development and validation of the addiction-like eating behaviour scale. Int J Obes. 2017;41(11):1710–7.

32. Potenza MN. Biological contributions to addictions in adolescents and adults: prevention, treatment, and policy implications. J Adolesc Health. 2013;52(2 Suppl 2):S22–32.
33. Moreno C, Tandon R. Should overeating and obesity be classified as an addictive disorder in DSM-5? Curr Pharm Des. 2011;17(12):1128–31.
34. Marlatt GA. The controlled-drinking controversy. A commentary. Am Psychol. 1983;38(10):1097–110.
35. Rodriguez-Martin BC, Gallego-Arjiz B. Overeaters anonymous: a mutual-help fellowship for food addiction recovery. Front Psychol. 2018;9:1491.
36. Russell-Mayhew S, von Ranson KM, Masson PC. How does overeaters anonymous help its members? A qualitative analysis. Eur Eat Disord Rev. 2010;18(1):33–42.
37. Freeland-Graves JH, Nitzke S, Academy of N Dietetics. Position of the academy of nutrition and dietetics: total diet approach to healthy eating. J Acad Nutr Diet. 2013;113(2):307–17.
38. Avery JJ, Avery JD, Mouallem J, Demner AR, Cooper J. Physicians' and Attorneys' beliefs and attitudes related to the brain disease model of addiction. Am J Addict. 2020;29(4):305–12.
39. Carter A, Hendrikse J, Lee N, Yucel M, Verdejo-Garcia A, Andrews ZB, et al. The neurobiology of "food addiction" and its implications for obesity treatment and policy. Annu Rev Nutr. 2016;36:105–28.
40. Pearl RL, Lebowitz MS. Beyond personal responsibility: effects of causal attributions for overweight and obesity on weight-related beliefs, stigma, and policy support. Psychol Health. 2014;29(10):1176–91.
41. Cosci F. Bulimia nervosa treated with an adapted version of Carroll's cognitive-behavioral approach for treatment of cocaine addiction. J Neuropsychiatry Clin Neurosci. 2014;26(4):E28–9.
42. Gearhardt AN, Brownell KD. Can food and addiction change the game? Biol Psychiatry. 2013;73(9):802–3.
43. Gearhardt AN, Grilo CM, DiLeone RJ, Brownell KD, Potenza MN. Can food be addictive? Public health and policy implications. Addiction. 2011;106(7):1208–12.
44. Carter A, Hardman CA, Burrows T. Food addiction and eating addiction: scientific advances and their clinical, social and policy implications. Nutrients. 2020;12(5)
45. Morin JP, Rodriguez-Duran LF, Guzman-Ramos K, Perez-Cruz C, Ferreira G, Diaz-Cintra S, et al. Palatable hyper-caloric foods impact on neuronal plasticity. Front Behav Neurosci. 2017;11:19.
46. Wiss DA, Criscitelli K, Gold M, Avena N. Preclinical evidence for the addiction potential of highly palatable foods: current developments related to maternal influence. Appetite. 2017;15:19–27.
47. Moran A, Musicus A, Soo J, Gearhardt AN, Gollust SE, Roberto CA. Believing that certain foods are addictive is associated with support for obesity-related public policies. Prev Med. 2016;90:39–46.
48. Frew E, Ng SW, Coast J, Hollingsworth B, Smith R. How can economics help tackle obesity? Obesity. 2018;26(7):1112–3.
49. Wilcox CE. Binge Eating Disorder. 2019. CMEtoGo.com: American Physician Institute.
50. Gearhardt AN, Yokum S, Orr PT, Stice E, Corbin WR, Brownell KD. Neural correlates of food addiction. Arch Gen Psychiatry. 2011;68(8):808–16.
51. Gearhardt AN, Corbin WR, Brownell KD. Food addiction: an examination of the diagnostic criteria for dependence. J Addict Med. 2009;3(1):1–7.
52. Cassin S, Leung S, Hawa R, Wnuk S, Jackson T, Sockalingam S. Food addiction is associated with binge eating and psychiatric distress among post-operative bariatric surgery patients and may improve in response to cognitive behavioural therapy. Nutrients. 2020;12(10):2905.
53. Cassin SE, Buchman DZ, Leung SE, Kantarovich K, Hawa A, Carter A, et al. Ethical, stigma, and policy implications of food addiction: a scoping review. Nutrients. 2019;11(4):710.
54. Loxton NJ, Dawe S, Cahill A. Does negative mood drive the urge to eat? The contribution of negative mood, exposure to food cues and eating style. Appetite. 2011;56(2):368–74.
55. Vartanian LR, Novak SA. Internalized societal attitudes moderate the impact of weight stigma on avoidance of exercise. Obesity. 2011;19(4):757–62.
56. Ivezaj V, White MA, Grilo CM. Examining binge-eating disorder and food addiction in adults with overweight and obesity. Obesity. 2016;24(10):2064–9.
57. Latner JD, Puhl RM, Murakami JM, O'Brien KS. Food addiction as a causal model of obesity. Effects on stigma, blame, and perceived psychopathology. Appetite. 2014;77:77–82.
58. O'Brien KS, Puhl RM, Latner JD, Lynott D, Reid JD, Vakhitova Z, et al. The effect of a food addiction explanation model for weight control and obesity on weight stigma. Nutrients. 2020;12(2)
59. Lee NM, Hall WD, Lucke J, Forlini C, Carter A. Food addiction and its impact on weight-based stigma and the treatment of obese individuals in the U.S. and Australia. Nutrients. 2014;6(11):5312–26.
60. Higgins GA, Zeeb FD, Fletcher PJ. Role of impulsivity and reward in the anti-obesity actions of 5-HT2C receptor agonists. J Psychopharmacol. 2017;31(11):1403–18.
61. Blundell JE, Dulloo AG, Salvador J, Fruhbeck G, BMI ESWGo. Beyond BMI–phenotyping the obesities. Obes Facts. 2014;7(5):322–8.
62. Dishman E. Precision Medicine. 2018. https://www.nih.gov/precision-medicine-initiative-cohort-program. Accessed 2018.
63. Lee NM, Lucke J, Hall WD, Meurk C, Boyle FM, Carter A. Public views on food addiction and obesity: implications for policy and treatment. PLoS One. 2013;8(9):e74836.

Part III

Clinical Evidence for Food Addiction

6 Clinical Evidence for the Validity of Food Addiction

6.1 Shared DSM Criteria

There are 11 criteria for a DSM-V diagnosis of a substance use disorder (SUD). These criteria can be categorized into four categories: impaired control, social impairment, risky use, and physiological criteria [3] (Box 6.1). Severity is classified as mild (2–3 symptoms), moderate (4–5 symptoms), or severe (> or = 6 symptoms), and symptom assessment should cover the previous 12 months [3]. Although not in the DSM-V criteria, SUD also, importantly, are vulnerable to relapse after long periods of sobriety [3].

Box 6.1 DSM-V Criteria for an SUD [3]

Impaired Control

1. Substance consumed in amounts or over longer periods of time than intended.
2. Persistent desire or unsuccessful attempts to decrease or limit substance use.
3. Significant amount of time spent acquiring, using, or recovering from a substance.
4. Strong craving to use the substance.

Social Impairment

5. Inability to fulfill obligations at work, school, or home due to use of a substance.
6. Continued use despite recurrent exacerbation of social or interpersonal problems.
7. Reduced engagement social, occupational, or recreational activities due to substance use.

Risky Use

8. Continued use of the substance in situations in which it is physically dangerous (e.g., driving under the influence).
9. Continued use despite physical or psychological problems that are caused or made worse by the substance.

C. E. Wilcox, *Food Addiction, Obesity, and Disorders of Overeating*,
https://doi.org/10.1007/978-3-030-83078-6_6

Physiological Criteria

10. Increased dose needed to achieve the desired effect and reduced effect when consumed (i.e., tolerance).
11. Negative physiological or psychological effects upon cessation (i.e., withdrawal).

Clinical distress or impairment must be evidenced by two or more of the above symptoms within a 12-month period.

People with obesity and eating disorders (EDs) experience impaired control over food, especially HP food [1, 7] (Chap. 11). Dieters usually fail to lose significant amounts of weight or maintain their weight loss, and, for some, dieting may ultimately lead to more weight gain, in the long run [1, 8]. Indeed, loss of control is a criteria in the DSM-V to diagnose binge eating disorder (BED) and bulimia nervosa (BN) (e.g., impaired control over food quantity of and length of time engaged in food consumption, consumption of large amounts of food in a short period of time, an inability to successfully stop or cut down on consumption despite an expressed desire to do so, and recurrent negative consequences) [1, 9, 10].

Food craving typically refers to an intense desire to consume a specific food [1, 11], is very commonly reported by people with obesity and eating disorders (ED)) [2], and occurs even in normal-weight individuals, with reports of 100% of women and 70% men experiencing a craving for at least one food in the past year [1]. Several standardized questionnaires to measure food cravings have been developed and show good internal consistency and construct validity [1]. More frequent and intense food cravings are associated with binge eating, increased food intake, self-reported FA symptoms, increased body mass index (BMI), BN, and BED [1, 12]. FA severity is also correlated with difficulty controlling eating and cravings and higher appetite ratings [3, 13, 14]. With more and more use, the reward system is primed, and craving increases. For example, in women who reported craving carbohydrates, a 100% carbohydrate sweetened beverage dispelled craving, but this quelling effect decreased over multiple exposures [3, 15]. That said, there may be a ceiling effect, as supported by several bodies of work. For example, in one study of morbidly obese individuals, as BMI increased, craving decreased [16, 17]. In the context of both food and alcohol or drug use, craving is often accompanied by rationalizations and justifications that lead the individual to engage in food or drug-seeking behavior that they had previously sworn against.

The SUD criterion of time spent obtaining, using, and recovering from use also translates to people who overeat, especially for those with BED and bulimia nervosa, in that bingeing is often a planned behavior which may require a great deal of effort to purchase and store foods ready for a binge episode [1]. Indeed there is a threshold for ED diagnosis based on this category, in that three episodes of binge eating per week are required to meet criteria for BED [1]. Moreover, people with BED often experience physical and emotional distress following a binge eating episode, and food addicts report feeling sleepy or "hung-over" [1, 7, 18] after overeating.

From the standpoint of social impairment, disorders of overeating and obesity are stigmatized (Chap. 5) resulting in social isolation. In one study, 60% of a sample of bariatric surgery candidates endorsed choosing to spend time eating over conducting other activities, and their addictive personality scores explained a significant amount of variance in social isolation [3, 19]. Those who meet criteria for FA score lower on physical, mental, and social aspects of health-related quality of life scales [1, 20] and report lower self-esteem, impaired sexual life, and poorer work performance. Interpersonal problems have also been associated with binge eating – a relationship which is likely to be bidirectional [1].

From the standpoint of risky use, many obese individuals continue to eat unhealthy foods even in the face of severe negative consequences, such as diabetes, heart disease, and stigmatization [9, 10]. In EDs, individuals continue to binge eat despite physical and emotional distress [1] and despite increased risk for severe neurological, cardiac, dental, and gastrointestinal medical consequences (Chap. 3). Furthermore, those who have undergone weight loss treatment often fail to lose weight or gain weight following intervention [1, 21], even after bariatric surgery [1, 22].

Numerous studies have shown that tolerance to HP food occurs [3, 23]. Neurobiologically, tolerance is manifested by reduced dopamine receptor density (in particular, the type-2 dopamine receptor, due to downregulation), and blunted dopamine and opioid release to natural rewards, both of which have been observed in animal models and humans with obesity and EDs [3, 23] (Chap. 8). Clinically, tolerance may manifest as anhedonia or hyposensitivity to reward in obese participants compared to controls [1, 24, 25]. For example, one study showed that although overweight women were more sensitive to reward than healthy-weight women, those who were obese were significantly less reward-sensitive than overweight women [1, 25]. Another study showed that those who regularly consumed ice cream exhibited a blunted reward-related neural response to a small portion of ice cream, relative to those who did not frequently eat ice cream [2, 26]. Finally, another interesting study supporting the existence increased tolerance over time reported that although sucrose has an analgesic effect in young infants, but this diminishes as they get past 18 months, which is the time when sugar consumption increases [1, 27]. Like with drugs of abuse, tolerance may lead animals and humans to consume progressively increased amounts of food, in an attempt to achieve its beneficial mood-enhancing effect [1, 3, 23–25]. For example, normal weight participants provided with chocolate for 3 weeks increased their intake over time while at the same time reporting a reduction in food liking [1, 28]. In a study of bariatric surgery candidates [3, 19], 69% reported increasing quantities of food to reach satiation over time, and those who endorsed this symptom also had higher scores on an addictive personality measure. In BED, as the illness duration grows longer, the frequency of binges, the amount of food consumed, the length of the episode, and the feeling of being out of control all increase [9, 10].

Withdrawal is defined by the presence of physical or psychological symptoms in response to substance deprivation and/or the use of the substance in order to relieve these symptoms [1]. Like with tolerance, numerous animal models have demonstrated withdrawal behaviors upon cessation of high sugar or high fat foods that mirror behaviors that occur during withdrawal from drugs, including teeth chattering, forepaw tremor, head shaking, and reduced body temperature as well as increased aggression and anxiety [1] (Chap. 8). Human studies also support the existence of food withdrawal [5, 6, 29] which is marked by affective, cognitive, and physical symptoms [30]. Anecdotal reports indicate that when individuals reduce their consumption of highly processed foods, they experience cravings and negative affect as well as fatigue, anxiety, depression, and agitation [1, 2, 7, 9, 31]. For example, a case study documented the reemergence of anxiety and panic symptoms when a patient went on the Atkins diet (a low-carbohydrate diet), and Atkins himself warned dieters that they may experience "fatigue, faintness, palpitations, headaches, and cold sweats" [9, 10]. Although the frequency of withdrawal symptoms in various clinical populations varies, withdrawal has been reported in up to 50% of individuals with obesity and BED [1, 31]. However, rates were lower in a study of 1414 participants who had at least one YFAS symptom in the last year, where 10% endorsed "withdrawal-like" effects in response to cessation of either high-fat savory foods (4%), high-fat sweet foods (3%), low-fat sugary foods (2%), or low-fat savory foods (1%) [3, 32]. Importantly, in humans, withdrawal may hinder dietary change [30]. People with withdrawal symptoms report the tendency to eat to avoid the emotional symptoms such as fatigue, anxiety, and depression [1, 7]. Another study of bariatric surgery candidates showed that higher scores on an addictive personality measure was related to higher levels of anxiety when they were not near food [3, 19].

A food withdrawal scale called the Highly Processed Food Withdrawal Scale (ProWS) has been developed and validated with the YFAS for use in adults [30, 33] and children [30], supporting the validity of an HP food withdrawal construct, although it's important to note that the original validation study was done on individuals who had been trying to diet, and the questions were retrospective, and so the possibility that some of the symptoms were due to a caloric deficit cannot be ruled out [2, 33]. The ProWS validity studies utilized items from the Wisconsin Smoking Withdrawal Scale and Cannabis Withdrawal Scale [2, 33] including psychological symptoms (e.g., craving, anxiety, irritability) and physical symptoms (e.g., headaches, sleep disruption). The time course of withdrawal from food has been measured to peak at 2–5 days, and then symptoms improved over time, similar to what is seen with many drugs of abuse [2, 33]. In adults, higher scores are related to higher addictive tendencies less self-reported success with dieting attempts and impaired dietary restraint in adults [2, 33]. In children, the scale shows discriminant validity with child food neophobia, and higher scores are associated with less success in reducing child highly processed food intake independent of BMI [30].

Although relapse has not been officially investigated in human studies of obesity and binge eating disorder, clearly the fact that people end up usually gaining back weight they lost (Chap. 4) indicates that a relapse-like phenomena exists in relation to food. Indeed, animal and neuroimaging studies show that the neurobiological underpinnings of relapse to SUD and overeating have significant overlap [3] (Chap. 8).

6.2 Yale Food Addiction Scale Development

The YFAS [9, 34] was originally published in 2009, and revised in 2016 (YFAS 2.0), and it is currently the only validated measure to operationalize FA and addictive-like eating behavior [2]. The original YFAS and the updated version have been translated and validated in many languages and for many different cultures [2, 34].

The original YFAS is a self-report questionnaire that screens for the seven DSM-IV [35] symptoms of substance dependence as applied to the addictive-like consumption of certain foods, prompting for peoples' experiences in relation to HP foods in particular (e.g., foods with high amounts of sugar, processed carbohydrates, fat or salt) [2, 9]. Like for SUD, a diagnosis is obtained if three symptoms are endorsed above a certain severity threshold plus clinically significant impairment or distress [35]. It asks about whether the symptoms have been experienced over the last year.

The advent of the DSM-V saw major changes in how SUD were evaluated, merging criteria for substance abuse and dependence into one diagnosis, adding craving as a criteria, removing legal consequences, listing eleven total criteria, and applying a severity spectrum (mild, moderate, severe) [36]. In response, the YFAS 2.0 was developed in 2016 to parallel these changes [2, 34]. Like the original YFAS, it produces both a continuous score based on the number criteria met, and a cutoff score, and like in the DSM-V, severity can be determined from the number of criteria met [34].

The validity of a test is established if it is shown to measure what it claims to measure. Construct validity has to do with whether a test captures a constellation of symptoms that truly exist in the real world [37]. In our case, a test of FA should measure a true biologically based set of addictive behavior patterns around food and eating and symptoms that are problematic for some individuals. A subtype of construct validity, named convergent validity, depends on the internal consistency of a measure and requires that the symptoms of a proposed syndrome cluster together in the sample [9, 34]. For example, in the case of FA, internal consistency of a measure of FA would be established if withdrawal symptoms also seem to occur in a population of people who report continued use despite negative consequences [9, 34]. A test of FA would also have convergent validity if it related something else to which it should theoretically relate, like weight gain or more severe binge eating [37, 38]. Finally, a good test needs to capture something that isn't already captured by our existing constructs or diagnoses, and not be redundant [39]. This is determined through tests of discriminant validity, another subtype of construct validity, or incremental validity [34, 38]. For example, a tool to determine FA needs to measure something that is not captured already by BED, bulimia nervosa, or obesity. There is no single test for construct validity, and the more evidence to support it, the better [37].

The original YFAS exhibited excellent internal consistency [2]. It also demonstrated adequate internal reliability, and good convergent validity, being associated with BMI and binge eating [9]. The YFAS 2.0 demonstrated even better internal consistency [2], loading onto a single factor, and also had good reliability, similar to the original YFAS [34].

The YFAS 2.0 is apparently more inclusive than the original YFAS, and, in a sample of more than 200 participants, individuals were more likely to meet criteria for FA on the YFAS 2.0 than the YFAS (16 versus 10%). This makes sense, since the DSM-V is more likely to diagnose SUD than the DSM-IV, as a consequence of the fact that it adds four new diagnostic criteria to the list of dependence and abuse criteria from DSM–IV and lowers the threshold for diagnosis from three to two symptoms. Indeed, some have argued that the YFAS is over-inclusive because of these high rates of positivity, but rates of ED are almost 20%, too. To narrow the range of positives, one could always use the severity thresholding (e.g., only clinically refer people with moderate or severe FA for treatment) in the case of limited resources, for example [9, 34]. Finally, FA as assessed by the YFAS 2.0 differed by weight class, in that obese participants had a higher prevalence of food addiction (24.6%) than overweight (16.7%) or normal weight (7.8%) participants, an improvement on the convergent validity from the original YFAS. Otherwise both scales were associated with BMI, binge eating frequency, and weight cycling [34].

Further support for convergent validity of the YFAS 2.0, in particular, can be inferred from the fact that scores on the YFAS 2.0 and other measures relevant to problematic eating behaviors were associated with several other important clinical items (disinhibition and impulsive eating, hunger, current BMI, highest lifetime BMI, and frequency of binge eating episodes) and a history of more frequent weight cycling (a weight loss and regain of 20 pounds or more, excluding pregnancy) [34]. Studies supporting the convergent validity of the FA construct continues to build, with each month seeing more publications in the area [3].

Whether FA is simply a reflection of BED, and therefore not providing anything new, is an area of continuing controversy [4, 39, 40] (Chap. 5): if FA is not distinct from BED, it could be argued that it is not a necessary construct [3, 41, 42] because it simply captures a more severe presentation of BED or does not add meaningfully to BED [2]. Indeed these arguments are supported by the fact that there is phenomenological overlap between the behaviors seen in BED and FA (e.g., excessive consumption of food, loss of control, continued use despite negative consequences post-binge distress, binges involved consumption of high fat, high sugar, highly processed foods, etc.) [34], that FA scores correlate highly with measures of binge eating and diagnoses of BN and BED [1, 2, 39, 41, 43, 44], and that there are high rates of FA in ED populations, as high as 100% in some studies of BN patients and 77% in BED [1, 45, 46] (Chap. 12).

However, despite these concerns, in the aforementioned validation papers, the YFAS scales show good discriminant and incremental validity, supporting arguments on the other side: that FA is distinguishable enough from already existing constructs like BED to provide something conceptually and even possibly clinically useful [9, 34]. Of note, the participants in the YFAS validation studies were drawn from a community, non-treatment-seeking population, instead of from a treatment-seeking sample, and for them, less than half of participants with an ED diagnosis met criteria for FA, and about half of participants with a FA diagnosis did not meet criteria for an ED diagnosis [34]. Only 42% of participants with BN and 47% of participants with BED also met criteria for a FA diagnosis, and 44% of participants with a FA diagnosis did not meet criteria for AN, BN, or BED [34]. In another study, 19% of overweight and obese participants, some of whom did engage in regular binge eating, were classified as food addicted according to the YFAS, but most of these did not meet criteria for BED [4, 47]. Therefore, it is likely that although EDs associated with binge eating and FA constructs overlap quite a bit in some populations, they are distinct entities, and degree of their overlap depends on the population in which it is measured [3, 48, 49].

Other evidence to support the discriminant validity of the FA measuring scales and which indicate that FA is a separate entity than BED/BN relate to the fact that patients differ slightly in their phenotypic presentations [45, 49, 50]. For example, grazing is reported by individuals with FA [45, 51], and bingeing is not required to meet diagnostic criteria for FA, whereas it is a criteria for BN and BED. Indeed, post bariatric surgery, one can meet criteria for FA, but it is physically difficult or impossible to binge (at least initially) [45, 51].

Finally, in discussions of YFAS discriminant validity, and the validity of the FA construct in general, it's important to mention some expert's concerns that the FA construct might simply be a byproduct of over-restricting [43]. Recall that in ED treatment communities, restrictive behavior is widely considered an important causal factor and contributor to ED behavior, in that it correlates with restriction in ED treatment populations [52]. However, that scores on the YFAS 2.0 and dietary restraint (i.e., the intention to restrict food for weight loss purposes) were *not* correlated and that dietary restraint was also not associated with FA scores on the original YFAS [53, 54] indicate that, at least in community populations, restrictive behavior is unlikely to be the sole contributor to the FA syndrome. Still, screening for a history of caloric restriction behaviors is essential in clinical settings, because a history of restriction could create a risk for false-positives in FA diagnoses and/or a negative outcome with abstinence-based approaches in food-plan development such as rebound bingeing [43] (Chaps. 12, 13, and 14).

6.3 SUD and Disordered Eating Co-occur

That SUD and some overeating problems tend to co-occur in the same people further supports the validity of the FA construct [3]. That said, SUD and obesity travel together less than SUD and BED/BN do, however [55]. Therefore, addictive models of overeating may apply more frequently to those with EDs associated with binge eating than obesity.

High rates of SUD in ED populations have been documented by numerous studies in teens and adults [39, 42, 56–58]; in one study, 50% of women affected with an ED were found to have a comorbid substance abuse or dependence diagnosis [58, 59]. Moreover, higher rates SUD are seen in people with binge and binge-purge ED, with one meta-analysis showing rates of alcohol use disorder (AUD) at 20%, more than 1.5 times higher than controls [60], and another one showing rates of SUD at 22% [43, 61]. Comparing the different ED diagnoses, BN has the strongest correlation with SUD, followed by BED, but rates of SUD in anorexia nervosa are almost the same as that of normal controls [58]. People with SUD also have higher ED rates. For example, one study showed that women with comorbid AUD and nicotine use disorder (NUD) report a higher prevalence of ED symptoms and ED than women with AUD or NUD only, who in turn had a higher prevalence than those without SUD [43, 62].

Individuals with elevated substance use and SUD also have higher rates of FA and vice versa [63]. These relationships have been documented in a large Dutch adolescent sample [43, 56, 58, 64], in men with heroin use disorder who had triple the odds of meeting criteria for BED or FA compared to controls [43, 65], in a large Italian sample of substance-using patients where the overall prevalence of FA was 20% (the rates were highest among cannabis users (31%) and the lowest among tobacco users (11%), and FA risk increased with the number of substances used) [43, 58], and among alcohol abusers (35% had FA, as opposed to 3% in the general population) [58, 59].

Rates of FA are also higher in people with behavioral addictions and general addictive personality scores. Food cravings were found to be higher in people with addictive personalities in a study of bariatric surgery candidates with BED, explaining a significant amount of the variance in cravings [3, 19]. Another study showed that addictive phone use in adolescents was associated with overeating behavior and higher BMI [66]. Finally, a higher prevalence of FA has been demonstrated among gamblers [58, 67] and people with exercise dependence [58, 68].

6.4 Sweet Preference, Addiction Transfer, and Cross-Sensitization

People with AUD and other SUD also have higher rates of sweet preference compared to normal controls, arguing for shared neurobiological underpinnings [69–73]. For example, heroin users reportedly seek convenient, sweet foods, and eat more sporadically with a more binge-like pattern [73, 74]. Furthermore, subjects on methadone often report high cravings for sugar [69, 73, 75], with reports that a third of their calorie intake is from sugar [73, 76]. Research in cocaine use disorder (CUD) is mixed with some data showing a preference for high fat and carbohydrate-rich foods, but not sugary foods [73, 77], and others reporting preferences for sweet taste [72, 73].

Sweet preference may also be linked to both FA and SUD via propensities for depression or impulsivity [73, 78, 79]. For example, young children who had both a family history of AUD and self-reported depressive symptoms showed the strongest preference for sweetness [73, 80]. Furthermore, a preference for sweetness combined with a novelty-seeking (impulsive) personality markedly increased the risk of suffering from AUD [73, 81].

Genetic factors may contribute to this overlap as well, and genetic factors may explain as much as 50% of the variation in both sugar consumption and substance consumption suggesting similar biological underpinnings [73]. In AUD in particular, men with a genetic link to AUD had a greater sweet preference than men without that link [73, 82].

Reasons for higher rates of sweet preference in SUD may also result from the effects of substances on the brain, as indicated by the fact that craving and sweet preference changes depending on where patients are in their recovery. In AUD, cravings for chocolate increased significantly in the month following alcohol cessation [73]. However, the sweet preference among subjects with AUD may decline following longer periods of abstinence [70, 73].

Some have posited that increased sweet cravings in SUD during recovery may be due to primed reward pathways from chronic substance use and the increased craving and motivational value of food during states of withdrawal [73, 83]. Relatedly, many animal studies also show that consuming sugar [73, 84, 85] and "bingeing" on fat-rich foods can alleviate opiate withdrawal in rats [73, 83]. The nutritional depletion seen in SUD is another important contributor [73, 86–88], since deficits in certain micronutrients and hunger or food deprivation can further prime reward pathways [73, 89]. Indeed, previous work has shown that AUD given nutrition counselling, who may have chosen to eat more food or at least more regularly, had less alcohol craving and more periods of abstinence [73].

Addiction transfer refers to the phenomena that when some people become abstinent from one substance of abuse, they switch to a new substance and can rapidly develop compulsive use of that new substance. Addiction transfer from drugs of abuse to HP food occurs in humans. For example, in a large longitudinal study from Australia, illicit substance users had significant risk of developing recurrent binge eating in addition to, or in place of, their substance use [43, 90]. Anecdotally, many individuals early in recovery from SUD report increased cravings for food, both sweet and fat [73], which can then segue into disordered eating behavior and binge eating, studies show [3, 58].

There is less evidence that obese individuals or individuals with BED in recovery switch to substances of abuse than there is in humans that people in recovery from substances switch to overuse of food [58]. For example, recurrent binge eating was not found to predict later substance use in a large longitudinal study in Australia [43, 90]. However, certain subgroups of bariatric surgery patients might be at risk of addiction transfer to drugs or alcohol [43]. For example, patients who have lost greater weight after the Roux-en-Y gastric bypass procedure have been found to be at enhanced risk of SUD [73, 91]. Furthermore, increases in alcohol intake have been reported in a group of patients who also had reductions in FA scores after weight loss surgery [58, 92]. Finally, those who report more problems with high glycemic index and high-sugar/low-fat foods before surgery were more likely to develop a new SUD post-surgery, indicating a possible subgroup of BA surgery candidates that had higher FA tendencies [3, 93]. Not all studies have shown this to happen post-surgery, however [94], indicating that addiction transfer may be a phenomena that occurs only in particular subgroups of people who struggle with overeating.

Addiction transfer could be secondary to shared reward and motivational pathways involving the opioidergic system, in particular [73] (Chap. 8). This is supported by work showing that sweet preference increases with exposure to opioids, that opiate antagonists decrease sweet preference, but that opiate agonist use acutely reduces cravings in heroin users [73, 76]. Further support comes from studies showing that individuals with AUD who initially have a greater liking for sweetness respond more robustly from the standpoint of drinking reduction when they take opioid antagonists such as naltrexone (commonly used as a relapse prevention treatment for AUD) [73, 95].

The dopamine system also plays an important role in addiction transfer, as evidenced by studies showing that cross-sensitization (cross-sensitization is a dopaminergic process and measures the ability of drug or food use to prime excitatory pathways for facilitating rapid development of addictive behavior around another substance) can occur between drugs and food, such that exposure to a drug will make an animal more sensitive to food and vice versa. Indeed, numerous studies have shown that sugar-binging rats or rats sensitized to palatable food such as high fat food or western diet reliably increase behavioral and locomotor responses to cocaine, amphetamine, and opioids and drug-associated cues or contexts [3, 9, 73, 96–99]. These studies have lead experts to propose a Gateway Theory of food, wherein overuse of palatable food should be examined as a vulnerability factor that might increase the later risk of SUD development [96].

6.5 Overlapping Neuropsychological, Emotional, and Personality Traits, Psychiatric Diagnoses, and Predisposing Conditions (Trauma and Stress)

SUDs are associated with numerous personality and neuropsychological traits or tendencies and psychiatric symptoms that are likely both made worse by excessive substance use and contribute to SUD development and maintenance and the vicious cycle and downward spiral of addiction [1, 73, 100–103]. Neuropsychological traits of note include heightened reward sensitivity, cognitive bias, impulsivity and executive dysfunction, negative urgency, proclivity towards negative affect (including emotion regulation difficulties), and alexithymia [1, 43, 60, 102–108] (Box 6.2).

Box 6.2 Neuropsychological and Emotional Traits and Tendencies Associated with SUD and Disordered Eating [1, 43, 100–102, 106–110]

- Reward sensitivity: the degree of subjective response to positive stimuli (e.g., food or drugs), also associated with sensation- and novelty-seeking
- Cognitive bias (e.g., attentional, approach, and affective bias): the tendency to unconsciously attend to and approach cues such as smell, sights, sounds, or environments associated with past and potential future experiences. Underlies drug, food, or aversive cue-elicited craving.

- Impulse or cognitive/executive control (impulsivity often refers to self-report scale scores and cognitive/executive control often refers to task performance, but terms are often used interchangeably): the ability to stay on task in the face of distractors, inhibit habitual responses, and make adaptive decisions. There are several subcategories/contributors:
  - Response inhibition (the ability to inhibiting a prepotent response like on a Go/No-go task)
  - Delay discounting (the ability to delay gratification)
  - Self-reported impulsivity (as assessed with the Barratt Impulsiveness Scale or through tests of risky decision-making)
  - Interference control (the ability to stay on task in the context of a distractor and suppress influence of irrelevant information like on a Stroop-like task depends on attention)
  - Working memory (the ability to hold information in memory in order to perform a task)
  - Negative urgency (the tendency to act rashly and impulsively when experiencing strong negative emotions, dependent on both impulse control and negative mood proclivity)
- Negative mood proclivity: Higher proclivity towards irritability, depression, anxiety, etc. There are several subcategories/contributors:
  - Emotion dysregulation [related to alexithymia (difficulty identifying one's emotions) and struggles with acceptance of what is and reframing)]
  - Heightened stress reactivity
  - Withdrawal intensity
  - Underlying psychiatric diagnosis

In terms of personality traits, high neuroticism, low conscientiousness, low agreeableness, high extraversion, high harm avoidance, and low self-directedness are associated with SUD [12]. Relatedly, posttraumatic stress disorder (PTSD) and depressive and anxiety disorders both result from and are known to increase risk of development of SUD and cause overuse of substances of abuse and impede recovery [43, 102, 111, 112]. Furthermore, attention deficit hyperactivity disorder (ADHD) can result from and fuel and worsen SUD, not surprising given the role of impulsivity in loss of control [43, 113, 114]. Finally, a history maltreatment or trauma in childhood, trauma in general, chronic stress states, and chronic uncontrollable feelings of stress increases SUD risk and severity [43, 102].

There is a growing and large body of literature to indicate that these same traits and diagnoses are seen at higher rates in some groups of obese individuals and in people with EDs and FA, such that they both result from or are made worse by and contribute to disordered eating. Likewise, a history of trauma and stress increase ED and obesity risk and severity [43, 63, 115].

From the standpoint of traits, reward sensitivity has been found to be positively associated with disordered eating in several studies and is associated with higher BMI and levels of food craving as well as preferences for foods high in fat and sugar [1, 116, 117]. If reward sensitivity is combined with poor impulse control (labeled the "hot-cold empathy gap" by some experts), then this can create an especially challenging situation for people who overeat [116, 118]. In terms of associations with FA scores in particular, reward eating and sensitivity to food cues are also associated with FA scores and diagnoses [12, 119, 120].

Attentional and approach bias to reward-related food cues also likely drive disordered eating [1, 4, 121], with higher attentional bias to food cues seen in unsuccessful restrained eaters, those with higher trait food craving, people with disordered eating patterns, and in those who are overweight or obese [1, 6, 110]. In terms of FA in particular, higher attentional bias for food cues has been found to be associated with higher FA scores or FA diagnoses in several studies [1, 4, 34, 46, 57, 116, 118, 121], and sad mood induction can increase this bias [16].

Impulsivity and impaired cognitive control have been identified as key shared mechanisms underlying both binge eating and addictive disorders [43, 109, 122]. Impulsivity is believed to be one of the most important and consistently identified traits contributing to disordered eating, obesity, and overweight as well as is the tendency to make poorer food choices, lack of physical activity, and greater likelihood of snacking on high fat foods [1, 3, 12, 16, 34, 43, 46, 57, 109, 117, 122–132]. Impulsivity levels often distinguish eating disordered populations, especially BED and BN, from non-eating disordered patients [43, 129, 130]. Higher scores on the Barratt Impulsiveness Scale (BIS), greater delay discounting, and impaired response inhibition are associated with higher rates of compulsive overeating, eating disorder psychopathology, and likelihood to engage in poor health behaviors [1, 11, 116, 118, 124, 133]. One study showed that reward sensitivity was associated with greater food intake but that impaired response inhibition was associated with being overweight [1], indicating that reward sensitivity may cause overeating, but inhibitory control impairment may maintain it. Higher FA scores and FA diagnoses are associated with higher levels of impulsivity, as well [1, 2, 12, 16, 34, 43, 57, 109, 124, 126–129, 131, 134], as measured with the BIS [109], tests of delay discounting [1, 11, 116, 118, 124, 126, 127], response inhibition tasks [1, 16, 124, 126, 127, 135], and other tasks of cognitive control [3, 103]. Studies show that FA may be a mediator between impulsivity and obesity, such that impulsivity leads to FA which then leads to obesity [43, 124]. On the other hand, not all studies have found associations between FA and all forms of impulsivity and executive or cognitive control [16, 109], with some reporting a stronger association between FA and self-report measures (like the BIS) than with task performance (like on a response inhibition task) [109].

Negative urgency, which depends on impulsivity and proclivity towards negative affect, is also commonly measured at higher levels in BED [60, 136], obesity [137], and other forms of disordered eating [12, 129, 130]. Negative urgency and lack of perseverance were shown to be strongly associated with FA, and tests of mediation indicated that, like with impulsivity in general, FA was a mediator of the effect of negative urgency on BMI [12]. Deficiencies in related areas such as the aforementioned hot-cold empathy gap [118] and intolerance of uncertainty [138] are increasingly recognized as important contributors to binge eating and loss of control around food. Finally, an important longitudinal study, important because it demonstrates causality more than a cross-sectional associative study, showed that negative urgency predicted increases in expectancies for reinforcement from eating which in turn predicted increases in binge eating behavior over several years [139]. In terms of FA in particular, individuals with high levels of negative urgency have been found to be at greater risk of later developing addictive eating patterns [60, 129, 130] and have higher levels of FA [12, 109].

A tendency towards irritability, anxiety, and depressed mood, made worse by heightened stress reactivity, and difficulty regulating emotions, is also related to and believed to cause and make worse binge eating-based eating disorders and obesity [2, 12, 53, 54, 125, 140, 141]. High psychological distress has been found to directly contribute to higher BMI by its effect on eating disorder attitudes, FA, and insomnia [142, 143]. Several studies using ecological momentary assessment, which is a method that allows for moment-to-moment tracking of behaviors and emotional states to get more at causality, identify negative affect as important predictors of binge eating behavior [141, 144]. Another longer longitudinal study confirmed the importance of negative affect as a contributor to eating disordered behavior, showing that negative affect predicted increases in thinness expectancies, which in turn predicted increases in purging several years later [139]. Socio-evaluative stress may play a particularly important role in BED [145]. Alexithymia, or difficulty identifying one's emotions, is also seen at higher rates in people with EDs [2, 12, 53, 54, 141, 143, 146]. Higher scores on the YFAS and FA-positive diagnoses are also associated with heightened negative affect due to low self-esteem (feeling ashamed or critical of oneself, upset, or worried due to one's eating habits) [103], higher levels of emotional eating [147], emotion dysregulation and alexithymia [2, 12, 53, 54, 141, 143, 146], and more frequent irrational beliefs, the latter of which were in turn related to higher depression and anxiety and emotional eating [148].

Finally, in terms of personality traits, mirroring much of what is seen in SUD populations, high extraversion, high neuroticism, high harm avoidance, low self-directedness, high novelty seeking, and low agreeableness have been found to be associated with FA and ED diagnoses [12, 129, 130, 146, 149].

As with SUD, obesity and EDs are associated with higher rates of psychiatric disorders and symptoms, and evidence suggests these associated psychiatric diagnoses cause heightened obesity and eating disorder severity and persistence. These associations have been seen for depression [137, 150, 151], anxiety [16, 43, 47, 103, 104, 134, 149, 150, 152–154], and social anxiety [43]. Rates of PTSD are also higher in ED populations, and higher rates of ED are seen in patients with PTSD [43]. Depression in particular may contribute to greater levels of shame and lower self-esteem people with obesity and disordered eating [103], as well as poorer quality of life [16], all of which could contribute to further disordered eating behavior and weight gain. Depression, anxiety, and PTSD can fuel overeating via self-soothing which is consistent with reports of "comfort food" consumption when under stress [43, 155]. Higher FA scores are also correlated with higher depression scores and a higher likelihood of an MDD diagnosis [2, 12, 16, 43, 137, 147, 150, 152, 156] as well as higher levels of anxiety and anxiety sensitivity [12, 43, 48, 149, 152–154, 157] and higher levels of PTSD symptomatology [43, 158]. In a study of surgery patients 6 month post-op complaining of loss of control eating, individuals with high FA scores also had high depression levels [147, 154, 159]. Irrational beliefs may be one source of the anxiety associated with FA [43, 148].

ADHD is also highly related to disordered eating, as has been discussed in several excellent systematic reviews [160–162]. Notably, these and other studies show strong associations between bingeing diagnoses (BED BN) and overeating behavior with ADHD in both childhood and adult populations [43, 160, 161, 163]. Restrictive behavior and anorexia nervosa, by contrast, are not highly correlated with ADHD [160, 161]. ADHD is posited to contribute both to higher eating disorder severity and treatment dropout [43, 164] via increased impulsivity, increased negative affect, or both [162]. Obesity is also associated with ADHD diagnoses and ADHD-related executive dysfunctions [151, 160], although, unlike in eating disorders, a large genome-wide association study suggests that higher BMI increases risk of developing ADHD but not the other way around [43, 165]. It is worth noting that stimulant medications (i.e., amphetamines) often used in the treatment of ADHD can also suppress appetite and are used in the treatment of both BED and obesity [43] (Chaps. 2 and 3). ADHD and FA, proper, have been found to be associated with one another as well [43, 163].

Like in SUD, there is a clear and positive association between adiposity, elevated BMI, and weight gain and a history of uncontrollable stressful events and chronic stress states such as job strain, unemployment, family caregiving, marital conflicts, and poverty [102]. The relationship between stress and weight is strongest among individuals who binge eat. Stress and adversity increase binge consumption of fast food snacks and calorie-dense and highly palatable foods, and stress-driven eating is more severe in obese women compared to lean women [102]. Perceived stress, per a self-report scale, is also correlated with BMI [166].

Like what is seen in SUD, childhood trauma and childhood maltreatment increase the risk of development of obesity [43, 158, 167–170] even after controlling for confounders [171], although in some cases studies show the link occurs via increased impulsivity [43, 170, 172] especially in the binge forms (BN, BED, binge eating without ED criteria) [43]. In a related area of research, higher attachment insecurity – as defined by failure to form trusting and reliable relationships with others and which often results from childhood trauma and poor parenting or at least poor child-parent emotional match – systematically characterized individuals with EDs and unhealthy eating behaviors from those without, in the general population [173].

Both chronic stress and childhood trauma also relate to FA scores and diagnoses. For example, self-reported perceived stress has been found to be associated with FA, and FA significantly mediated the relationship between perceived stress and BMI [166]. Childhood trauma and maltreatment, early life adversity, and psychological and sexual abuse have also been highlighted by several authors as a likely precursor to FA as well [12, 43, 48, 153, 154, 157, 158, 167–169, 171, 174] with childhood physical abuse and childhood sexual abuse increasing risk for FA by as much as 90% [43, 167]. Highlighting the importance of childhood, earlier onset of PTSD predicts a stronger association between PTSD and FA [43, 158].

6.6 Conclusion

In summary, there is a rapidly ballooning body of clinical evidence indicating that people can develop an "addictive" relationship to certain foods and that the FA construct is likely a valid one.

References

1. Adams RC, Sedgmond J, Maizey L, Chambers CD, Lawrence NS. Food addiction: implications for the diagnosis and treatment of overeating. Nutrients. 2019;11(9):2086.
2. Schulte EM, Wadden TA, Allison KC. An evaluation of food addiction as a distinct psychiatric disorder. Int J Eat Disord. 2020;53(10):1610–22.
3. Gordon EL, Ariel-Donges AH, Bauman V, Merlo LJ. What is the evidence for "food addiction?" a systematic review. Nutrients. 2018;10(4):477.
4. Meule A. A critical examination of the practical implications derived from the food addiction concept. Curr Obes Rep. 2019;8(1):11–7.
5. Tobore TO. Towards a comprehensive theory of obesity and a healthy diet: the causal role of oxidative stress in food addiction and obesity. Behav Brain Res. 2020;384:112560.
6. Morin JP, Rodriguez-Duran LF, Guzman-Ramos K, Perez-Cruz C, Ferreira G, Diaz-Cintra S, et al. Palatable hyper-caloric foods impact on neuronal plasticity. Front Behav Neurosci. 2017;11:19.
7. Ifland JR, Preuss HG, Marcus MT, Rourke KM, Taylor WC, Burau K, et al. Refined food addiction: a classic substance use disorder. Med Hypotheses. 2009;72(5):518–26.
8. Guise S. Mini habits for weight loss: stop dieting. form new habits. Change your lifestyle without suffering. Selective Entertainment LLC; 2016.
9. Gearhardt AN, Corbin WR, Brownell KD. Preliminary validation of the Yale Food Addiction Scale. Appetite. 2009;52(2):430–6.
10. Gearhardt AN, Corbin WR, Brownell KD. Food addiction: an examination of the diagnostic criteria for dependence. J Addict Med. 2009;3(1):1–7.
11. Kekic M, McClelland J, Campbell I, Nestler S, Rubia K, David AS, et al. The effects of prefrontal cortex transcranial direct current stimulation (tDCS) on food craving and temporal discounting in women with frequent food cravings. Appetite. 2014;78:55–62.
12. Jimenez-Murcia S, Aguera Z, Paslakis G, Munguia L, Granero R, Sanchez-Gonzalez J, et al. Food addiction in eating disorders and obesity: analysis of clusters and implications for treatment. Nutrients. 2019;11(11):2633.
13. Burmeister JM, Hinman N, Koball A, Hoffmann DA Carels RA. Food addiction in adults seeking weight loss treatment. Implications for psychosocial health and weight loss. Appetite. 2013;60(1):103–10.
14. Davis C, Levitan RD, Kaplan AS, Kennedy JL, Carter JC. Food cravings, appetite, and snack-food consumption in response to a psychomotor stimulant drug: the moderating effect of "food-addiction". Front Psychol. 2014;5:403.
15. Spring B, Schneider K, Smith M, Kendzor D, Appelhans B, Hedeker D, et al. Abuse potential of carbohydrates for overweight carbohydrate cravers. Psychopharmacology. 2008;197(4):637–47.
16. Sarkar S, Kochhar KP, Khan NA. Fat addiction: psychological and physiological trajectory. Nutrients. 2019;11(11):2785.
17. Gearhardt AN, Boswell RG, White MA. The association of "food addiction" with disordered eating and body mass index. Eat Behav. 2014;15(3):427–33.
18. Russell-Mayhew S, von Ranson KM, Masson PC. How does overeaters anonymous help its members? A qualitative analysis. Eur Eat Disord Rev: the journal of the Eating Disorders Association. 2010;18(1):33–42.
19. Lent MR, Swencionis C. Addictive personality and maladaptive eating behaviors in adults seeking bariatric surgery. Eat Behav. 2012;13(1):67–70.
20. Chao AM, Shaw JA, Pearl RL, Alamuddin N, Hopkins CM, Bakizada ZM, et al. Prevalence and psychosocial correlates of food addiction in persons

with obesity seeking weight reduction. Compr Psychiatry. 2017;73:97–104.
21. Pietilainen KH, Saarni SE, Kaprio J, Rissanen A. Does dieting make you fat? A twin study. Int J Obes. 2012;36(3):456–64.
22. Toussi R, Fujioka K, Coleman KJ. Pre- and post-surgery behavioral compliance, patient health, and postbariatric surgical weight loss. Obesity. 2009;17(5):996–1002.
23. Johnson PM, Kenny PJ. Dopamine D2 receptors in addiction-like reward dysfunction and compulsive eating in obese rats. Nat Neurosci. 2010;13(5):635–41.
24. Volkow ND, Wang GJ, Fowler JS, Telang F. Overlapping neuronal circuits in addiction and obesity: evidence of systems pathology. Philos Trans R Soc Lond Ser B Biol Sci. 2008;363(1507):3191–200.
25. Davis C, Strachan S, Berkson M. Sensitivity to reward: implications for overeating and overweight. Appetite. 2004;42(2):131–8.
26. Burger KS, Stice E. Frequent ice cream consumption is associated with reduced striatal response to receipt of an ice cream-based milkshake. Am J Clin Nutr. 2012;95(4):810–7.
27. Slater R, Cornelissen L, Fabrizi L, Patten D, Yoxen J, Worley A, et al. Oral sucrose as an analgesic drug for procedural pain in newborn infants: a randomised controlled trial. Lancet. 2010;376(9748):1225–32.
28. Hetherington MM, Pirie LM, Nabb S. Stimulus satiation: effects of repeated exposure to foods on pleasantness and intake. Appetite. 2002;38(1):19–28.
29. Garcia-Garcia I, Horstmann A, Jurado MA, Garolera M, Chaudhry SJ, Margulies DS, et al. Reward processing in obesity, substance addiction and non-substance addiction. Obes Rev. 2014;15(11):853–69.
30. Parnarouskis L, Schulte EM, Lumeng JC, Gearhardt AN. Development of the highly processed food withdrawal scale for children. Appetite. 2020;147:104553.
31. Cassin SE, von Ranson KM. Is binge eating experienced as an addiction? Appetite. 2007;49(3):687–90.
32. Markus CR, Rogers PJ, Brouns F, Schepers R. Eating dependence and weight gain; no human evidence for a 'sugar-addiction' model of overweight. Appetite. 2017;114:64–72.
33. Schulte EM, Smeal JK, Lewis J, Gearhardt AN. Development of the highly processed food withdrawal scale. Appetite. 2018;131:148–54.
34. Gearhardt AN, Corbin WR, Brownell KD. Development of the Yale Food Addiction Scale Version 2.0. Psychol Addict Behav. 2016;30(1):113–21.
35. American Psychiatric Association. Diagnostic and statistical manual of mental disorders (DSM-IV-TR). 4th ed. Washington, DC: American Psychiatric Association; 2000.
36. American Psychiatric Association. Diagnostic and statistical manual of mental disorders (DSM-V). 5th ed. Washington, DC: American Psychiatric Association; 2013.
37. McLeod S. What is validity? Simply psychology. 2013. https://www.simplypsychology.org/validity.html. Accessed 21 Mar 2021.
38. Trochim WMK. Conjointly, Sydney, Australia. 2020. https://conjointly.com/kb/convergent-and-discriminant-validity/. Accessed 21 Mar 2021.
39. Onaolapo AY, Onaolapo OJ. Food additives, food and the concept of 'food addiction': is stimulation of the brain reward circuit by food sufficient to trigger addiction? Pathophysiology. 2018;25(4):263–76.
40. Davis C, Curtis C, Levitan RD, Carter JC, Kaplan AS, Kennedy JL. Evidence that 'food addiction' is a valid phenotype of obesity. Appetite. 2011;57(3):711–7.
41. Leigh SJ, Morris MJ. The role of reward circuitry and food addiction in the obesity epidemic: an update. Biol Psychol. 2018;131:31–42.
42. Ziauddeen H, Fletcher PC. Is food addiction a valid and useful concept? Obes Rev. 2013;14(1):19–28.
43. Wiss D, Brewerton T. Separating the signal from the noise: how psychiatric diagnoses can help discern food addiction from dietary restraint. Nutrients. 2020;12(10):2937.
44. Schreiber LR, Odlaug BL, Grant JE. The overlap between binge eating disorder and substance use disorders: diagnosis and neurobiology. J Behav Addict. 2013;2(4):191–8.
45. Hauck C, Cook B, Ellrott T. Food addiction, eating addiction and eating disorders. Proc Nutr Soc. 2020;79(1):103–12.
46. Meule A, Gearhardt AN. Food addiction in the light of DSM-5. Nutrients. 2014;6(9):3653–71.
47. Ivezaj V, White MA, Grilo CM. Examining binge-eating disorder and food addiction in adults with overweight and obesity. Obesity. 2016;24(10):2064–9.
48. Burrows T, Skinner J, McKenna R, Rollo M. Food addiction, Binge eating disorder, and obesity: is there a relationship? Behav Sci. 2017;7(3):54.
49. Davis C. A commentary on the associations among 'food addiction', binge eating disorder, and obesity: overlapping conditions with idiosyncratic clinical features. Appetite. 2017;115:3–8.
50. Hone-Blanchet A, Fecteau S. Overlap of food addiction and substance use disorders definitions: analysis of animal and human studies. Neuropharmacology. 2014;85:81–90.
51. Yoder R, MacNeela P, Conway R, Heary C. How do individuals develop alcohol use disorder after bariatric surgery? A grounded theory exploration. Obes Surg. 2018;28(3):717–24.
52. Wiedemann AA, Carr MM, Ivezaj V, Barnes RD. Examining the construct validity of food addiction severity specifiers. Eat Weight Disord. 2020;26:1503.
53. Gearhardt AN, White MA, Masheb RM, Grilo CM. An examination of food addiction in a racially diverse sample of obese patients with binge eating disorder in primary care settings. Compr Psychiatry. 2013;54(5):500–5.
54. Gearhardt AN, White MA, Masheb RM, Morgan PT, Crosby RD, Grilo CM. An examination of the food

addiction construct in obese patients with binge eating disorder. Int J Eat Disord. 2012;45(5):657–63.
55. Ivezaj V, Stoeckel LE, Avena NM, Benoit SC, Conason A, Davis JF, et al. Obesity and addiction: can a complication of surgery help us understand the connection? Obes Rev. 2017;18(7):765–75.
56. Denoth F, Siciliano V, Iozzo P, Fortunato L, Molinaro S. The association between overweight and illegal drug consumption in adolescents: is there an underlying influence of the sociocultural environment? PLoS One. 2011;6(11):e27358.
57. Pursey KM, Stanwell P, Gearhardt AN, Collins CE, Burrows TL. The prevalence of food addiction as assessed by the Yale Food Addiction Scale: a systematic review. Nutrients. 2014;6(10):4552–90.
58. Tinghino B, Lugoboni F, Amatulli A, Biasin C, Bramani Araldi M, Cantiero D, et al. The FODRAT study (FOod addiction, DRugs, Alcohol and Tobacco): first data on food addiction prevalence among patients with addiction to drugs, tobacco and alcohol. Eat Weight Disord. 2020;26:449.
59. Harrop EN, Marlatt GA. The comorbidity of substance use disorders and eating disorders in women: prevalence, etiology, and treatment. Addict Behav. 2010;35(5):392–8.
60. Bogusz K, Kopera M, Jakubczyk A, Trucco EM, Kucharska K, Walenda A, et al. Prevalence of alcohol use disorder among individuals who binge eat: a systematic review and meta-analysis. Addiction. 2021;116(1):18–31.
61. Bahji A, Mazhar MN, Hudson CC, Nadkarni P, MacNeil BA, Hawken E. Prevalence of substance use disorder comorbidity among individuals with eating disorders: a systematic review and meta-analysis. Psychiatry Res. 2019;273:58–66.
62. Munn-Chernoff MA, Few LR, Matherne CE, Baker JH, Men VY, McCutcheon VV, et al. Eating disorders in a community-based sample of women with alcohol use disorder and nicotine dependence. Drug Alcohol Depend. 2020;212:107981.
63. Eskander N, Chakrapani S, Ghani MR. The risk of substance use among adolescents and adults with eating disorders. Cureus. 2020;12(9):e10309.
64. Mies GW, Treur JL, Larsen JK, Halberstadt J, Pasman JA, Vink JM. The prevalence of food addiction in a large sample of adolescents and its association with addictive substances. Appetite. 2017;118:97–105.
65. Canan F, Karaca S, Sogucak S, Gecici O, Kuloglu M. Eating disorders and food addiction in men with heroin use disorder: a controlled study. Eat Weight Disord. 2017;22(2):249–57.
66. Domoff SE, Sutherland EQ, Yokum S, Gearhardt AN. Adolescents' addictive phone use: associations with eating behaviors and adiposity. Int J Environ Res Public Health. 2020;17(8):2861.
67. Jimenez-Murcia S, Granero R, Wolz I, Bano M, Mestre-Bach G, Steward T, et al. Food addiction in gambling disorder: frequency and clinical outcomes. Front Psychol. 2017;8:473.
68. Hauck C, Schipfer M, Ellrott T, Cook B. The relationship between food addiction and patterns of disordered eating with exercise dependence: in amateur endurance athletes. Eat Weight Disord. 2020;25(6):1573–82.
69. Fenn JM, Laurent JS, Sigmon SC. Increases in body mass index following initiation of methadone treatment. J Subst Abus Treat. 2015;51:59–63.
70. Krahn D, Grossman J, Henk H, Mussey M, Crosby R, Gosnell B. Sweet intake, sweet-liking, urges to eat, and weight change: relationship to alcohol dependence and abstinence. Addict Behav. 2006;31(4):622–31.
71. Leggio L, Addolorato G, Cippitelli A, Jerlhag E, Kampov-Polevoy AB, Swift RM. Role of feeding-related pathways in alcohol dependence: a focus on sweet preference, NPY, and ghrelin. Alcohol Clin Exp Res. 2011;35(2):194–202.
72. Janowsky DS, Pucilowski O, Buyinza M. Preference for higher sucrose concentrations in cocaine abusing-dependent patients. J Psychiatr Res. 2003;37(1):35–41.
73. Jeynes KD, Gibson EL. The importance of nutrition in aiding recovery from substance use disorders: a review. Drug Alcohol Depend. 2017;179:229–39.
74. Neale J, Nettleton S, Pickering L, Fischer J. Eating patterns among heroin users: a qualitative study with implications for nutritional interventions. Addiction. 2012;107(3):635–41.
75. Peles E, Schreiber S, Sason A, Adelson M. Risk factors for weight gain during methadone maintenance treatment. Subst Abus. 2016;37(4):613–8.
76. Mysels DJ, Sullivan MA. The relationship between opioid and sugar intake: review of evidence and clinical applications. J Opioid Manag. 2010;6(6):445–52.
77. Ersche KD, Stochl J, Woodward JM, Fletcher PC. The skinny on cocaine: insights into eating behavior and body weight in cocaine-dependent men. Appetite. 2013;71:75–80.
78. Leggio L, Zywiak WH, Fricchione SR, Edwards SM, de la Monte SM, Swift RM, et al. Intravenous ghrelin administration increases alcohol craving in alcohol-dependent heavy drinkers: a preliminary investigation. Biol Psychiatry. 2014;76(9):734–41.
79. Gibson EL. The psychobiology of comfort eating: implications for neuropharmacological interventions. Behav Pharmacol. 2012;23(5–6):442–60.
80. Children's hedonic response to the smell of alcohol: effects of parental drinking habits, 2000.
81. Lange LA, Kampov-Polevoy AB, Garbutt JC. Sweet liking and high novelty seeking: independent phenotypes associated with alcohol-related problems. Alcohol Alcohol. 2010;45(5):431–6.
82. Kampov-Polevoy AB, Garbutt JC, Khalitov E. Family history of alcoholism and response to sweets. Alcohol Clin Exp Res. 2003;27(11):1743–9.
83. Bocarsly ME, Berner LA, Hoebel BG, Avena NM. Rats that binge eat fat-rich food do not show somatic signs or anxiety associated with opiate-

like withdrawal: implications for nutrient-specific food addiction behaviors. Physiol Behav. 2011;104(5):865–72.
84. Colantuoni C, Schwenker J, McCarthy J, Rada P, Ladenheim B, Cadet JL, et al. Excessive sugar intake alters binding to dopamine and mu-opioid receptors in the brain. Neuroreport. 2001;12(16):3549–52.
85. Avena NM, Rada P, Hoebel BG. Sugar and fat bingeing have notable differences in addictive-like behavior. J Nutr. 2009;139(3):623–8.
86. Hebebrand J, Albayrak O, Adan R, Antel J, Dieguez C, de Jong J, et al. "Eating addiction", rather than "food addiction", better captures addictive-like eating behavior. Neurosci Biobehav Rev. 2014;47:295–306.
87. Rogers PJ. Food and drug addictions: similarities and differences. Pharmacol Biochem Behav. 2017;153:182–90.
88. Westwater ML, Fletcher PC, Ziauddeen H. Sugar addiction: the state of the science. Eur J Nutr. 2016;55(Suppl 2):55–69.
89. Hetherington MM, Cunningham K, Dye L, Gibson EL, Gregersen NT, Halford JC, et al. Potential benefits of satiety to the consumer: scientific considerations. Nutr Res Rev. 2013;26(1):22–38.
90. Lu HK, Mannan H, Hay P. Exploring relationships between recurrent binge eating and illicit substance use in a non-clinical sample of women over two years. Behav Sci. 2017;7(3):46.
91. Reslan S, Saules KK, Greenwald MK, Schuh LM. Substance misuse following Roux-en-Y gastric bypass surgery. Subst Use Misuse. 2014;49(4):405–17.
92. Murray SM, Tweardy S, Geliebter A, Avena NM. A longitudinal preliminary study of addiction-like responses to food and alcohol consumption among individuals undergoing weight loss surgery. Obes Surg. 2019;29(8):2700–3.
93. Fowler L, Ivezaj V, Saules KK. Problematic intake of high-sugar/low-fat and high glycemic index foods by bariatric patients is associated with development of post-surgical new onset substance use disorders. Eat Behav. 2014;15(3):505–8.
94. Chiappetta S, Stier C, Hadid MA, Malo N, Theodoridou S, Weiner R, et al. Remission of food addiction does not induce cross-addiction after sleeve gastrectomy and gastric bypass: a prospective cohort study. Obes Facts. 2020;13(3):307–20.
95. Laaksonen E, Lahti J, Sinclair JD, Heinala P, Alho H. Predictors for the efficacy of naltrexone treatment in alcohol dependence: sweet preference. Alcohol Alcohol. 2011;46(3):308–11.
96. Blanco-Gandia MC, Minarro J, Rodriguez-Arias M. Common neural mechanisms of palatable food intake and drug abuse: knowledge obtained with animal models. Curr Pharm Des. 2020;26(20):2372–84.
97. Avena NM, Hoebel BG. A diet promoting sugar dependency causes behavioral cross-sensitization to a low dose of amphetamine. Neuroscience. 2003;122(1):17–20.
98. Gosnell BA. Sucrose intake enhances behavioral sensitization produced by cocaine. Brain Res. 2005;1031(2):194–201.
99. Clasen MM, Riley AL, Davidson TL. Hippocampal-dependent inhibitory learning and memory processes in the control of eating and drug taking. Curr Pharm Des. 2020;26(20):2334–52.
100. Koob GF, Powell P, White A. Addiction as a coping response: Hyperkatifeia, deaths of despair, and COVID-19. Am J Psychiatry. 2020;177(11):1031–7.
101. Kwako LE, Momenan R, Litten RZ, Koob GF, Goldman D. Addictions Neuroclinical assessment: a neuroscience-based framework for addictive disorders. Biol Psychiatry. 2015;80:179.
102. Sinha R. Role of addiction and stress neurobiology on food intake and obesity. Biol Psychol. 2018;131:5–13.
103. Lacroix E, von Ranson KM. Prevalence of social, cognitive, and emotional impairment among individuals with food addiction. Eat Weight Disord. 2020;26:1253.
104. Hardy R, Fani N, Jovanovic T, Michopoulos V. Food addiction and substance addiction in women: common clinical characteristics. Appetite. 2018;120:367–73.
105. Hershberger AR, Um M, Cyders MA. The relationship between the UPPS-P impulsive personality traits and substance use psychotherapy outcomes: a meta-analysis. Drug Alcohol Depend. 2017;178:408–16.
106. Wilcox CE, Dekonenko CJ, Mayer AR, Bogenschutz MP, Turner JA. Cognitive control in alcohol use disorder: deficits and clinical relevance. Rev Neurosci. 2014;25:1–24.
107. Wilcox CE, Pommy JM, Adinoff B. Neural circuitry of impaired emotion regulation in substance use disorders. Am J Psychiatr. 2016;173:344.
108. Kwako LE, Schwandt ML, Ramchandani VA, Diazgranados N, Koob GF, Volkow ND, et al. Neurofunctional domains derived from deep behavioral phenotyping in alcohol use disorder. Am J Psychiatry. 2019;176(9):744–53.
109. Maxwell AL, Gardiner E, Loxton NJ. Investigating the relationship between reward sensitivity, impulsivity, and food addiction: a systematic review. Eur Eat Disord Rev: the journal of the Eating Disorders Association. 2020;28(4):368–84.
110. Wiers CE, Zhao J, Manza P, Murani K, Ramirez V, Zehra A, et al. Conscious and unconscious brain responses to food and cocaine cues. Brain Imaging Behav. 2021;15(1):311–9.
111. Wilcox CE, Bogenschutz MB. Psychopharmacologies for alcohol and drug use disorders. In: McCrady BS, Epstein EE, editors. Addictions: a comprehensive guidebook. 2nd ed. New York: Oxford University Press; 2013. p. 526–50.
112. Vujanovic AA, Farris SG, Bartlett BA, Lyons RC, Haller M, Colvonen PJ, et al. Anxiety sensitivity in the association between posttraumatic stress and substance use disorders: a systematic review. Clin Psychol Rev. 2018;62:37–55.

113. Paraskevopoulou M, van Rooij D, Schene AH, Scheres APJ, Buitelaar JK, Schellekens AFA. Effects of substance misuse and family history of substance use disorder on delay discounting in adolescents and young adults with attention-deficit/hyperactivity disorder. Eur Addict Res. 2020;26(4–5):295–305.
114. Blevins D, Choi CJ, Pavlicova M, Martinez D, Mariani JJ, Grabowski J, et al. Impulsiveness as a moderator of amphetamine treatment response for cocaine use disorder among ADHD patients. Drug Alcohol Depend. 2020;213:108082.
115. Gibson-Smith D, Bot M, Brouwer IA, Visser M, Penninx B. Diet quality in persons with and without depressive and anxiety disorders. J Psychiatr Res. 2018;106:1–7.
116. Appelhans BM, Woolf K, Pagoto SL, Schneider KL, Whited MC, Liebman R. Inhibiting food reward: delay discounting, food reward sensitivity, and palatable food intake in overweight and obese women. Obesity. 2011;19(11):2175–82.
117. Nederkoorn C, Braet C, Van Eijs Y, Tanghe A, Jansen A. Why obese children cannot resist food: the role of impulsivity. Eat Behav. 2006;7(4):315–22.
118. Appelhans BM, French SA, Pagoto SL, Sherwood NE. Managing temptation in obesity treatment: a neurobehavioral model of intervention strategies. Appetite. 2016;96:268–79.
119. Lin Z, Qu S. Legend of weight loss: a crosstalk between the bariatric surgery and the brain. Obes Surg. 2020;30(5):1988–2002.
120. Loxton NJ, Tipman RJ. Reward sensitivity and food addiction in women. Appetite. 2017;115:28–35.
121. Val-Laillet D, Aarts E, Weber B, Ferrari M, Quaresima V, Stoeckel LE, et al. Neuroimaging and neuromodulation approaches to study eating behavior and prevent and treat eating disorders and obesity. NeuroImage Clin. 2015;8:1–31.
122. Schulte EM, Tuttle HM, Gearhardt AN. Belief in food addiction and obesity-related policy support. PLoS One. 2016;11(1):e0147557.
123. Benard M, Camilleri GM, Etile F, Mejean C, Bellisle F, Reach G, et al. Association between impulsivity and weight status in a general population. Nutrients. 2017;9(3):217.
124. VanderBroek-Stice L, Stojek MK, Beach SRH, van Dellen MR, Mac Killop J. Multidimensional assessment of impulsivity in relation to obesity and food addiction. Appetite. 2017;112:59–68.
125. Giel KE, Teufel M, Junne F, Zipfel S, Schag K. Food-related impulsivity in obesity and Binge eating disorder-a systematic update of the evidence. Nutrients. 2017;9(11):1170.
126. Meule A, Blechert J. Interactive and indirect effects of trait impulsivity facets on body mass index. Appetite. 2017;118:60–5.
127. Meule A, de Zwaan M, Muller A. Attentional and motor impulsivity interactively predict 'food addiction' in obese individuals. Compr Psychiatry. 2017;72:83–7.
128. Davis C, Mackew L, Levitan RD, Kaplan AS, Carter JC, Kennedy JL. Binge Eating Disorder (BED) in relation to addictive behaviors and personality risk factors. Front Psychol. 2017;8:579.
129. Wolz I, Granero R, Fernandez-Aranda F. A comprehensive model of food addiction in patients with binge-eating symptomatology: the essential role of negative urgency. Compr Psychiatry. 2017;74:118–24.
130. Wolz I, Hilker I, Granero R, Jimenez-Murcia S, Gearhardt AN, Dieguez C, et al. "Food addiction" in patients with eating disorders is associated with negative urgency and difficulties to focus on long-term goals. Front Psychol. 2016;7:61.
131. Higgins GA, Zeeb FD, Fletcher PJ. Role of impulsivity and reward in the anti-obesity actions of 5-HT2C receptor agonists. J Psychopharmacol. 2017;31(11):1403–18.
132. Churchill S, Jessop DC. Reflective and non-reflective antecedents of health-related behaviour: exploring the relative contributions of impulsivity and implicit self-control to the prediction of dietary behaviour. Br J Health Psychol. 2011;16(Pt 2):257–72.
133. DeHart WB, Snider SE, Pope DA Bickel WK. A reinforcer pathology model of health behaviors in individuals with obesity. Health Psychol. 2020;39(11):966–74.
134. Wenzel KR, Weinstock J, McGrath AB. The clinical significance of food addiction. J Addict Med. 2020;14(5):e153–e9.
135. Rodrigue C, Ouellette AS, Lemieux S, Tchernof A, Biertho L, Begin C. Executive functioning and psychological symptoms in food addiction: a study among individuals with severe obesity. Eat Weight Disord. 2018;23(4):469–78.
136. Davis HA, Smith GT. An integrative model of risk for high school disordered eating. J Abnorm Psychol. 2018;127(6):559–70.
137. Ben-Porat T, Weiss R, Sherf-Dagan S, Rottenstreich A, Kaluti D, Khalaileh A, et al. Food addiction and Binge eating during one year following sleeve gastrectomy: prevalence and implications for postoperative outcomes. Obes Surg. 2021;31(2):603–11.
138. Brown M, Robinson L, Campione GC, Wuensch K, Hildebrandt T, Micali N. Intolerance of uncertainty in eating disorders: a systematic review and meta-analysis. Eur Eat Disord Rev: the journal of the Eating Disorders Association. 2017;25(5):329–43.
139. Pearson CM, Smith GT. Bulimic symptom onset in young girls: a longitudinal trajectory analysis. J Abnorm Psychol. 2015;124(4):1003–13.
140. Ouwens MA, van Strien T, van Leeuwe JF. Possible pathways between depression, emotional and external eating. A structural equation model. Appetite. 2009;53(2):245–8.
141. Schaefer LM, Smith KE, Anderson LM, Cao L, Crosby RD, Engel SG, et al. The role of affect in the maintenance of binge-eating disorder: evidence from an ecological momentary assessment study. J Abnorm Psychol. 2020;129(4):387–96.

142. Lin CY, Cheung P, Imani V, Griffiths MD, Pakpour AH. The mediating effects of eating disorder, food addiction, and insomnia in the association between psychological distress and being overweight among Iranian adolescents. Nutrients. 2020;12(5):1371.
143. Westwood H, Kerr-Gaffney J, Stahl D, Tchanturia K. Alexithymia in eating disorders: systematic review and meta-analyses of studies using the Toronto Alexithymia Scale. J Psychosom Res. 2017;99:66–81.
144. Smith KE, Mason TB, Schaefer LM, Juarascio A, Dvorak R, Weinbach N, et al. Examining intra-individual variability in food-related inhibitory control and negative affect as predictors of binge eating using ecological momentary assessment. J Psychiatr Res. 2020;120:137–43.
145. Fernandes J, Ferreira-Santos F, Miller K, Torres S. Emotional processing in obesity: a systematic review and exploratory meta-analysis. Obes Rev. 2018;19(1):111–20.
146. Brunault P, Ducluzeau PH, Courtois R, Bourbao-Tournois C, Delbachian I, Reveillere C, et al. Food addiction is associated with higher neuroticism, lower conscientiousness, higher impulsivity, but lower extraversion in obese patient candidates for bariatric surgery. Subst Use Misuse. 2018;53(11):1919–23.
147. Bourdier L, Fatseas M, Maria AS, Carre A, Berthoz S. The psycho-affective roots of obesity: results from a French study in the general population. Nutrients. 2020;12(10):2962.
148. Nolan LJ, Jenkins SM. Food addiction is associated with irrational beliefs via trait anxiety and emotional eating. Nutrients. 2019;11(8):1711.
149. Tang CS, Gan Y, Ko J, Kwon JH, Wu A, Yan E, et al. The associations among emotional factors, personality traits, and addiction-like eating: a study on university students in six Asian countries/regions. Int J Eat Disord. 2021;54(2):125–31.
150. Piccinni A, Bucchi R, Fini C, Vanelli F, Mauri M, Stallone T, et al. Food addiction and psychiatric comorbidities: a review of current evidence. Eat Weight Disord. 2020;26:1049.
151. Weiss F, Barbuti M, Carignani G, Calderone A, Santini F, Maremmani I, et al. Psychiatric aspects of obesity: a narrative review of pathophysiology and psychopathology. J Clin Med. 2020;9(8):2344.
152. Kiyici S, Koca N, Sigirli D, Aslan BB, Guclu M, Kisakol G. Food addiction correlates with psychosocial functioning more than metabolic parameters in patients with obesity. Metab Syndr Relat Disord. 2020;18(3):161–7.
153. Burrows T, Kay-Lambkin F, Pursey K, Skinner J, Dayas C. Food addiction and associations with mental health symptoms: a systematic review with meta-analysis. J Hum Nutr Diet. 2018;31(4):544–72.
154. Burrows T, Collins R, Rollo M, Leary M, Hides L, Davis C. The feasibility of a personality targeted intervention for addictive overeating: FoodFix. Appetite. 2021;156:104974.
155. Tomiyama AJ, Dallman MF, Epel ES. Comfort food is comforting to those most stressed: evidence of the chronic stress response network in high stress women. Psychoneuroendocrinology. 2011;36(10):1513–9.
156. Nicolau J, Romerosa JM, Rodriguez I, Sanchis P, Bonet A, Arteaga M, et al. Associations of food addiction with metabolic control, medical complications and depression among patients with type 2 diabetes. Acta Diabetol. 2020;57(9):1093–100.
157. Burrows T, Hides L, Brown R, Dayas CV, Kay-Lambkin F. Differences in dietary preferences, personality and mental health in Australian adults with and without food addiction. Nutrients. 2017;9(3):285.
158. Mason SM, Flint AJ, Roberts AL, Agnew-Blais J, Koenen KC, Rich-Edwards JW. Posttraumatic stress disorder symptoms and food addiction in women by timing and type of trauma exposure. JAMA Psychiat. 2014;71(11):1271–8.
159. Ivezaj V, Wiedemann AA, Lawson JL, Grilo CM. Food addiction in sleeve gastrectomy patients with loss-of-control eating. Obes Surg. 2019;29(7):2071–7.
160. Kaisari P, Dourish CT, Higgs S. Attention Deficit Hyperactivity Disorder (ADHD) and disordered eating behaviour: a systematic review and a framework for future research. Clin Psychol Rev. 2017;53:109–21.
161. Nazar BP, Bernardes C, Peachey G, Sergeant J, Mattos P, Treasure J. The risk of eating disorders comorbid with attention-deficit/hyperactivity disorder: a systematic review and meta-analysis. Int J Eat Disord. 2016;49(12):1045–57.
162. El Archi S, Cortese S, Ballon N, Reveillere C, De Luca A, Barrault S, et al. Negative affectivity and emotion dysregulation as mediators between ADHD and disordered eating: a systematic review. Nutrients. 2020;12(11):3292.
163. Brunault P, Frammery J, Montaudon P, De Luca A, Hankard R, Ducluzeau PH, et al. Adulthood and childhood ADHD in patients consulting for obesity is associated with food addiction and binge eating, but not sleep apnea syndrome. Appetite. 2019;136:25–32.
164. Testa G, Baenas I, Vintro-Alcaraz C, Granero R, Aguera Z, Sanchez I, et al. Does ADHD symptomatology influence treatment outcome and dropout risk in eating disorders? A longitudinal study. J Clin Med. 2020;9(7):2305.
165. Martins-Silva T, Vaz JDS, Hutz MH, Salatino-Oliveira A, Genro JP, Hartwig FP, et al. Assessing causality in the association between attention-deficit/hyperactivity disorder and obesity: a Mendelian randomization study. Int J Obes. 2019;43(12):2500–8.
166. Lin YS, Tung YT, Yen YC, Chien YW. Food addiction mediates the relationship between perceived stress and body mass index in Taiwan young adults. Nutrients. 2020;12(7):1951.

167. Mason SM, Flint AJ, Field AE, Austin SB, Rich-Edwards JW. Abuse victimization in childhood or adolescence and risk of food addiction in adult women. Obesity. 2013;21(12):E775–81.
168. Mason SM, Santaularia NJ, Berge JM, Larson N, Neumark-Sztainer D. Is the childhood home food environment a confounder of the association between child maltreatment exposure and adult body mass index? Prev Med. 2018;110:86–92.
169. Palmisano GL, Innamorati M, Vanderlinden J. Life adverse experiences in relation with obesity and binge eating disorder: a systematic review. J Behav Addict. 2016;5(1):11–31.
170. Molendijk ML, Hoek HW, Brewerton TD, Elzinga BM. Childhood maltreatment and eating disorder pathology: a systematic review and dose-response meta-analysis. Psychol Med. 2017:1–15.
171. Wiss DA, Brewerton TD. Adverse childhood experiences and adult obesity: a systematic review of plausible mechanisms and meta-analysis of cross-sectional studies. Physiol Behav. 2020;223:112964.
172. McMullin SD, Shields GS, Slavich GM, Buchanan TW. Cumulative lifetime stress exposure predicts greater impulsivity and addictive behaviors. J Health Psychol. 2020:1359105320937055.
173. Faber A, Dube L, Knauper B. Attachment and eating: a meta-analytic review of the relevance of attachment for unhealthy and healthy eating behaviors in the general population. Appetite. 2018;123:410–38.
174. Khalil H, Ellwood L, Lord H, Fernandez R. Pharmacological treatment for obesity in adults: an umbrella review. Ann Pharmacother. 2020;54(7):691–705.

Part IV

Basic Biology of Food Addiction, and Its Overlap with Substance Use Disorders

Neurobiology and Cognitive Neuroscience of Substance Use Disorders

7

7.1 Overview of Substance Use Disorders

The purpose of this chapter is to provide an overview of what we know about the neurobiological mechanisms of substance use disorders (SUD) and their related neuropsychological underpinnings (reward-processing, conditioning, craving, impulse control, negative urgency, attentional bias, and emotion regulation) and to understand how individuals progress from early experimentation with drug or alcohol use, to craving, and then to impaired decision-making around drug use, compulsive use, and loss of control. When we speak about "drugs," we are talking about any of the following: cocaine, opiates, alcohol, nicotine, cannabis, and caffeine, since addictive behavior can develop towards any of these substances [1]. Conditioned learning plays a key role in the development of the disorder, and pleasure or relief provided by use drugs of abuse affects the brain chemistry to cause a vicious cycle (Box 7.1, Fig. 7.1).

Box 7.1 Terms Related to Conditioned Learning [2–4]

- Negative Reinforcement: the process by which removal of an aversive stimulus (or aversive state, in the case of addiction) increases the probability of a response.
- Positive Reinforcement: the process by which addition of pleasant or euphoric state increases probability of a response.
- Classical Conditioning: a type of learning that involves the acquisition of an automatic response elicited by a stimulus (i.e., dog salivates when food and bell ringing are paired together, then salivates even when food taken away in response to bell ringing). Learning strengthens the links between a stimulus and a response.
- Operant Conditioning: a type of learning through rewards and punishment that results in an association being made between a behavior and a consequence for that behavior. Learning strengthens the links between a behavior and a consequence.
- Reward: stimulus intended to encourage and increase a behavior or response.
- Punishment: stimulus intended to discourage and decrease a behavior or response.

The use of the drugs and the immediate neurochemical consequences "stamp in" the experience of taking the drug and solidify its future use [2, 3, 5–8]. The other known physiological effects of drugs on the brain, including tolerance and

C. E. Wilcox, *Food Addiction, Obesity, and Disorders of Overeating*,
https://doi.org/10.1007/978-3-030-83078-6_7

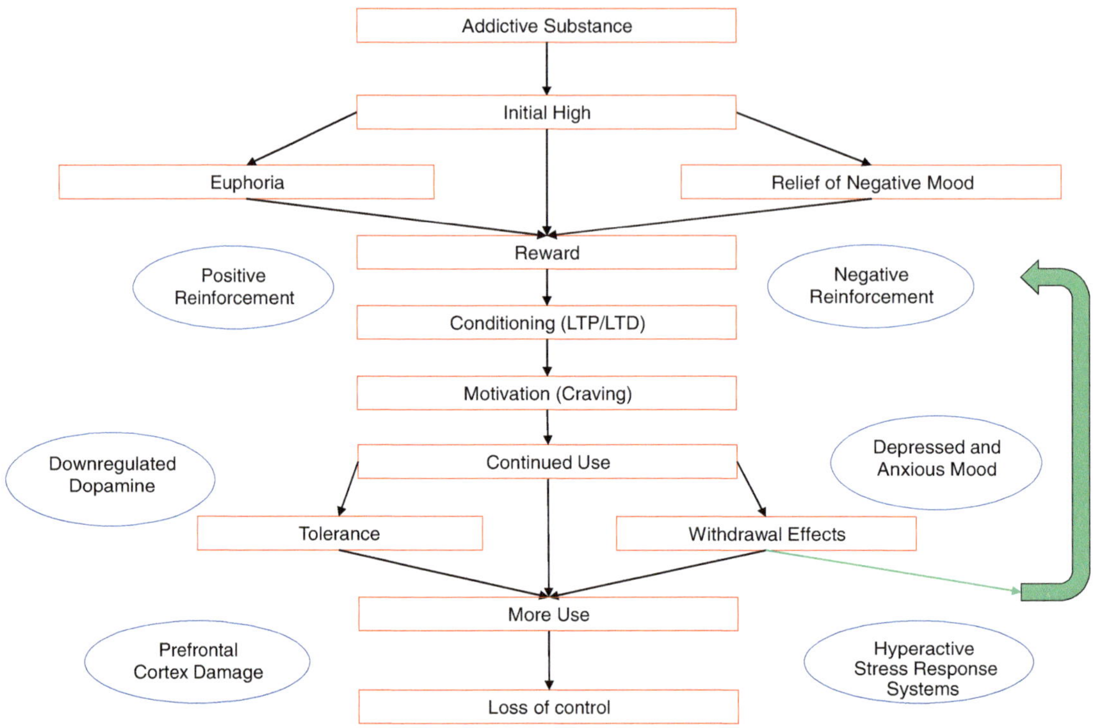

Fig. 7.1 This figure depicts the conditioning processes that cause and perpetuate substance use disorders. Red boxes – stage of addiction process. Blue circles – neurobiological/psychological consequences of and contributors to the addiction process (LTP long-term potentiation, LTD long-term depression)

withdrawal, play a major role in perpetuation of the disorder as well via the associated negative affect states. SUD involve several key neurotransmitter systems [dopamine (DA), norepinephrine, glutamate, opioids] and brain regions (striatum, prefrontal cortex, including anterior cingulate cortex and orbitofrontal cortex, amygdala, insula, cerebellum, visual cortex), as has been demonstrated through studies done in animals and humans, the latter mostly determined through neuroimaging studies [1, 5–11].

7.2 Core Brain Regions

The dopaminergic system, or the "mesolimbic dopamine system," refers to the network of neurons projecting from the midbrain ventral tegmental area (VTA) ("meso = mid-brain") to the ventral striatum [in which the nucleus accumbens (NAc) resides], as well as amygdala (both "limbic"), and is a key pathway in the "liking" process (dopaminergic projections from NAc to ventral tegmental area (VTA) are also important, but less discussed) [12–14]. The "nigrostriatal system" refers to the system of DA neurons projecting from the substantia nigra to the dorsal striatum (caudate and putamen), and this is involved in action initiation and drug-seeking behaviors. Habit formation and learning and conditioning occur via the effects of DA in both the mesolimbic and mesostriatal system, but the mesostriatal system is especially important in the movement-based aspects of habit (e.g., it is this system that is damaged in Parkinson's disease). The "mesocortical system" refers to the system of DA neurons projecting from the VTA to the prefrontal cortex (PFC) ("cortical") and is also involved in the "liking" process [15–17]. The PFC is broken down into many important brain areas including the anterior cingulate, orbitofrontal, dorsolateral, and ventromedial (abbreviated ACC, OFC, DLPFC, and vmPFC, respectively), all of which play important roles in decision-

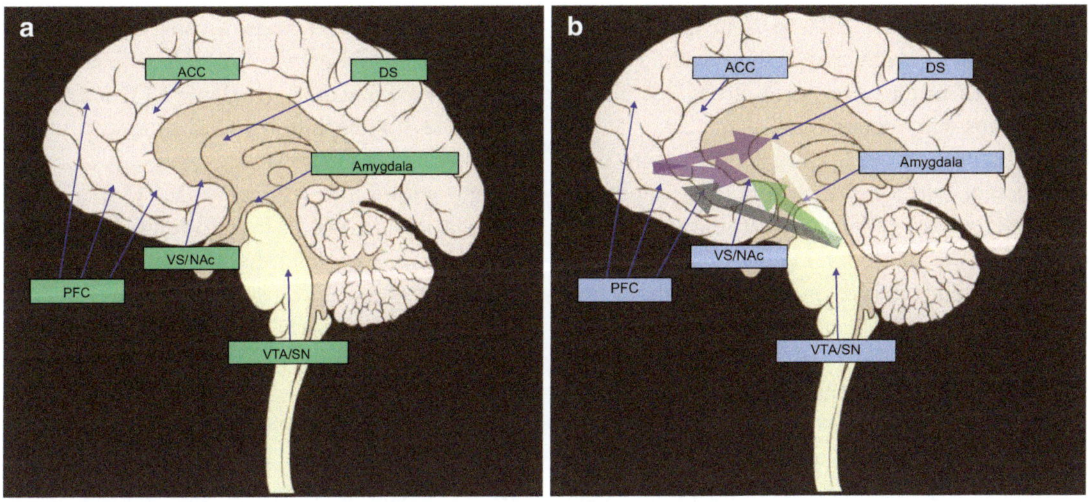

Fig. 7.2 (**a**) This figure shows the approximate locations of several important brain regions which are involved in the initiation, development, and perpetuation of substance use disorders and includes brain regions involved in reward, stress response, and executive control. ACC anterior cingulate cortex, PFC prefrontal cortex; includes anterior cingulate, orbitofrontal, dorsolateral, and ventromedial (ACC, OFC, DLPFC, VMPFC, respectively), DS dorsal striatum, includes caudate and putamen, VS/NAc ventral striatum and nucleus accumbens; nucleus accumbens resides in the ventral striatum, VTA/SN ventral tegmental area and substantia nigra. (**b**) This figure depicts the three key dopaminergic pathways. Mesolimbic system – network of dopamine (DA) neurons projecting from VTA to the VS, where the NAc resides; key pathway in "liking" process (green). Nigrostriatal system – network of DA neurons projecting from the SN to the DS; involved in action-initiation and drug-seeking behaviors (white). Mesocortical system – network of DA neurons projecting from the VTA to the PFC; also involved in the "liking" process (black). Frontostriatal circuits – network of projections from PFC into the VS and DS; works with cue-related DA release to drive drug-seeking behavior (purple)

making, cue processing, and action initiation (Fig. 7.2a, b). For example, DLPFC is involved in working memory (the ability to hold information in memory in order to perform a task) and impulse control, whereas vmPFC and ACC are more directly linked with limbic centers and sensory areas and respond to drug-related sensory cues [10, 11, 18]. Lateral OFC is involved in decision-making, whereas medial OFC tends to be more cue-reactive and immediately responsive to reward [10, 11, 18]. Other important brain areas in reward involve the insula, which is a relay that processes bodily sensations like gustatory and gut-related pleasure and links higher-order decision-making regions [19]. Opioid, glutamate, and GABA receptors exist throughout the brain, including the VTA and NAc, where their actions play key roles at many of the stages of the addiction process. For example, neurons projecting from cortex to the striatum release glutamate into dorsal striatum, which importantly affects the power of a drug-related cue to affect attention and behavior around drug-seeking and use [20, 21].

7.3 Reward

Drugs and pleasurable experience cause release of DA into the NAc and other brain regions (e.g., basolateral amygdala) [5, 22, 23], otherwise known as "reward" or "liking" [13, 14]. The mesolimbic DA system plays a key role in this process, as does the mesocortical system. The more rewarding the drug is evaluated to be, and the greater the self-reported pleasantness, the greater the release of extracellular DA in the NAc [1, 5, 7, 22, 23]. Pharmacological blockade of DA receptors and lesions of the mesolimbic dopaminergic system reduce the reward value of drugs of abuse [24–27]. A tendency towards reward sensitivity is mediated in part by a hypersensitive DA system [28, 29]. The dopaminergic projections that link VTA to NAc and VTA to PFC are crucial pathways of the reward system. DA neurons in the VTA form strong reciprocal connections with regions such as the NAc, lateral hypothalamus, and PFC [30]. The striatum (dorsal striatum and NAc) serves a very important role in the reward pathway by serving as the main integration site for dopaminergic inputs from the VT and glutamatergic inputs from the PFC, amygdala, hippocampus, and thalamus [30].

Opioids are also released to reward in the NAc and VTA with consumption of a rewarding substance, mediate "liking," and play a key role in the subjective experience of pleasure [13, 14, 27]. Some posit that endogenous opioids, rather than DA, play the most important role in mediating the reward component of drug and alcohol use [17]. For example, the μ opioid blockers naloxone and naltrexone reduce the pleasure experienced with alcohol consumption [27]; however, DA antagonists reduce cocaine-enhanced brain-stimulation reward in rats [31]. Opioid peptide release in the VTA plays a key role in modulating the quantity and quality of DA release into the ventral striatum [32].

7.4 Conditioning: Positive Reinforcement

As drug use progresses, repeated drug use causes the drug use behavior to become linked with the stimuli and events that preceded and accompany drug use, such as the drug-using environment [1, 33], or visual, auditory, or olfactory drug cues. Habits develop as a result of the DA-mediated conditioning and positive reinforcement from drugs' euphoric effects [15, 34]. Higher levels of reward lead to more powerful learning and conditioning processes at the neurobiological level, which contributes to greater future motivation to obtain a reward upon exposure to familiar reward-related cues (Fig. 7.1).

Conditioning requires long-term potentiation (LTP) and long-term depression (LTD), which is a phenomenon of neural plasticity known to underlie the learning, consolidation, and refinement of both adaptive and maladaptive behaviors [34–36]. There is a huge diversity of cellular plasticity mechanisms [34]. Those include Hebbian-type plasticity, (includes LTP and LTD), as well as homeostatic sync scaling and meta-plasticity (modifications that maintain synaptic strength within a functional range) [34, 37, 38]. DA is a key player in reward-related learning, and dopamine agonists induce reward learning (explaining why Parkinson's patients who get L-Dopa, a dopamine precursor, can develop behavioral addictions) [39, 40], and D1 receptors may be key for this process [17, 26]. Glutamate, via its effects on N-methyl-D-aspartate (NMDA) receptors, is the other key player; blockade of NMDA receptors, which blocks LTP and LTD [34, 37], also prevents many behavioral adaptations normally associated with drug reinforcement, such as conditioned-place preference, behavioral sensitization, and self-administration [17, 34]. Sensitization (a process in which repeated administration of drugs causes increased motor and/or behavioral responses to their stimulant and rewarding effects that also parallels LTP and is seen as a marker of conditioning in animal models) is also mediated by the interacting effects of glutamate and DA in mesolimbic and mesocortical circuits [17, 34].

7.5 Motivation: Positive Reinforcement

After conditioning has occurred, motivation to obtain a rewarding substance ("wanting"), often associated with craving, increases in the context of exposure to environments or cues associated with previous experiences of pleasantness and euphoria [13, 14, 41]. Greater sensitivity to cues, as is demonstrated in hundreds of imaging and self-report studies in humans, is related to greater craving and then greater seeking [13, 14, 19, 28, 41, 42]. Incentive-sensitization theory posits repeated intake results in an increased incentive salience for drugs of abuse, which also contributes to loss of control (Fig. 7.1) [13, 14, 41].

Motivation to obtain a rewarding substance is mediated by DA release into the dorsal striatum in response to drug cues [16, 34], with increased release of DA into the striatum in response to drug cues associated with greater drug-seeking [15, 16, 34]). Furthermore, glutamate release into dorsal and ventral striatum from projections from the PFC into the dorsal and ventral striatum "frontostriatal circuits" (Fig. 7.2b) (specifically their binding to AMPA receptors [15]) works in concert with cue-related DA release to drive further drug-seeking behavior [16, 17, 34]. Opioids, via their effects in the NAc, VTA, and extended amygdala, also likely play a role in motivation, with several studies showing that naltrexone blocks the brain's response to alcohol cues and craving for future use, mediating relapse prevention [27]. These exert their effects through binding in the striatum, VTA, and extended amygdala.

A significant amount of our understanding of the neurobiology of motivation is due in large part to animal studies in which animals are trained to engage in a behavior to procure a substance and then trained that the substance is no longer available (extinguished), so drug-seeking behaviors disappear. Then, the behavior (as measured through self-administration, a return to environments where drugs were previously used as a conditioned place preference, or working hard on a task that previously produced a drug) is "reinstated" by presentation of numerous amounts of possible cues including drug cue (something that reminds the person of prior use, such as a context, a visual cue, a sound, a smell), stress (which we will discuss below more in the negative reinforcement section), and the drug itself (e.g., re-experiencing the cocaine use feeling will trigger intense drug use seeking and a binge). These reinstatement paradigms model these types of triggered relapse [9].

Neuroimaging studies in humans also support many of these theories, with hundreds of trials now showing brain activation in regions, such as the dorsal and ventral striatum, PFC, amygdala, insula, and visual cortex to drug cues, being linked to craving, development, and persistence of the disorder [1, 10, 27, 32–37, 39–46]. These drug-cue-related neuroimaging findings relate directly to studies showing cognitive biases (approach, attentional, and affective [28]) to drug cues in SUD and their ability to affect drug-seeking behavior. With repeated use, drug cues become more and more powerful in their ability to divert attention of the brain and motivational systems towards them, leading both consciously and unconsciously to craving and use of a drug [1, 47].

The chronicity of conditioning effects from substances are evident in both animal and human studies, as evidenced by relapse and the ability of drug-related cues to trigger engagement in compulsive drug-seeking behavior in long-term abstinent individuals with SUD [48]. That being said, there is good news here, too. Extinction processes, either through nutritional support, therapy, or simple abstinence, can train the brain to not respond to the cues so it becomes second nature over time. In fact, abstinence results in brain growth, and brain volume can begin to normalize even after 1 month of sobriety [10]. Ask anyone in recovery from SUD who will tell you that the more time sober reduces craving and leads to an increased ease resisting temptation to use [10].

7.6 Tolerance: Downregulation of Dopamine and Opioid System

As use progresses, the individual will experience less pleasure from the food ("liking") but will simultaneously experience an increased desire ("wanting") for the food, driving further reward seeking and consumption [13, 14, 28, 41]. Recall "tolerance" is the experience that individuals with SUD face where the more they use the drug, the more they need to achieve the same rewarding effect. Downregulation of DA and opioid systems mediates this effect, with studies showing progressively less release of DA and opioids to the drug of abuse [49], and reductions in presynaptic DA synthesis capacity, and DA receptor density [which could be types 1, 2, or 3 receptors (D1, D2, D3)] in the striatum [5, 22, 23, 28, 50–52]. These changes are also associated with a reduction in the subjective pleasure experienced with use of the drug and trouble experiencing reward from normal activities [15, 16, 34, 53], which also may increase motivation to continue using and may contribute to loss of control in a desperate attempt to experience pleasure again (Fig. 7.1) [15, 16, 34].

7.7 Withdrawal and Hyperkatifeia

Withdrawal is induced by sudden cessation of chronic drug use and is usually characterized by signs and symptoms that are subjectively opposite to the acute positively perceived effects of the drug [6–8]. Hyperkatifeia is defined as an increase in intensity of the constellation of negative emotional or motivational signs and symptoms of withdrawal from drugs of abuse [6–8]. Excessive use of any substance of abuse leads to brain changes, such that upon substance cessation, the individual begins to enter into a state of intense dysphoria, associated with irritability, emotional and physical pain, malaise, sleep disturbances, anxiety, hypohedonia and elevated craving for drug use, as well as various other physical symptoms [2]. Withdrawal occurs in the early days of drug cessation; but also "protracted withdrawal," which is associated with dysphoria lasting for weeks to months and heightened vulnerability to craving and relapse, especially under stress for example, can mimic the withdrawal state [6–8, 46].

The withdrawal state is mediated by changes in several neurotransmitters and neural systems including brain glucocorticoid, corticotrophin-releasing factor, and noradrenergic activity in the limbic and emotional regions such as the extended amygdala and locus coeruleus [2, 6–8, 45]. Opioids also play an important role in these experiences and associated behaviors via their actions in the VTA, NAc, and extended amygdala [2]. Other neurotransmitter systems, including dynorphin, vasopressin, hypocretin, and substance P, and neuroimmune systems are also recruited by excessive alcohol consumption and drug use, producing aversive or stress-like states, also contributing to hyperkatifeia [6–8].

7.8 Conditioning and Motivation: Negative Reinforcement

The learned behavior to engage in an action to relieve physical or psychological discomfort is referred to as negative reinforcement [2]. Alcohol and other substances can initially dampen stress-related brain function and reduce emotional discomfort, which can contribute to learning to continue to use the drug to relieve negative affect (Fig. 7.1) [7, 8]. Neuroadaptations subsequently lead to the need for escalating doses to have the same relieving effect, and then repeated withdrawals lead to even more emotional discomfort when the drug wears off [6–8].

Because stress and negative affect states are so similar to the experience of withdrawal, drug-seeking is triggered by stress, depression, or anxiety, for example [3]. Emotional dysregulation, inefficient utilization of emotion regulation strategies, and a tendency towards dysphoric affect states have been noted as predictors for SUD that can make recovery more challenging [46, 54]. Although hyperkatifeia is most likely to manifest during the withdrawal/negative affect stage, it can also infiltrate other stages of the addiction cycle to promote or facilitate craving, a more rapid progression to loss of control and relapse [6–8].

It is believed by many experts that the negative reinforcement conditioning is as equally important as the positive in the development of addiction. For example, one study found that positive reinforcement that was associated with alcohol consumption did not differ as a function of the presence of alcohol dependence, but negative reinforcement behavior that was associated with alcohol consumption became stronger as alcohol dependence developed [6–8, 55]. However, like we see with positive reinforcement, extinction processes can also occur, making stress and negative affect less likely to trigger drug-seeking the more time someone has been sober [10].

7.9 Impulsivity and Executive Function Deficits

Lastly, but not least importantly, overuse of substances both causes and contributes to and results from impaired global impulse control, which can make it impossible to stay with a commitment to not use in the face of a strong craving, for example [1, 10, 28, 29, 34, 56–58]. In addition to driving reward-seeking behavior, frontostriatal circuits are also involved in processes of impulse control and inhibition of habitual responses [59], with DLPFC, dorsal ACC, parietal cortex and lateral OFC playing important roles [10, 17]. The hippocampus (and related learning and memory systems) also plays a role in cognitive, inhibitory control mechanisms and decision-making [60].

Deficiencies in functioning in these circuits and behavioral domains have been demonstrated time and again in numerous animal studies and in humans in many neuroimaging and neuropsychological testing studies in SUD models [10, 46, 61]. In humans, this commonly manifests in fMRI studies as reduced activation in circuits (PFC) involved in cognitive control during tasks requiring these brain functions [10, 11]. Moreover, as mentioned above, positron emission topography (PET) imaging studies show lower striatal D2 receptor availability in people with SUD, which is also believed to underlie some of the deficits in impulse control [16, 22, 23, 51, 52]. The DA system is well understood to play an important role in inhibitory control [28, 29], as well as in the ability to delay rewards [57, 58], whereas increased receptor availability may be protective against development of addictive behavior [28, 62]. It appears that D2 receptor availability might have a direct impact on prefrontal function, as demonstrated in studies showing that low D2 receptor density is associated with reduced prefrontal perfusion in cocaine use disorders [22, 63]. Additionally, studies show that an intensive exercise regimen reduces impulsivity and increases D2 and D3 receptor density (45), further supporting the importance of D2 receptor density in impulse control.

The combination of impaired impulse control and strong negative reinforcement conditioning is also posited to underlie the negative urgency trait (as discussed in Chap. 6), a trait which is also strongly associated with SUD [7, 8].

7.10 Benefits of Understanding the Neurobiology

Our rapid advancement in understanding the brain chemistry of SUD in the last several decades has significantly impacted and improved our ability to treat them over the last several years. For example, by understanding that SUDs are chronic, relapsing disorders, driven by long-standing brain changes, we now treat people with relapse prevention treatments, including medication, in some cases for years, instead of only using medications for days to reduce withdrawal, as we had done in the past. We also now know that preventing exposure to the substance of abuse reduces conditioned learning and enhances extinction, which may explain why abstinence is so important for some people and for some substances. Behavioral and pharmacologic interventions to target negative affect, impulsivity, cue reactivity, DA receptor density, and neuroinflammation are of growing interest to researchers and clinicians because of our deepening understanding of the underlying neuroscience. Furthermore, it has led to a reduction in stigma regarding addiction, with a greater appreciation that addiction is a disease just like cancer or diabetes, and not a fault in someone's willpower, nor a sign of character flaw or weakness. If similar circuitry drives food seeking, as the growing literature indicates, similar benefits might be observed to take place in the binge eating disorder, food addiction, and obesity treatment fields.

7.11 Conclusion

In conclusion, neurobiological processes exacerbated by conditioned learning play a role in the manifestation of SUD. These concepts provide insight to improve the treatment of SUD and disordered eating.

References

1. Carter A, Hendrikse J, Lee N, Yucel M, Verdejo-Garcia A, Andrews ZB, et al. The neurobiology of "food addiction" and its implications for obesity treatment and policy. Annu Rev Nutr. 2016;36:105–28.
2. Wise RA, Koob GF. The development and maintenance of drug addiction. Neuropsychopharmacology. 2014;39(2):254–62.
3. Jeynes KD, Gibson EL. The importance of nutrition in aiding recovery from substance use disorders: a review. Drug Alcohol Depend. 2017;179:229–39.
4. Kirsch I, Lynn SJ, Vigorito M, Miller RR. The role of cognition in classical and operant conditioning. J Clin Psychol. 2004;60(4):369–92.
5. Volkow ND, Wang GJ, Tomasi D, Baler RD. Obesity and addiction: neurobiological overlaps. Obes Rev. 2013;14(1):2–18.
6. Koob GF, Le Moal M. Review. Neurobiological mechanisms for opponent motivational processes in addiction. Philos Trans R Soc Lond Ser B Biol Sci. 2008;363(1507):3113–23.
7. Koob GF. Neurobiology of opioid addiction: opponent process, Hyperkatifeia, and negative reinforcement. Biol Psychiatry. 2020;87(1):44–53.
8. Koob GF, Powell P, White A. Addiction as a coping response: Hyperkatifeia, deaths of despair, and COVID-19. Am J Psychiatry. 2020;177(11):1031–7.
9. Bossert JM, Marchant NJ, Calu DJ, Shaham Y. The reinstatement model of drug relapse: recent neurobiological findings, emerging research topics, and translational research. Psychopharmacology. 2013;229(3):453–76.
10. Wilcox CE, Dekonenko CJ, Mayer AR, Bogenschutz MP, Turner JA. Cognitive control in alcohol use disorder: deficits and clinical relevance. Rev Neurosci. 2014:1–24.
11. Wilcox CE, Pommy JM, Adinoff B. Neural circuitry of impaired emotion regulation in substance use disorders. Am J Psychiatr. 2016;173:344.
12. Bond CW, Trinko R, Foscue E, Furman K, Groman SM, Taylor JR, et al. Medial nucleus Accumbens projections to the ventral tegmental area control food consumption. J Neurosci. 2020;40(24):4727–38.
13. Morales I, Berridge KC. 'Liking' and 'wanting' in eating and food reward: brain mechanisms and clinical implications. Physiol Behav. 2020;227:113152.
14. Robinson MJ, Fischer AM, Ahuja A, Lesser EN, Maniates H. Roles of "wanting" and "liking" in motivating behavior: gambling, food, and drug addictions. Curr Top Behav Neurosci. 2016;27:105–36.
15. Novelle MG, Dieguez C. Food addiction and binge eating: lessons learned from animal models. Nutrients. 2018;10(1):71.
16. Val-Laillet D, Aarts E, Weber B, Ferrari M, Quaresima V, Stoeckel LE, et al. Neuroimaging and neuromodulation approaches to study eating behavior and prevent and treat eating disorders and obesity. NeuroImage Clin. 2015;8:1–31.
17. Onaolapo AY, Onaolapo OJ. Food additives, food and the concept of 'food addiction': is stimulation of the brain reward circuit by food sufficient to trigger addiction? Pathophysiology. 2018;25(4):263–76.
18. Seabrook LT, Borgland SL. The orbitofrontal cortex, food intake and obesity. J Psychiatry Neurosci. 2020;45(5):304–12.
19. Gordon EL, Lent MR, Merlo LJ. The effect of food composition and behavior on neurobiological response to food: a review of recent research. Curr Nutr Rep. 2020;9(2):75–82.
20. Vanderschuren LJ, Di Ciano P, Everitt BJ. Involvement of the dorsal striatum in cue-controlled cocaine seeking. J Neurosci. 2005;25(38):8665–70.
21. Yager LM, Garcia AF, Wunsch AM, Ferguson SM. The ins and outs of the striatum: role in drug addiction. Neuroscience. 2015;301:529–41.
22. Volkow ND, Wang GJ, Fowler JS, Tomasi D, Telang F. Addiction: beyond dopamine reward circuitry. Proc Natl Acad Sci U S A. 2011;108(37):15037–42.
23. Wang GJ, Volkow ND, Thanos PK, Fowler JS. Imaging of brain dopamine pathways: implications for understanding obesity. J Addict Med. 2009;3(1):8–18.
24. Avena NM, Rada P, Hoebel BG. Evidence for sugar addiction: behavioral and neurochemical effects of intermittent, excessive sugar intake. Neurosci Biobehav Rev. 2008;32(1):20–39.
25. Colantuoni C, Rada P, McCarthy J, Patten C, Avena NM, Chadeayne A, et al. Evidence that intermittent, excessive sugar intake causes endogenous opioid dependence. Obes Res. 2002;10(6):478–88.
26. Colantuoni C, Schwenker J, McCarthy J, Rada P, Ladenheim B, Cadet JL, et al. Excessive sugar intake alters binding to dopamine and mu-opioid receptors in the brain. Neuroreport. 2001;12(16):3549–52.
27. Gearhardt AN, Corbin WR, Brownell KD. Preliminary validation of the Yale Food Addiction Scale. Appetite. 2009;52(2):430–6.
28. Adams RC, Sedgmond J, Maizey L, Chambers CD, Lawrence NS. Food addiction: implications for the diagnosis and treatment of overeating. Nutrients. 2019;11(9):2086.
29. Jentsch JD, Pennington ZT. Reward, interrupted: inhibitory control and its relevance to addictions. Neuropharmacology. 2014;76 Pt B:479–86.
30. Onaolapo AY, Onaolapo OJ. Food additives, food and the concept of 'food addiction': is stimulation of

the brain reward circuit by food sufficient to trigger addiction? Pathophysiology. 2018;25(4):263–76.

31. Peng XQ, Ashby CR Jr, Spiller K, Li X, Li J, Thomasson N, Millan MJ, Mocaër E, Muńoz C, Gardner EL, Xi ZX. The preferential dopamine D3 receptor antagonist S33138 inhibits cocaine reward and cocaine-triggered relapse to drug-seeking behavior in rats. Neuropharmacology. 2009;56(4):752–60.
32. Hernandez J, Perez L, Soto R, Le N, Gastelum C, Wagner EJ. Nociceptin/orphanin FQ neurons in the arcuate nucleus and ventral tegmental area act via Nociceptin opioid peptide receptor signaling to inhibit proopiomelanocortin and A10 dopamine neurons and thereby modulate ingestion of palatable food. Physiol Behav. 2021;228:113183.
33. Hyman SE, et al. Neural mechanisms of addiction: The role of reward-related learning and memory. Annu Rev Neurosci. 2006;29:565.
34. Morin JP, Rodriguez-Duran LF, Guzman-Ramos K, Perez-Cruz C, Ferreira G, Diaz-Cintra S, et al. Palatable hyper-caloric foods impact on neuronal plasticity. Front Behav Neurosci. 2017;11:19.
35. Citri A, Malenka RC. Synaptic plasticity: multiple forms, functions, and mechanisms. Neuropsychopharmacology. 2008;33(1):18–41.
36. Sehgal M, Song C, Ehlers VL, Moyer JR Jr. Learning to learn - intrinsic plasticity as a metaplasticity mechanism for memory formation. Neurobiol Learn Mem. 2013;105:186–99.
37. Malenka RC, Bear MF. LTP and LTD: an embarrassment of riches. Neuron. 2004;44(1):5–21.
38. Pérez-Otaño I, Ehlers MD. Homeostatic plasticity and NMDA receptor trafficking. Trends Neurosci. 2005;28(5):229–38.
39. Gibson AS, Keefe KA, Furlong TM. Accelerated habitual learning resulting from L-dopa exposure in rats is prevented by N-acetylcysteine. Pharmacol Biochem Behav. 2020;198:173033.
40. Hadad NA, Knackstedt LA. Addicted to palatable foods: comparing the neurobiology of Bulimia Nervosa to that of drug addiction. Psychopharmacology. 2014;231(9):1897–912.
41. Berridge KC. 'Liking' and 'wanting' food rewards: brain substrates and roles in eating disorders. Physiol Behav. 2009;97(5):537–50.
42. Sinha R, Jastreboff AM. Stress as a common risk factor for obesity and addiction. Biol Psychiatry. 2013;73(9):827–35.
43. Hone-Blanchet A, Fecteau S. Overlap of food addiction and substance use disorders definitions: analysis of animal and human studies. Neuropharmacology. 2014;85:81–90.
44. Gordon EL, Ariel-Donges AH, Bauman V, Merlo LJ. What is the evidence for "food addiction?" a systematic review. Nutrients. 2018;10(4):477.
45. Sinha R. Role of addiction and stress neurobiology on food intake and obesity. Biol Psychol. 2018;131:5–13.
46. Bogusz K, Kopera M, Jakubczyk A, Trucco EM, Kucharska K, Walenda A, et al. Prevalence of alcohol use disorder among individuals who binge eat: a systematic review and meta-analysis. Addiction. 2021;116(1):18–31.
47. Wiers CE, Zhao J, Manza P, Murani K, Ramirez V, Zehra A, et al. Conscious and unconscious brain responses to food and cocaine cues. Brain Imaging Behav. 2021;15(1):311–9.
48. Chen J, Wang F, Zhu J, Li Y, Liu W, Xue J, Shi H, Li W, Li Q, Wang W. Assessing effect of long-term abstinence on coupling of three core brain networks in male heroin addicts: a resting-state functional magnetic resonance imaging study. Addict Biol. 2020;3:e12982.
49. Tobore TO. Towards a comprehensive theory of obesity and a healthy diet: the causal role of oxidative stress in food addiction and obesity. Behav Brain Res. 2020;384:112560.
50. Blum K, Braverman ER, Holder JM, Lubar JF, Monastra VJ, Miller D, et al. Reward deficiency syndrome: a biogenetic model for the diagnosis and treatment of impulsive, addictive, and compulsive behaviors. J Psychoactive Drugs. 2000;32 Suppl:i-iv:1–112.
51. Wilcox CE, Braskie MN, Kluth JT, Jagust WJ. Overeating behavior and striatal dopamine with 6-[F]-Fluoro-L-m-Tyrosine PET. J Obes. 2010;2010:909348.
52. Robertson CL, Ishibashi K, Chudzynski J, Mooney LJ, Rawson RA, Dolezal BA, et al. Effect of exercise training on striatal Dopamine D2/D3 receptors in methamphetamine users during behavioral treatment. Neuropsychopharmacology. 2016;41(6):1629–36.
53. Jimenez-Murcia S, Aguera Z, Paslakis G, Munguia L, Granero R, Sanchez-Gonzalez J, et al. Food addiction in eating disorders and obesity: analysis of clusters and implications for treatment. Nutrients. 2019;11(11):2633.
54. Koob GF. The dark side of emotion: the addiction perspective. Eur J Pharmacol. 2015;753:73–87.
55. Cho SB, Su J, Kuo SI, Bucholz KK, Chan G, Edenberg HJ, et al. Positive and negative reinforcement are differentially associated with alcohol consumption as a function of alcohol dependence. Psychol Addict Behav. 2019;33(1):58–68.
56. Wiss DA, Criscitelli K, Gold M, Avena N. Preclinical evidence for the addiction potential of highly palatable foods: current developments related to maternal influence. Appetite. 2017;15:19–27.
57. Trifilieff P, Martinez D. Blunted dopamine release as a biomarker for vulnerability for substance use disorders. Biol Psychiatry. 2014;76(1):4–5.
58. Trifilieff P, Martinez D. Imaging addiction: D2 receptors and dopamine signaling in the striatum as biomarkers for impulsivity. Neuropharmacology. 2014;76 Pt B:498–509.
59. Wiss D, Brewerton T. Separating the signal from the noise: how psychiatric diagnoses can help discern food addiction from dietary restraint. Nutrients. 2020;12(10):2937.
60. Clasen MM, Riley AL, Davidson TL. Hippocampal-dependent inhibitory learning and memory processes

in the control of eating and drug taking. Curr Pharm Des. 2020;26(20):2334–52.
61. Fritz M, Klawonn AM, Zahr NM. Neuroimaging in alcohol use disorder: from mouse to man. J Neurosci Res. 2019.
62. Volkow ND, et al. High levels of dopamine D-2 receptors in unaffected members of alcoholic families - Possible protective factors. Arch Gen Psychiatry. 2006;63:999.
63. Domingo-Rodriguez L, Ruiz de Azua I, Dominguez E, Senabre E, Serra I, Kummer S, et al. A specific prelimbic-nucleus accumbens pathway controls resilience versus vulnerability to food addiction. Nat Commun. 2020;11(1):782.

Neurobiology and Cognitive Neuroscience of Hedonic Eating

8

8.1 Reward and Hedonic Liking

As occurs with drugs and alcohol, foods that are rich in both sugar and fat stimulate excessive eating in rodent models and produce pleasure and euphoria [1, 2]. This corresponds to the "like" component of the incentive salience model (Chap. 7) [2, 3].

Intake of these foods also stimulates the brain reward system in similar ways as do alcohol and drugs of abuse [1, 4–11]. For one, HP food causes potent release of dopamine (DA) into the nucleus accumbens (NAc; recall this structure resides in the ventral striatum) and basolateral amygdala (BLA) from neurons whose cell bodies reside in the ventral tegmental area (VTA) [1, 2, 4, 12–25]. Further support for above is highlighted in a review article comparing animal models of SUD and bulimia nervosa, which reports consistent palatable food-related increases in extracellular DA, type 1 dopamine receptor (D1) binding, and DA synthesis in both groups of disorders [26, 27]. Furthermore, there is evidence that neuronal projections from the NAc projecting to the VTA also regulate food intake [22] (Fig. 8.1).

Like with drugs of abuse, studies show that greater release of DA in ventral striatal brain areas to food intake, correlates with self-reported pleasantness and perceived value of food [1, 29, 30]. People with obesity report greater pleasure with tasty meals than those with normal weight [2, 3], and the more rewarding the food is evaluated to be, the greater the release of extracellular DA in the NAc [24]. As is observed in drug use disorders, overeating disorders and obesity are associated with elevated preference for sweet and fat foods, and heightened reward sensitivity [4, 13], which is partially mediated by greater DA release to reward [31]. Like in SUD, DA also plays a role in modulating food-seeking behavior which may in part result from its effects on palatability. For example, the DA release to HP food leads to further overconsumption, as seen in a study in an animal model of Parkinsonism which showed that DA drives binge-like consumption palatable food [32]. Recall that DA also plays a very important role in the strength of downstream conditioning effects [33], which will be discussed below.

The endogenous opioid system has also been implicated in hedonic liking for palatable and calorically dense food [4, 21, 34], like is seen with alcohol and drugs of abuse. Palatable foods robustly stimulate endogenous opioid release [4, 23, 24, 35, 36], in addition to DA, causing widespread activation of μ-opioid receptors in the VTA, NAc, and other brain regions [4–6, 9, 10, 24, 37]. Opioid peptide release in the VTA further modulates DA function, often stimulating DA release into the ventral striatum [2, 38, 39], as well.

Like with DA, endogenous opioid release mediates hedonic liking and triggers binge eating. Systemic or intra-NAc administration of

C. E. Wilcox, *Food Addiction, Obesity, and Disorders of Overeating*,
https://doi.org/10.1007/978-3-030-83078-6_8

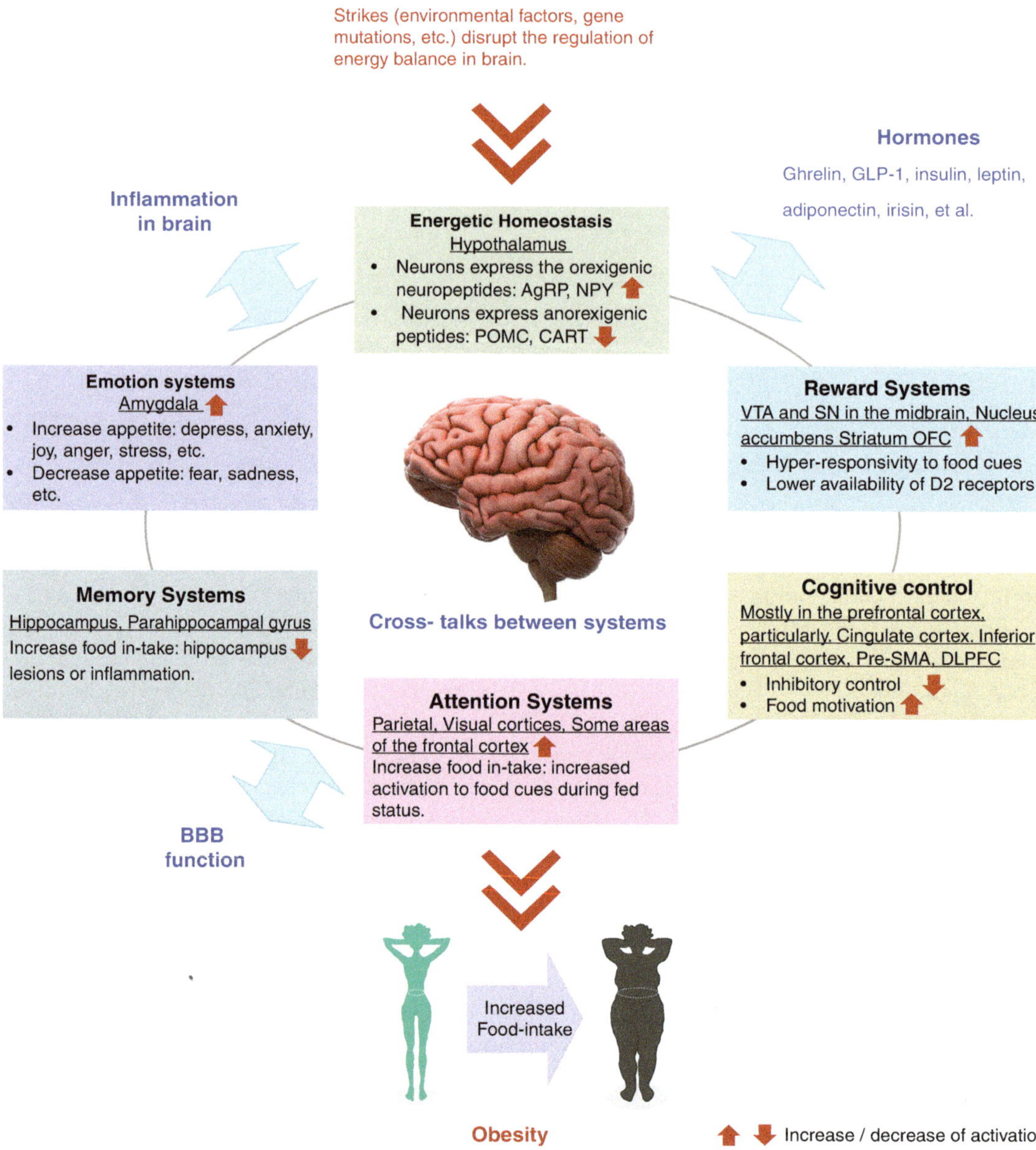

Fig. 8.1 Brain regulation of eating. Brain regulation of eating involves almost all of the neural systems and is influenced by inflammation in the brain, hormones, and blood-brain barrier (BBB) functions. Strikes from the environmental or gene mutations disrupt the normal regulation of energy balance in the brain, and result in obesity. AgRP agouti-related peptide, CART cocaine and amphetamineregulated transcript, D2 receptors dopamine 2 receptors, DLPFC dorsolateral prefrontal cortex, GLP-1 glucagon-like peptide-1, NPY neuropeptide Y, OFC orbitofrontal cortex, POMC proopiomelanocortin, pre-SMA pre-supplementary motor area, SN substantia nigra, VTA ventral tegmental area. (Reproduced from Ref. [28])

μ-opioid agonists increases the consumption of fats, high sucrose foods, binge eating, and other "liking" reactions [2, 4, 34, 40–42]. These hedonic effects are blocked by μ-opioid antagonists like naltrexone, in animals [34, 40]. These effects are also blocked in humans; for example, GSK1521498, another μ-opioid antagonist, reduced hedonic preferences for high-calorific foods and reduced calorific intake [23, 35, 43] in binge eating, obese people. Naloxone [24, 37,

41] and naltrexone [4] have also been found to reduce consumption and preference for sweet high-fat foods in both normal weight and obese binge eaters as well, but effects are too weak for routine clinical use. Opiate-like effects of sugar on gene expression in reward areas of the rat brain has also been observed [4].

In human neuroimaging studies, food consumption also activates the brain [1, 25] in a similar manner as drugs of abuse [12, 16, 17, 20, 44, 45]. For example, high calorie drinks were found to activate orbitofrontal cortex (OFC) and inferior frontal gyrus [both parts of the prefrontal cortex (PFC)] as well as temporal and frontal parietal regions to a greater degree than low-calorie drinks in an adolescent sample [46, 47]. In other work, chocolate milkshake tasting produced activation in the right middle and inferior frontal gyri (also PFC) and insula [47, 48].

Neuroimaging studies in humans also show that reward-related activation is more extensive and robust in those with overeating tendencies than in others [12, 25, 47]. For example, greater activation in ventral striatum and insular cortex to HP food was found to correlate with greater intake of high-fat/high-sugar snacks [47, 49], and greater blood oxygen-dependent (BOLD) responses [measured with functional MRI scanning (fMRI)] to high-calorie beverages in the NAc and amygdala was measured in adolescents with greater body mass index (BMI) [46, 47]. Response to taste stimuli was also found to be stronger in insula, anterior cingulate cortex (ACC), OFC, amygdala, NAc, and dorsal striatum in obese individuals compared to controls [50, 51]. Relatedly greater perfusion [measured with positron emission tomography scanning (PET)] in the ventral striatum to fructose was also observed in those with obesity compared to controls [47, 52, 53], while greater activation in the amygdala, insula, paracingulate gyrus (PFC), and putamen to sucrose was observed in obese children compared to non-obese children [47, 54, 55]. Finally, similar patterns are seen in people with binge eating disorder (BED), with neuroimaging studies showing greater activation in posterior cingulate cortex, and medial OFC in individuals with binge eating-related disorders during a food reward task [47, 56, 57].

Regarding food addiction (FA) scores in particular, heightened ACC reactivity to milkshake has been found to correlate with higher FA scores [17, 47]. Also, enhanced activation of dorsolateral PFC and caudate (but reduced activation in lateral OFC, an area associated with both decision-making and integration of sensory information) [57] was observed in individuals with higher Yale Food Addiction Scale (YFAS) scores compared to controls [17, 41].

Early work indicates that the degree of brain reactivity to the taste or consumption of HP foods may also have predictive value, from a clinical perspective. For example, variability in NAc response over hungry versus sated or fixed meal versus ad libitum eating sessions to HP food intake not only relates to higher variance in food intake and glucose levels to food intake but also predicts higher BMI 1 year later [47, 58].

Likely related to their reward value, HP foods also activate brain regions specifically involved in gustation and taste. For example, sugar versus Truvia consumption was found to be associated with greater nucleus tractus solitarius activation (a brain region that receives visceral input and controls homeostasis) [47]. Obese participants have also demonstrated increased resting and HP food induced activity in gustatory and somatosensory regions [13, 59, 60], suggesting a heightened sensitivity to palatable food, even in non-reward-related homeostatic pathways. Similarly, the hypothalamus (the primary structure involved in homeostatic eating) is recruited with food reward, with one study showing greater perfusion [measured with positron emission tomography scanning (PET)] glucose administration in those with obesity compared to controls [47, 52, 53].

8.2 Conditioning: Positive Reinforcement

Recall that conditioning is a key component of the addictive process. During conditioning, which is a learning-process, the brain increasingly comes to associate cues or emotional experiences with use of a drug. As a result of these brain changes, the behavior of drug use becomes more and more habitual and compulsive, and drug related sensory cues can more rapidly trigger drug seeking behavior (Chap. 7). Conditioning through positive reinforcement occurs with palatable food in the same way as it does with drugs of abuse, especially with sucrose [1, 4, 12, 19, 41, 61, 62]. For example, rats with limited access to a sucrose diet show a progressive escalation in their response to the diet and develop excessive food intake within a short period of time [1, 63]. Like with drugs of abuse, animals also develop conditioned place preference to sucrose (meaning they choose to be in places where they are more likely to receive sucrose), indicating rapid development of conditioning and a variety of other increased food-seeking behaviors [1, 13, 24, 63–66]. In one study, chocolate induced a persistent conditioned place preference response similar in magnitude to that observed for drugs in monkeys [41, 61] which persisted for at least 15 days. Even humans show conditioning effects – people who reported craving carbohydrates endorsed increased "liking" for a pure carbohydrate beverage over time, compared to a control high-protein beverage, indicating conditioning [41].

As discussed in Chap. 7, conditioning occurs through long-term potentiation (LTP) and long-term depression (LTD) induced by HP food, like substances of abuse [2, 3, 67]. LTP is dependent on both DA and glutamate release into the striatum [1, 12, 26, 29], like with drugs of abuse, which occurs with HP food consumption. Elevated initial reward responsiveness to food and associated DA may predispose individuals to develop a future tendency to overeat [29], which is likely, in part, because of the role that DA plays in the conditioning process, driving more intense learning to respond to drug-related sensory cues.

Binge eating can also cause positive reinforcement learning via its effect on the DA system [68]. A history of sugar bingeing and deprivation results in decreased DA levels in the NAc following fasting and then enhanced release upon consumption of sweet food [26]. It is surmised that the degree of change in DA release from the deprived state to the stimulated one results in a more powerful chemical conditioning effect [1, 10, 26]. Repeated intake of foods that are high in sugar results in increased D1 receptor binding (in the shell and core of the NA) changes which are similar to those associated with a number of drugs of abuse [1, 10, 26].

8.3 Motivation: Positive Reinforcement

Like in SUD, the experience of "want" has also been described in the context of the incentive salience model for palatable food consumption [2, 6, 69]; increased "wanting" results from conditioning as we discussed in the previous section. Conditioned palatable food cues (which can be olfactory, visual, taste, sounds, etc. [1, 12, 34, 68, 70, 71]) trigger craving for the food which then causes greater motivation to seek and consume it, often regardless of the cost. Recall that motivation can either be to procure something rewarding (reward motivation or positive reinforcement) or to get rid of something negative (like a negative affective state, referred to as "relief motivation" or "negative reinforcement" which will be discussed below) [2, 8, 68]. The conditioned properties of HP food cues and contexts are similar to those of drugs, with their heightened incentive salience promoting drug- and food-seeking behavior [3, 72], in a manner that overrides homeostatic feeding mechanisms and leads an animal or human to eat beyond their energy needs [73].

This process of positive reinforcement has an important clinical role in disorders associated with overeating or binge eating. For example, the intensity of craving induced by HP food cues is heightened among those with elevated BMI [13, 74–76] and in obese individuals [34, 77]. Furthermore, the degree of cue-induced craving also predicts later energy intake and weight gain in clinical populations, in one study accounting for approximately 11% of the variance in these outcomes [13, 78]. Interestingly, women have greater food cue reactivity compared to men [1]. Indeed most flavor preferences are learned [1]: just one taste can trigger a binge (the taste of the food itself being a powerful conditioned cue for some individuals).

Like is seen in SUD, conditioned cue responding is also driven by processes involving DA [34, 77] and glutamate [12, 68, 70], with dorsal striatum and frontostriatal pathways playing a particularly important role [12, 29]. First of all, increased DA transmission into dorsal striatum with exposure to HP food cues drives concomitant increases in motivation to procure food [68, 79, 80]. This is demonstrated through numerous studies. For example, animals with previous exposure to HP food, who showed greater persistence in lever pressing compared to controls, suggesting a habit-based strategy, also showed enhanced activation of the dorsolateral striatum to food cues, and D1 antagonism rescued behavior to the level of controls [81]. Blockade of glutamate AMPA receptors also blocks cue-triggered food seeking in over-motivated rodents to the level of controls [12, 81]. The effects of AMPA blockade on conditioned responding has been replicated in several studies [41, 82] during several paradigms [41]. Furthermore, glutamatergic adaptations in the NAc following a history of binge eating prime the postsynaptic neurons in this region to respond more strongly to cues associated with palatable food [26] and to dopamine. Indeed, the glutamate AMPA system might in some cases be more important than the DA system for this particular cue-elicited driven drug- or food-seeking behavior. In one study, as compared to sucrose, the D1 and type 2 dopamine (D2) receptor antagonists were not able to attenuate the fat-conditioned flavor preference [40, 83].

Finally, as is seen in animal models of SUD, the endogenous opioid system also plays an important role in reward-based motivation [4, 34, 40, 41]. Rats conditioned on sugar sweetened pellets no longer responded to a conditioned cue when given an opiate antagonist (naltrexone) [41, 82]. By contrast, intra-NAc administration of μ-opioid agonists increased the consumption of fats in another study, an effect which was also blocked by the administration of naltrexone [34, 40]. Stimulation of μ-opioid receptors in the striatum also promotes the intake of sucrose and repeated intake of foods that are high in sugar results in increased μ-opioid receptor binding in the ACC, hippocampus, NAc shell, and locus coeruleus [1, 10]. Finally, in humans with obesity and binge eating, GSK1521498, a μ-opioid receptor antagonist, reduced responses to high-calorie food images in the putamen, a region in the dorsal striatum, which is, as a reminder, a brain region recognized as central to motivational components of hedonic feeding [23, 35, 41, 84].

Like is observed in individuals with SUD, cue reactivity (e.g., craving, or activation in reward and other brain regions that control motivated behavior) appears to be greater in clinical populations that overeat or binge eat as well. For example, cue-induced craving is heightened in obese individuals relative to controls and in individuals with higher BMIs and those who report binge eating or FA symptoms [1, 13, 29, 30, 34, 59, 60, 68, 79, 80, 85–88]. Cue reactivity is also associated with higher food cravings [41, 73], general hyperphagia [34], and weight gain [6, 13, 68, 89]. For example, one study showed that greater high-fat food cravings and high-fat food choice were associated with greater dorsal ACC activation [47, 90]. Hyperresponsiveness in the lateral OFC, insula, amygdala, frontal operculum, and striatum was seen during anticipation of palatable food [1, 59, 60, 87] and in response to pictures of palatable foods [1, 91] in obese compared to control subjects. In studies using food pictures, women with binge eating displayed hyperresponsivity of the dorsal ACC [47] and ventral striatum [8, 92] compared to controls. In a study that used a food reward task, women with bulimia or BED showed increased food cue-related activity in the PFC and OFC [47, 56] and stronger activation of the ventral striatum in response to food pictures than healthy controls [8, 92]. Finally, individuals with FA or higher YFAS scores demonstrated greater chocolate cake cue reactivity [17, 93] in the hypothalamus, thalamus, midbrain, and putamen (part of the dorsal striatum) [47, 94], and another showed elevated activity in the superior frontal to images of highly processed foods [47, 95]. Self-reported lipid consumption was also found to be correlated with activation in the OFC, temporal gyrus, PFC, and post central gyrus in the high YFAS participants [47, 94]. Other more susceptible states, such as alcohol intoxication and sleep debt, will increase the brain's food cue reactivity as well [96, 97].

As brain reactivity to substance cues predict clinical outcome, so do responses to HP food cues (reviewed in [29]). One example of such a study showed that cue-triggered neural activity in the NAc correlated positively with weight gain during the following 6 months in 48 female college students [51, 98]. A similar study showed that elevated midbrain, thalamus, hypothalamus, and ventral striatum responsivity to milk shake taste also predicted future weight gain [29]. In a third study, elevated dorsal striatum responsivity to palatable food images also showed greater future weight gain, but only in participants who were at genetic risk for higher DA signaling capacity at the D4 receptor by virtue of having a particular TaqIA polymorphism [29, 59, 71, 88]. Finally, a study in obese individuals undergoing a weight loss treatment found that those with greater pretreatment activation in response to high-calorie food vs. control pictures in NAc, insula, ACC, superior occipital cortex, inferior and superior parietal lobule, and PFC were also least successful in losing weight over a 12-week psychosocial treatment program. Furthermore, those who were less successful at maintaining weight loss at 9-month follow-up showed greater posttreatment activation in insula, VTA, putamen, and fusiform gyrus [28, 51, 99].

Further compelling evidence for the clinical importance of brain activation to food cues is indicated by the fact that interventions to reduce weight also reduce brain reactivity [29]. For example, one study showed that activation in the medial PFC to food cues reduced after patients were given recommendations to reduce high-calorie foods with high bulk low-calorie foods [51, 99]. Another study reported a similar effect of an intervention of three meals and two snacks that totaled up to 1600 kcal per day (50% carbohydrates, 30% fats, and 20% proteins) for 3 months [47, 94]; this intervention resolved chocolate cake cue-elicited differences in activation in the hypothalamus, thalamus, midbrain, and putamen between a high YFAS and low YFAS group (e.g., the high YFAS group looked more similar to the low YFAS group after 3 months) [47, 94] and correlations between lipid consumption and activation in the OFC, temporal, prefrontal cortex, and post central gyrus in the high YFAS participants were no longer present [47, 94]. Bariatric surgery as an intervention may have particularly pronounced dampening effects on cue-elicited brain activation, effects which likely outshine those of simple dietary psychosocial ones (Chap. 10).

Like with substances of abuse, conditioning effects from HP food intake are chronic and can lead to relapse months or years into recovery. In one study, just 3 days of a binge/compensate pattern of eating sweetened vegetable shortening still had a significant impact on rats' motivation for sucrose over 1 month later [41]. Relatedly, there is persistence of heightened neural responses to a meal in post-obese individuals many weeks after weight loss [100].

8.4 Food Reward, Conditioning, and Reward Motivation: Additional Factors

There are several additional factors that can influence reward, conditioning and motivation that warrant mention. For one, the presence or absence of binge consumption of food may be especially important for development of conditioning and compulsive use of food, perhaps in a way that is more important than it is for the conditioning effects of drugs and alcohol. For example, rats given intermittent and excessive access to sugar solution increase their intake significantly over time, and this is accompanied by neurochemical changes that are similar to those seen with administration of drugs of abuse [6, 10, 13, 64]. However, when palatable food is administered continuously (as opposed to in binge fashion) in some animal models of obesity, the neurochemical consequences are different, indicating that for FA to develop, binge use might be an especially important component [2]. Whether this is true needs further study, however.

Second, the rapidity of onset of the food's neurochemical effect is important for conditioning to occur and for compulsive use of food to develop. This explains why HP foods in particular are more likely to be addictive than others: foods reported to be more addictive are also more rapidly digested and absorbed, whereas foods high in fiber and protein are generally not considered addictive [12, 18]. This is related to the glucostatic theory, which theorizes that the intensity of sugar spikes after eating and the glycemic index of foods are of high importance in driving food palatability and in upsetting natural satiety mechanisms [101, 102]. Drugs of abuse also show greater "addictiveness" with more rapid onset (which is why smoking a drug leads to more rapid development of out-of-control use than will taking it orally) [103].

Third, whereas most drugs of abuse activate the reward system primarily through direct pharmacological effects [24], pleasurable food activates the brain through indirect mechanisms, which ultimately stimulate DA release into the NAc. Regardless of whether the mechanism is direct or indirect, however, as long as a drug or particular food causes release of DA into the NAc, it can reinforce future consummatory behavior towards itself by causing conditioning [4, 11, 14, 15].

In terms of food (and incidentally alcohol, which operates both directly and indirectly via the hedonic eating system to stimulate dopamine release), there are two primary hedonic components that drive DA release. The first results from sensory signals such as taste, is of rapid onset, and primarily depends on the food's palatability. The second component results from post-prandial ingestion processes (such as glucose blood levels changing in the brain), is of slow onset, and is dependent on the amount of energy consumed, rather than the palatability [1, 11, 12, 14, 15].

Regarding the first component, simply the taste or texture of a food can induce a hedonic response regardless of the homeostatic need for the food [1, 104]: sugar and fat are both sensed by the mouth and have inherent palatability based on taste alone [1, 12, 104], regardless of their effects on blood sugar levels. For example, fat binding to receptors in the mouth triggers intracellular signaling mechanisms mediated by G-proteins which directly activate reward processes via downstream effects on both the VTA and gustatory brain regions [1, 40]. Primary taste pathways go through the thalamus and then terminate in the OFC, insula, and amygdala [1].

Regarding the second component, rodents can learn to identify food as rewarding independently of its taste simply as a result of its caloric value [1, 12, 105]. This is because sugar and fat are sensed by gut chemosensors, and sugar is sensed by chemosensors in post-absorptive sites (like the liver, pancreas, and brain), all of which give positive feedback signals to strengthen innate or preexisting sugar- and fat-conditioned flavor preferences [1]. Indeed, intragastric or intraduodenal infusion (bypassing taste pathways) of sugars can enhance conditioned taste preference for sugar in humans, in part mediated by ghrelin release from the gut and DA release into NAc [12, 105]. Furthermore, activation of reward regions occurs following infusion of glucose or fructose into the brain [1, 4, 93, 106]. These studies demonstrate that the brain is exquisitely sensitive to the effect of energy or its absence [1, 4, 93, 106].

8.5 Tolerance and Downregulation of DA and Opioid Systems

With repeated binges or overeating episodes, tolerance to the rewarding effects of HP food develops (Chap. 6) [3, 107] in a manner that directly parallels that observed in SUD after continued excessive use of a substance. Recall that tolerance is defined as the need to consume more and more food over time to achieve the same pleasurable effect and is part of the diagnostic criteria for FA and SUD. This effect has also been seen in humans (Chap. 6) and has also been observed in several animal models (e.g., rats on daily intermittent sucrose slowly increase their sugar consumption over time) [10, 13, 24, 64]. This tolerance is associated with less and less release of DA and opioids to palatable food and increasingly less and less experience of subjective pleasure [24, 34, 88, 108, 109]. This tolerance effect may also increase motivation to eat palatable foods in an attempt to try to experience more reward, which results in people increasingly choosing higher fat and more sugary foods over healthier options and which may contribute to further loss of control [12, 13, 29, 70, 110]. One interesting illustrative study found that rats fed regularly on a cafeteria-style diet (which is a more inherently palatable diet than normal chow) showed reduced baseline levels of mesolimbic DA activity which were only brought up to normal levels by cafeteria foods, but not their normal chow [13, 110].

Tolerance results from changes in brain DA function. Downregulation in post-synaptic D2 receptor density in the NAc shell and dorsal striatum has also been measured in numerous studies in animals overexposed to high-fat, high-sugar foods [1, 88, 111], or even just a high-fat/low sucrose diet (primarily lard) [41, 112]. This occurs especially when HP food is administered in an intermittent rather than continuous manner [10, 41] but can also be seen in rats that volitionally overate highly palatable foods (bacon, sausage, cheesecake, pound cake, frosting, chocolate) [41, 111]. Sucrose intake lowers dopamine D2/D3 receptor availability in porcine brain as well [113]. Low D2 density and overexposure to these HP foods can lead over time to elevated reward thresholds in some animal models, and these thresholds got higher as the rats gained more weight [41, 111].

Human imaging studies also show lower striatal D2 receptor availability in severely obese individuals compared to controls, and D2 density, especially in striatum, is significantly and negatively correlated with BMI, paralleling numerous studies across a wide variety of drug use disorders showing that more drug use and greater SUD severity is associated with lower D2 and D3 density [13, 24, 26, 29, 37, 109, 113–119] . This low D2 density might be genetic (the Taq1A polymorphism can affect D2 density and is associated with obesity and SUD) or the low D2 density could be caused by downregulation due to overuse of drugs or HP food [120] or both. Several studies have measured lower presynaptic dopamine synthesis capacity in the striatum in human subjects with higher BMIs as well which may contribute to a chronically blunted dopamine release to pleasurable stimuli [117].

The effects of D2 blockade on eating behavior supports theories that lower D2 activity contributes to higher body weight and overeating behavior. The administration of D2 antagonists has been shown to increase meal size, meal duration, and body weight, whereas treatment with D2 agonists can reduce hyperphagia and prevent weight gain in animals [1, 13]. The effects of such pharmaceutical interventions in human studies, however, have been fairly mixed. The use of antipsychotic medication which blocks D2 receptors is indeed typically associated with weight gain [13], and some D2 agonists have been found to reduce body weight [13], but not consistently enough to culminate in development of a therapeutic medication that acts via this mechanism.

In addition to blunted dopamine receptor activity and reduced dopamine release, blunted μ-opioid system functioning is also observed to occur over time. Specifically, blunting in opioid release causes reduced experiences of pleasure to rewards like food [12, 24, 34, 68, 70, 88, 109, 111]. In addition, chronic overexposure to HP food lowers μ-opioid receptor availability, as shown in studies of effects of sucrose on μ-opioid receptor density in porcine brain [113].

How downregulation or hypofunction in the DA system (e.g., reduced presynaptic dopamine synthesis capacity, reduced DA release, low D2 receptor density) and endogenous opioid system (reduced endogenous opioid release, reduced μ-opioid receptor density) causes FA or SUD symptoms to get worse is not clear. However, there are several potential mechanisms. For one, it might cause more negative-reinforcement eating, as indicated by one study which showed that emotional eating (e.g., eating for relief of negative affect) and not external eating (e.g., eating for reward motivations) was related to hypofunctioning dorsal striatal dopamine systems [86, 121]. Second, it may cause a "reward deficiency syndrome" [37, 114, 120]. This would lead to less and less experience of pleasure with reward consumption, as well as higher levels of general dysphoria, both of which would cause further and further consumption of the substance or food to achieve previous levels of reward-related pleasure [13, 114]. This model is supported by animal studies showing that lower D2 density is associated with reward dysfunction and elevated reward thresholds [41, 111]. Third, low D2 density in the striatum is also likely linked to impaired impulse control (discussed below).

Despite the growing evidence that low D2 receptor density is linked to chronic obesity and other forms of overeating, not all studies have shown this to be true, and the reasons for this are unclear. For example, in one study, rats placed on a 12-week high-fat diet of primarily hydrogenated coconut oil, maltodextrin, sucrose, and casein had significantly higher DeltaFosB (a signaling consequence of DA receptor activation), higher D2 receptor expression, and lower D1 receptor expression in the NAc. These changes were observed before the onset of obesity and were linked to behaviors suggestive of anhedonia [41, 122, 123]. Another study found that rats given a low-fat/high-sucrose diet did not have reduced D2 expression in the NAc [41, 112]. A third study showed that increased D2 receptor expression in the mPFC-NAc pathway, rather than decreased, promoted the compulsive feeding, addiction-like phenotype [31]. More research needs to be done to resolve these discrepancies.

8.6 Withdrawal

Similar to what is seen with drugs of abuse, suddenly reducing or stopping consumption of high amounts of HP food can induce withdrawal symptoms in humans (Chap. 6). This occurs as a result of brain changes induced by repeated overconsumption of HP foods.

Animal studies also show that sudden cessation of sweet food availability (frequency or quantity) after training animals to overuse or binge on it also induces withdrawal-like behavior [2, 6, 11, 12, 18, 21, 34, 40, 68, 70, 111]. Indeed, the behaviors observed in these animal studies are eerily similar to the behavior observed during opioid withdrawal: numerous studies report increases in anxiety behavior, teeth chattering, forepaw tremor, head shaking, reduced body temperature, aggression [10, 11, 13, 24, 95], poor appetite [41], greater motivation for sucrose and high-fat foods [41, 122, 123], elevated startle response [41], and impaired performance on a cognitive task testing impulse control [41]. Rats given so-called Western diet (higher in fat and carbohydrates than normal chow) during adolescence had also posttraumatic stress responsivity as adults [12, 116, 124] and anxiety [41, 122, 123] at higher levels. Fat models of bingeing have also been developed but have not had the same features of opiate-like withdrawal [2, 6, 40]; although when animals were deprived of high-fat diet after bingeing, an increased anxiety stress response to higher levels of palatable food-seeking have been observed [2].

Changes in the opioid system are likely to mediate much of the food withdrawal phenomena, with administration of μ-opioid agonists showing reduction in food withdrawal symptoms [11]. Changes in brain stress response systems from overeating and yo-yo dieting also contribute to the food withdrawal syndrome [68]. Indeed like with SUD, the neurochemical effects or mediators of withdrawal look much like those associated with the stress response; excessive HP food consumption over time leads to altered extrahypothalamic corticotrophin-releasing factor activity in the extended amygdala, noradrenergic system and hypothalamic pituitary axis functioning, and altered cortisol release such that upon sudden cessation of high levels of these kinds of food, there is rebound response in all of these systems in the opposite direction [41, 68, 122, 123].

8.7 Conditioning and Motivation: Negative Reinforcement

Recall that negative reinforcement is the learned behavior to engage in an action to relieve physical or psychological pain (Chap. 7). It leads a person or animal to habitually and sometimes even compulsively behave in a manner that has previously provided relief whenever this particular pain is re-experienced [125]. Both HP food and substances of abuse have strongly negative reinforcing properties, as they will quickly and efficiently relieve negative affect, anxiety and dysphoria, dampen stress-related brain function, and reduce emotional discomfort. People who consume drugs for this purpose are often referred to as having relief motivations (as opposed to reward motivations, where people consume the drug for positive reinforcement) [8, 68]. In the case of food, relief motivation is often referred to as "emotional eating" or "stress eating." A major contributor to the negative reinforcement learning comes from an animal or a person's experiences during withdrawal: using a drug or food that they have recently stopped relieves all sorts of negative affective experiences, teaching them that it's a good "go-to" when feeling down (e.g., the drug or food does not have any inherently soothing properties, but the brain is tricked into thinking it does, when it experiences the relief of the effect of its own withdrawal) [12]. Indeed, bingeing on fat-rich foods can alleviate withdrawal from opioids, not just food, showing what a powerful effect these kinds of food can have on brain chemistry linked to negative affective states [4, 24, 126]. Binge or heavy HP food consumption followed by cessation, like is seen in yo-yo dieting, results in adaptations in brain reward pathways that lead to greater and greater intensity of withdrawal and more and more learning that overeating relieves dysphoria, and wanting and craving for foods high in sugar and fat become strongly linked to the avoidance of negative emotional states [2, 68, 69].

Once negative reinforcement learning has occurred, stress and negative affect can easily trigger relapse to hedonic eating in the same way as it can in SUD. Like in SUD, in obesity and BED, HP food consumption is strongly influenced by emotional states [4, 127, 128]. Furthermore, as we have seen in previous chapters (Chap. 6), anxiety, depression, posttraumatic stress disorder, and a history of childhood trauma [116, 129] are risk factors for development of disordered eating. A tendency towards negative affective states, due to heightened stress reactivity or poor use of emotion regulation skills, predict and contribute to obesity and binge eating [8, 130, 131] because it makes food a more powerful negative reinforcer. Inefficient utilization of emotion regulation strategies may increase arousal, negative affect, and craving, which may be followed by more use of food to regulate affect, leading to further negative conditioning, thus fueling a vicious cycle of dependence [8, 130, 131]. One day, this tendency towards emotional eating may be measurable: one study showed that stress-induced reductions in brain activation in several areas (PFC, ACC, amygdala) identified individuals more likely to experience an increase in stress before binge eating [132].

The neurochemical basis of eating for relief of negative affect, or stress or emotional eating, is still being worked out. Indeed, the opioid system, the HPA axis, CRF, and noradrenergic systems, all of which play an important role in withdrawal, may also be responsible for the soothing effect of HP food. For example, bingeing on palatable food by stressed and food-restricted rats was found to be enhanced by μ-opioid agonists [4, 42]. High cortisol levels have been observed in women who engage in more emotional eating [41, 133] and that eating was blocked by naltrexone. However, one interesting study showed that eating in response to negative affect also positively correlated with striatal D2 binding on a PET scan, independent of BMI category (i.e., healthy or obese), suggesting that emotional eating may be related to low D2 functioning [41] as well. Another study showed that emotional eating and not external eating (e.g., cue-driven positive-reinforcement-based eating) were related to the hypo-functioning of dopamine-related reward systems located in the dorsal striatum of the brain [86, 121]. More work needs to be done to understand these mechanisms (and ultimately their treatments) more definitively.

8.8 Impulse Control and Executive Function Deficits

Like is seen with SUD, people with obesity and eating disorders and FA are more likely to have diminished inhibitory control, and executive function deficits, as well as global impulsivity, decision-making deficits around HP food consumption, and loss of control of eating, the latter of which is one of the DSM criteria for FA and BED (Chaps. 6 and 7) [12, 13, 19, 109, 134–136].

Findings from multiple neuroimaging studies have suggested that people with elevated body weight, compulsive or binge eating behaviors, and FA also have evidence of deficient functioning in areas of the brain associated with executive control, inhibition, and self-awareness [47]. For example, one study showed that people with increased BMI and poor food choices also had reductions in frontal gray matter volume and impaired executive functioning [13]. Another study found that greater vegetable intake correlated with greater activity during a decision-making task in the left superior frontal gyrus, while greater intake of high-fat/high-sugar snacks correlated with reduced activity in the left frontal pole (both PFC areas which are important in executive function) in healthy adolescents and young adults [41]. Other works have also found a negative correlation between BMI and activity in PFC [13], including one that reported lower brain activation in another frontal area and thalamus during response inhibition in subjects with obesity and FA compared to controls [40, 137]. Among children with obesity, similar effects were seen with reduced recruitment of several brain regions involved in inhibitory control, including the medial, lateral frontal, and temporal regions, compared to children without obesity [46]. In response to glucose or fructose administration, adolescents with obesity had decreased perfusion during PET scanning in the PFC, whereas adolescents without obesity had the opposite response [53], and also in adolescents, decreased activation of dorsolateral and ventrolateral PFC was also observed in the obese individuals compared to controls when trying to inhibit behavioral responses to high-calorie food images [40, 138]; both studies indicate impaired executive function in the obese adolescent individuals. Furthermore, individuals with BED and/or bulimia also show decreased basal metabolism in PFC on PET scans [29] and decreased activation in lateral PFC circuits and frontostriatal circuits during cognitive tasks [8, 26, 116, 119, 139]. Finally, reduced activation during the inhibitory portion of a Go/No-go task was also observed in the middle temporal gyrus, occipital gyrus, precuneus, and inferior frontal gyrus in adolescents with YFAS-diagnosed FA compared to those without [140].

The association between disordered eating and executive dysfunction/impulsivity is likely bidirectional [13, 141, 142]. In preclinical research, there is growing evidence that excessive consumption of HP food has long-lasting problematic effects on many of the relevant circuits that are involved in cognitive control, inhibitory control, and impulse control [12, 19]. Prenatal periods, childhood, and adolescence may be particularly vulnerable periods, where the effects of dietary environmental insults can lead to large changes in executive control [12, 19]. Furthermore, a large genome-wide association study in humans suggests that higher BMI increases the risk of developing attention deficit hyperactivity disorder (ADHD), a disorder associated with impulsivity and other neurocognitive deficits, but not the other way around [116, 143]. Obesity-promoting HP food-based diets also disrupt memory and learning and cognitive flexibility through affecting hippocampal functioning in a similar manner to drugs of abuse [12, 142]. Negative energy balance for 2 weeks (>1 kg wt loss) resulted in restored hippocampal function in one study [34], indicating that some of these adverse cognitive effects may be reversible.

On the other hand, impaired executive function could also theoretically contribute to greater intake of HP food by causing loss of control. The combination of impaired impulse control plus strong negative reinforcement conditioning is posited to underlie the negative urgency trait (discussed in Chap. 6), which is strongly associated with dysregulated eating of all kinds [144, 145].

Whether people are at a heightened risk of developing obesity, BED or FA due to inhibitory control deficits or executive dysfunction is not yet clear, although studies show that impulsivity as a trait (measured usually through self-report) is predictive of development of loss of control around food [13, 17, 146, 147] (Chap. 6). However, several studies show that impaired inhibitory control, executive function, and related fMRI-based markers of brain function predict greater later binge use of alcohol, for example (e.g., [148]). No doubt as more studies come out in the obesity, BED, and FA realms; they will show similar findings. It is already becoming clear, however, that impaired functioning in inhibitory and cognitive control circuits predicts poorer clinical outcomes in people who already have obesity and disordered eating. For example, greater dorsolateral PFC activation in obese individuals when instructed to "resist craving" predicted better weight loss success following gastric bypass surgery [40]. Furthermore, successful dieting has been found to be positively associated with heightened PFC activation to a meal [13, 149]. Finally, patients who are less successful at losing weight after surgery have shown to have reduced activation of the brain regions involved in inhibition (e.g., PFC) but no significant differences in activation in the reward areas compared with their more successful weight loss counterparts [28, 150].

In addition to hypo-functioning prefrontal circuits, dopamine alterations (such as low D2) especially in dorsal striatum, which we have discussed in the context of reward deficiency and tolerance above, also likely contribute to the patterns of diminished inhibitory control [13, 136] and impulsivity seen in disordered eating and SUD (Chap. 7). For one, higher striatal DA signaling at D2 receptors in animals is associated with greater willingness to expend effort to reach goals [146, 147]. D2 receptor availability in the striatum might have a direct impact on prefrontal function, and studies in obese individuals both reduced D2 receptor density and reduced perfusion of DLPFC and OFC and several other cortical areas [13, 31, 109]. Studies in healthy-weight participants have also demonstrated a positive correlation between striatal dopamine receptor availability and inhibitory control performance on a stop-signal task [13]. Both exercise and gastric bypass surgery result in increased D2/D3 receptor availability [13, 151], which may indicate a mechanism by which these interventions work to improve outcomes; if future studies show that these effects on the DA receptors lead to weight loss via their effects on cognitive control circuits, executive function, or inhibitory control, then we will have more certainty about this [28, 152].

8.9 Conclusion

In conclusion, food consumption is regulated by the hedonic system, and people eat for pleasure and comfort, which are the same motivations people have for using substances of abuse. Excessive use of HP food, in particular, results in changes in brain circuits which mirror those seen in response to drugs of abuse, contributing to the cyclical pattern that leads to the downward spiral of addiction. These brain changes cause the DSM criteria for FA and SUD such as loss of control, withdrawal, tolerance, and craving which were discussed in the clinical sense in Chap. 6.

References

1. Onaolapo AY, Onaolapo OJ. Food additives, food and the concept of 'food addiction': is stimulation of the brain reward circuit by food sufficient to trigger addiction? Pathophysiology. 2018;25(4):263–76.
2. Blanco-Gandia MC, Minarro J, Rodriguez-Arias M. Common neural mechanisms of palatable food intake and drug abuse: knowledge obtained with animal models. Curr Pharm Des. 2020;26(20):2372–84.
3. Berridge KC. 'Liking' and 'wanting' food rewards: brain substrates and roles in eating disorders. Physiol Behav. 2009;97(5):537–50.
4. Jeynes KD, Gibson EL. The importance of nutrition in aiding recovery from substance use disorders: a review. Drug Alcohol Depend. 2017;179:229–39.
5. Leggio L, Addolorato G, Cippitelli A, Jerlhag E, Kampov-Polevoy AB, Swift RM. Role of feeding-related pathways in alcohol dependence: a focus on sweet preference, NPY, and ghrelin. Alcohol Clin Exp Res. 2011;35(2):194–202.
6. Avena NM, Rada P, Hoebel BG. Sugar and fat bingeing have notable differences in addictive-like behavior. J Nutr. 2009;139(3):623–8.
7. Burrows T, Skinner J, McKenna R, Rollo M. Food addiction, binge eating disorder, and obesity: is there a relationship? Behav Sci. 2017;7(3):54.
8. Bogusz K, Kopera M, Jakubczyk A, Trucco EM, Kucharska K, Walenda A, et al. Prevalence of alcohol use disorder among individuals who binge eat: a systematic review and meta-analysis. Addiction. 2021;116(1):18–31.

9. Mysels DJ, Sullivan MA. The relationship between opioid and sugar intake: review of evidence and clinical applications. J Opioid Manag. 2010;6(6):445–52.
10. Colantuoni C, Schwenker J, McCarthy J, Rada P, Ladenheim B, Cadet JL, et al. Excessive sugar intake alters binding to dopamine and mu-opioid receptors in the brain. Neuroreport. 2001;12(16):3549–52.
11. Avena NM, Rada P, Hoebel BG. Evidence for sugar addiction: behavioral and neurochemical effects of intermittent, excessive sugar intake. Neurosci Biobehav Rev. 2008;32(1):20–39.
12. Morin JP, Rodriguez-Duran LF, Guzman-Ramos K, Perez-Cruz C, Ferreira G, Diaz-Cintra S, et al. Palatable hyper-caloric foods impact on neuronal plasticity. Front Behav Neurosci. 2017;11:19.
13. Adams RC, Sedgmond J, Maizey L, Chambers CD, Lawrence NS. Food addiction: implications for the diagnosis and treatment of overeating. Nutrients. 2019;11(9):2086.
14. Avena NM, Bocarsly ME, Hoebel BG. Animal models of sugar and fat bingeing: relationship to food addiction and increased body weight. Methods Mol Biol. 2012;829:351–65.
15. Avena NM, Gold JA, Kroll C, Gold MS. Further developments in the neurobiology of food and addiction: update on the state of the science. Nutrition. 2012;28(4):341–3.
16. Schulte EM, Tuttle HM, Gearhardt AN. Belief in food addiction and obesity-related policy support. PLoS One. 2016;11(1):e0147557.
17. Gearhardt AN, Yokum S, Orr PT, Stice E, Corbin WR, Brownell KD. Neural correlates of food addiction. Arch Gen Psychiatry. 2011;68(8):808–16.
18. Schulte EM, Avena NM, Gearhardt AN. Which foods may be addictive? The roles of processing, fat content, and glycemic load. PLoS One. 2015;10(2):e0117959.
19. Wiss DA, Criscitelli K, Gold M, Avena N. Preclinical evidence for the addiction potential of highly palatable foods: current developments related to maternal influence. Appetite. 2017;15:19–27.
20. Jimenez-Murcia S, Aguera Z, Paslakis G, Munguia L, Granero R, Sanchez-Gonzalez J, et al. Food addiction in eating disorders and obesity: analysis of clusters and implications for treatment. Nutrients. 2019;11(11):2633.
21. Avena NM, Bocarsly ME, Hoebel BG, Gold MS. Overlaps in the nosology of substance abuse and overeating: the translational implications of "food addiction". Curr Drug Abuse Rev. 2011;4(3):133–9.
22. Bond CW, Trinko R, Foscue E, Furman K, Groman SM, Taylor JR, et al. Medial nucleus Accumbens projections to the ventral tegmental area control food consumption. J Neurosci. 2020;40(24):4727–38.
23. Higgins GA, Sellers EM, Fletcher PJ. From obesity to substance abuse: therapeutic opportunities for 5-HT2C receptor agonists. Trends Pharmacol Sci. 2013;34(10):560–70.
24. Gearhardt AN, Corbin WR, Brownell KD. Preliminary validation of the Yale Food Addiction Scale. Appetite. 2009;52(2):430–6.
25. Carter A, Hendrikse J, Lee N, Yucel M, Verdejo-Garcia A, Andrews ZB, et al. The neurobiology of "food addiction" and its implications for obesity treatment and policy. Annu Rev Nutr. 2016;36:105–28.
26. Hadad NA, Knackstedt LA. Addicted to palatable foods: comparing the neurobiology of Bulimia Nervosa to that of drug addiction. Psychopharmacology. 2014;231(9):1897–912.
27. Volkow ND, Wang GJ, Fowler JS, Tomasi D, Baler R. Food and drug reward: overlapping circuits in human obesity and addiction. Curr Top Behav Neurosci. 2012;11:1–24.
28. Lin Z, Qu S. Legend of weight loss: a crosstalk between the bariatric surgery and the brain. Obes Surg. 2020;30(5):1988–2002.
29. Val-Laillet D, Aarts E, Weber B, Ferrari M, Quaresima V, Stoeckel LE, et al. Neuroimaging and neuromodulation approaches to study eating behavior and prevent and treat eating disorders and obesity. NeuroImage Clin. 2015;8:1–31.
30. Small DM, Jones-Gotman M, Dagher A. Feeding-induced dopamine release in dorsal striatum correlates with meal pleasantness ratings in healthy human volunteers. NeuroImage. 2003;19(4):1709–15.
31. Domingo-Rodriguez L, Ruiz de Azua I, Dominguez E, Senabre E, Serra I, Kummer S, et al. A specific prelimbic-nucleus accumbens pathway controls resilience versus vulnerability to food addiction. Nat Commun. 2020;11(1):782.
32. Mineo D, Cacace F, Mancini M, Vannelli A, Campanelli F, Natale G, et al. Dopamine drives binge-like consumption of a palatable food in experimental Parkinsonism. Mov Disord. 2019;34(6):821–31.
33. Flagel SB, Clark JJ, Robinson TE, Mayo L, Czuj A, Willuhn I, et al. A selective role for dopamine in stimulus-reward learning. Nature. 2011;469(7328):53–7.
34. Tobore TO. Towards a comprehensive theory of obesity and a healthy diet: the causal role of oxidative stress in food addiction and obesity. Behav Brain Res. 2020;384:112560.
35. Higgins GA, Zeeb FD, Fletcher PJ. Role of impulsivity and reward in the anti-obesity actions of 5-HT2C receptor agonists. J Psychopharmacol. 2017;31(11):1403–18.
36. Nieto MM, Wilson J, Cupo A, Roques BP, Noble F. Chronic morphine treatment modulates the extracellular levels of endogenous enkephalins in rat brain structures involved in opiate dependence: a microdialysis study. J Neurosci. 2002;22(3):1034–41.
37. Tinghino B, Lugoboni F, Amatulli A, Biasin C, Bramani Araldi M, Cantiero D, et al. The FODRAT study (FOod addiction, DRugs, Alcohol and Tobacco): first data on food addiction prevalence among patients with addiction to drugs, tobacco and alcohol. Eat Weight Disord. 2020;26(2):449–55.

38. Hernandez J, Perez L, Soto R, Le N, Gastelum C, Wagner EJ. Nociceptin/orphanin FQ neurons in the arcuate nucleus and ventral tegmental area act via Nociceptin opioid peptide receptor signaling to inhibit proopiomelanocortin and A10 dopamine neurons and thereby modulate ingestion of palatable food. Physiol Behav. 2021;228:113183.
39. Hernandez NS, Schmidt HD. Central GLP-1 receptors: novel molecular targets for cocaine use disorder. Physiol Behav. 2019;206:93–105.
40. Sarkar S, Kochhar KP, Khan NA. Fat addiction: psychological and physiological trajectory. Nutrients. 2019;11(11):2785.
41. Gordon EL, Ariel-Donges AH, Bauman V, Merlo LJ. What is the evidence for "food addiction?" A systematic review. Nutrients. 2018;10(4):477.
42. Boggiano MM, Chandler PC, Viana JB, Oswald KD, Maldonado CR, Wauford PK. Combined dieting and stress evoke exaggerated responses to opioids in binge-eating rats. Behav Neurosci. 2005;119(5):1207–14.
43. Ziauddeen H, Chamberlain SR, Nathan PJ, Koch A, Maltby K, Bush M, et al. Effects of the mu-opioid receptor antagonist GSK1521498 on hedonic and consummatory eating behaviour: a proof of mechanism study in binge-eating obese subjects. Mol Psychiatry. 2013;18(12):1287–93.
44. Davis C, Loxton NJ, Levitan RD, Kaplan AS, Carter JC, Kennedy JL. 'Food addiction' and its association with a dopaminergic multilocus genetic profile. Physiol Behav. 2013;118:63–9.
45. Contreras-Rodriguez O, Burrows T, Pursey KM, Stanwell P, Parkes L, Soriano-Mas C, et al. Food addiction linked to changes in ventral striatum functional connectivity between fasting and satiety. Appetite. 2019;133:18–23.
46. Feldstein Ewing SW, Claus ED, Hudson KA, Filbey FM, Yakes Jimenez E, Lisdahl KM, et al. Overweight adolescents' brain response to sweetened beverages mirrors addiction pathways. Brain Imaging Behav. 2017;11(4):925–35.
47. Gordon EL, Lent MR, Merlo LJ. The effect of food composition and behavior on neurobiological response to food: a review of recent research. Curr Nutr Rep. 2020;9(2):75–82.
48. Imperatori C, Fabbricatore M, Innamorati M, Farina B, Quintiliani MI, Lamis DA, et al. Modification of EEG functional connectivity and EEG power spectra in overweight and obese patients with food addiction: an eLORETA study. Brain Imaging Behav. 2015;9(4):703–16.
49. Kelley AE. Ventral striatal control of appetitive motivation: role in ingestive behavior and reward-related learning. Neurosci Biobehav Rev. 2004;27(8):765–76.
50. Szalay C, Aradi M, Schwarcz A, Orsi G, Perlaki G, Nemeth L, et al. Gustatory perception alterations in obesity: an fMRI study. Brain Res. 2012;1473:131–40.
51. Schlogl H, Horstmann A, Villringer A, Stumvoll M. Functional neuroimaging in obesity and the potential for development of novel treatments. Lancet Diabetes Endocrinol. 2016;4(8):695–705.
52. Jastreboff AM, Lacadie C, Seo D, Kubat J, Van Name MA, Giannini C, et al. Leptin is associated with exaggerated brain reward and emotion responses to food images in adolescent obesity. Diabetes Care. 2014;37(11):3061–8.
53. Jastreboff AM, Sinha R, Arora J, Giannini C, Kubat J, Malik S, et al. Altered brain response to drinking glucose and fructose in obese adolescents. Diabetes. 2016;65(7):1929–39.
54. Boutelle KN, Wierenga CE, Bischoff-Grethe A, Melrose AJ, Grenesko-Stevens E, Paulus MP, et al. Increased brain response to appetitive tastes in the insula and amygdala in obese compared with healthy weight children when sated. Int J Obes. 2015;39(4):620–8.
55. Garcia-Garcia I, Horstmann A, Jurado MA, Garolera M, Chaudhry SJ, Margulies DS, et al. Reward processing in obesity, substance addiction and non-substance addiction. Obes Rev. 2014;15(11):853–69.
56. Simon JJ, Skunde M, Walther S, Bendszus M, Herzog W, Friederich HC. Neural signature of food reward processing in bulimic-type eating disorders. Soc Cogn Affect Neurosci. 2016;11(9):1393–401.
57. Seabrook LT, Borgland SL. The orbitofrontal cortex, food intake and obesity. J Psychiatry Neurosci. 2020;45(5):304–12.
58. Kroemer NB, Sun X, Veldhuizen MG, Babbs AE, de Araujo IE, Small DM. Weighing the evidence: variance in brain responses to milkshake receipt is predictive of eating behavior. NeuroImage. 2016;128:273–83.
59. Stice E, Spoor S, Bohon C, Small DM. Relation between obesity and blunted striatal response to food is moderated by TaqIA A1 allele. Science. 2008;322(5900):449–52.
60. Stice E, Davis K, Miller NP, Marti CN. Fasting increases risk for onset of binge eating and bulimic pathology: a 5-year prospective study. J Abnorm Psychol. 2008;117(4):941–6.
61. Duarte RB, Patrono E, Borges AC, Cesar AA, Tomaz C, Ventura R, et al. Consumption of a highly palatable food induces a lasting place-conditioning memory in marmoset monkeys. Behav Process. 2014;107:163–6.
62. Davis C, Curtis C, Levitan RD, Carter JC, Kaplan AS, Kennedy JL. Evidence that 'food addiction' is a valid phenotype of obesity. Appetite. 2011;57(3):711–7.
63. Velazquez-Sanchez C, Santos JW, Smith KL, Ferragud A, Sabino V, Cottone P. Seeking behavior, place conditioning, and resistance to conditioned suppression of feeding in rats intermittently exposed to palatable food. Behav Neurosci. 2015;129(2):219–24.

64. Rada P, Avena NM, Hoebel BG. Daily bingeing on sugar repeatedly releases dopamine in the accumbens shell. Neuroscience. 2005;134(3):737–44.
65. Colantuoni C, Rada P, McCarthy J, Patten C, Avena NM, Chadeayne A, et al. Evidence that intermittent, excessive sugar intake causes endogenous opioid dependence. Obes Res. 2002;10(6):478–88.
66. Avena NM, Hoebel BG. A diet promoting sugar dependency causes behavioral cross-sensitization to a low dose of amphetamine. Neuroscience. 2003;122(1):17–20.
67. Morales I, Berridge KC. 'Liking' and 'wanting' in eating and food reward: brain mechanisms and clinical implications. Physiol Behav. 2020;227:113152.
68. Sinha R. Role of addiction and stress neurobiology on food intake and obesity. Biol Psychol. 2018;131:5–13.
69. Hoebel BG, Avena NM, Bocarsly ME, Rada P. Natural addiction: a behavioral and circuit model based on sugar addiction in rats. J Addict Med. 2009;3(1):33–41.
70. Novelle MG, Dieguez C. Food addiction and binge eating: lessons learned from animal models. Nutrients. 2018;10(1):71.
71. Stice E, Burger K, Yokum S. Caloric deprivation increases responsivity of attention and reward brain regions to intake, anticipated intake, and images of palatable foods. NeuroImage. 2013;67:322–30.
72. Sinha R, Jastreboff AM. Stress as a common risk factor for obesity and addiction. Biol Psychiatry. 2013;73(9):827–35.
73. Kinasz KR, Ross DA, Cooper JJ. Eat to live or live to eat? The neurobiology of appetite regulation. Biol Psychiatry. 2017;81(9):e73–e5.
74. Meule A. Food cravings in food addiction: exploring a potential cut-off value of the food cravings questionnaire-trait-reduced. Eat Weight Disord. 2018;23(1):39–43.
75. Styn MA, Bovbjerg DH, Lipsky S, Erblich J. Cue-induced cigarette and food craving: a common effect? Addict Behav. 2013;38(3):1840–3.
76. Mahler SV, de Wit H. Cue-reactors: individual differences in cue-induced craving after food or smoking abstinence. PLoS One. 2010;5(11):e15475.
77. Ferrario CR. Food addiction and obesity. Neuropsychopharmacology. 2017;42(1):361.
78. Boswell RG, Kober H. Food cue reactivity and craving predict eating and weight gain: a meta-analytic review. Obes Rev. 2016;17(2):159–77.
79. Kelley AE, Schiltz CA, Landry CF. Neural systems recruited by drug- and food-related cues: studies of gene activation in corticolimbic regions. Physiol Behav. 2005;86(1–2):11–4.
80. Small DM, Zatorre RJ, Dagher A, Evans AC, Jones-Gotman M. Changes in brain activity related to eating chocolate: from pleasure to aversion. Brain. 2001;124(Pt 9):1720–33.
81. Furlong TM, Jayaweera HK, Balleine BW, Corbit LH. Binge-like consumption of a palatable food accelerates habitual control of behavior and is dependent on activation of the dorsolateral striatum. J Neurosci. 2014;34(14):5012–22.
82. Le Merrer J, Stephens DN. Food-induced behavioral sensitization, its cross-sensitization to cocaine and morphine, pharmacological blockade, and effect on food intake. J Neurosci. 2006;26(27):7163–71.
83. Dela Cruz JA, Coke T, Bodnar RJ. Simultaneous detection of c-Fos activation from mesolimbic and Mesocortical dopamine reward sites following naive sugar and fat ingestion in rats. J Vis Exp. 2016;114
84. Cambridge VC, Ziauddeen H, Nathan PJ, Subramaniam N, Dodds C, Chamberlain SR, et al. Neural and behavioral effects of a novel mu opioid receptor antagonist in binge-eating obese people. Biol Psychiatry. 2013;73(9):887–94.
85. Volkow ND, Wang GJ, Fowler JS, Logan J, Jayne M, Franceschi D, et al. "Nonhedonic" food motivation in humans involves dopamine in the dorsal striatum and methylphenidate amplifies this effect. Synapse. 2002;44(3):175–80.
86. Volkow ND, Wang GJ, Maynard L, Jayne M, Fowler JS, Zhu W, et al. Brain dopamine is associated with eating behaviors in humans. Int J Eat Disord. 2003;33(2):136–42.
87. Rothemund Y, Preuschhof C, Bohner G, Bauknecht HC, Klingebiel R, Flor H, et al. Differential activation of the dorsal striatum by high-calorie visual food stimuli in obese individuals. NeuroImage. 2007;37(2):410–21.
88. Stice E, Yokum S, Bohon C, Marti N, Smolen A. Reward circuitry responsivity to food predicts future increases in body mass: moderating effects of DRD2 and DRD4. NeuroImage. 2010;50(4):1618–25.
89. Lutter M, Nestler EJ. Homeostatic and hedonic signals interact in the regulation of food intake. J Nutr. 2009;139(3):629–32.
90. Smith KE, Mason TB, Schaefer LM, Juarascio A, Dvorak R, Weinbach N, et al. Examining intra-individual variability in food-related inhibitory control and negative affect as predictors of binge eating using ecological momentary assessment. J Psychiatr Res. 2020;120:137–43.
91. Stoeckel LE, Weller RE, Cook EW 3rd, Twieg DB, Knowlton RC, Cox JE. Widespread reward-system activation in obese women in response to pictures of high-calorie foods. NeuroImage. 2008;41(2):636–47.
92. Lee JE, Namkoong K, Jung YC. Impaired prefrontal cognitive control over interference by food images in binge-eating disorder and bulimia nervosa. Neurosci Lett. 2017;651:95–101.
93. Gearhardt AN, Corbin WR, Brownell KD. Development of the Yale Food Addiction Scale Version 2.0. Psychol Addict Behav. 2016;30(1):113–21.
94. Guzzardi MA, Garelli S, Agostini A, Filidei E, Fanelli F, Giorgetti A, et al. Food addiction dis-

tinguishes an overweight phenotype that can be reversed by low calorie diet. Eur Eat Disord Rev. 2018;26(6):657–70.
95. Schulte EM, Wadden TA, Allison KC. An evaluation of food addiction as a distinct psychiatric disorder. Int J Eat Disord. 2020;53(10):1610–22.
96. Adams S, Wijk E. Effects of acute alcohol consumption on food intake and pictorial Stroop response to high-calorie food cues. Alcohol Alcohol. 2020;56(3):275–83.
97. Katsunuma R, Oba K, Kitamura S, Motomura Y, Terasawa Y, Nakazaki K, et al. Unrecognized sleep loss accumulated in daily life can promote brain hyperreactivity to food cue. Sleep. 2017;40(10):1–10.
98. Demos KE, Heatherton TF, Kelley WM. Individual differences in nucleus accumbens activity to food and sexual images predict weight gain and sexual behavior. J Neurosci. 2012;32(16):5549–52.
99. Murdaugh DL, Cox JE, Cook EW 3rd, Weller RE. fMRI reactivity to high-calorie food pictures predicts short- and long-term outcome in a weight-loss program. NeuroImage. 2012;59(3):2709–21.
100. DelParigi A, Chen K, Salbe AD, Hill JO, Wing RR, Reiman EM, et al. Persistence of abnormal neural responses to a meal in postobese individuals. Int J Obes Relat Metab Disord. 2004;28(3):370–7.
101. Sethi Dalai S, Sinha A, Gearhardt AN. Low carbohydrate ketogenic therapy as a metabolic treatment for binge eating and ultraprocessed food addiction. Curr Opin Endocrinol Diabetes Obes. 2020;27(5):275–82.
102. San-Cristobal R, Navas-Carretero S, Martinez-Gonzalez MA, Ordovas JM, Martinez JA. Contribution of macronutrients to obesity: implications for precision nutrition. Nat Rev Endocrinol. 2020;16(6):305–20.
103. Galanter M, Kleber HD, editors. Textbook of substance abuse treatment. 4th ed. Washington DC/London, England: American Psychiatric Publishing Inc; 2008.
104. Berthoud HR. Metabolic and hedonic drives in the neural control of appetite: who is the boss? Curr Opin Neurobiol. 2011;21(6):888–96.
105. de Araujo IE, Ferreira JG, Tellez LA, Ren X, Yeckel CW. The gut-brain dopamine axis: a regulatory system for caloric intake. Physiol Behav. 2012;106(3):394–9.
106. Hetherington MM, Cunningham K, Dye L, Gibson EL, Gregersen NT, Halford JC, et al. Potential benefits of satiety to the consumer: scientific considerations. Nutr Res Rev. 2013;26(1):22–38.
107. Kessler RM, Hutson PH, Herman BK, Potenza MN. The neurobiological basis of binge-eating disorder. Neurosci Biobehav Rev. 2016;63:223–38.
108. Volkow ND, Wang GJ, Fowler JS, Tomasi D, Telang F. Addiction: beyond dopamine reward circuitry. Proc Natl Acad Sci U S A. 2011;108(37):15037–42.
109. Volkow ND, Wang GJ, Fowler JS, Telang F. Overlapping neuronal circuits in addiction and obesity: evidence of systems pathology. Philos Trans R Soc Lond Ser B Biol Sci. 2008;363(1507):3191–200.
110. Geiger BM, Haburcak M, Avena NM, Moyer MC, Hoebel BG, Pothos EN. Deficits of mesolimbic dopamine neurotransmission in rat dietary obesity. Neuroscience. 2009;159(4):1193–9.
111. Johnson PM, Kenny PJ. Dopamine D2 receptors in addiction-like reward dysfunction and compulsive eating in obese rats. Nat Neurosci. 2010;13(5):635–41.
112. Adams WK, Sussman JL, Kaur S, D'Souza AM, Kieffer TJ, Winstanley CA. Long-term, calorie-restricted intake of a high-fat diet in rats reduces impulse control and ventral striatal D2 receptor signalling – two markers of addiction vulnerability. Eur J Neurosci. 2015;42(12):3095–104.
113. Winterdahl M, Noer O, Orlowski D, Schacht AC, Jakobsen S, Alstrup AKO, et al. Sucrose intake lowers mu-opioid and dopamine D2/3 receptor availability in porcine brain. Sci Rep. 2019;9(1):16918.
114. Wang GJ, Volkow ND, Logan J, Pappas NR, Wong CT, Zhu W, et al. Brain dopamine and obesity. Lancet. 2001;357(9253):354–7.
115. Leigh SJ, Morris MJ. The role of reward circuitry and food addiction in the obesity epidemic: an update. Biol Psychol. 2016;131:31–42.
116. Wiss D, Brewerton T. Separating the signal from the noise: how psychiatric diagnoses can help discern food addiction from dietary restraint. Nutrients. 2020;12(10):2937.
117. Wilcox CE, Braskie MN, Kluth JT, Jagust WJ. Overeating behavior and striatal dopamine with 6-[F]-Fluoro-L-m-tyrosine PET. J Obes. 2010;2010:909348.
118. Wang GJ, Volkow ND, Thanos PK, Fowler JS. Imaging of brain dopamine pathways: implications for understanding obesity. J Addict Med. 2009;3(1):8–18.
119. Kaye WH, Wierenga CE, Bailer UF, Simmons AN, Wagner A, Bischoff-Grethe A. Does a shared neurobiology for foods and drugs of abuse contribute to extremes of food ingestion in anorexia and bulimia nervosa? Biol Psychiatry. 2013;73(9):836–42.
120. Blum K, Braverman ER, Holder JM, Lubar JF, Monastra VJ, Miller D, et al. Reward deficiency syndrome: a biogenetic model for the diagnosis and treatment of impulsive, addictive, and compulsive behaviors. J Psychoactive Drugs. 2000;32(Suppl):i–iv, 1–112.
121. Ouwens MA, van Strien T, van Leeuwe JF. Possible pathways between depression, emotional and external eating. A structural equation model. Appetite. 2009;53(2):245–8.
122. Sharma S, Fernandes MF, Fulton S. Adaptations in brain reward circuitry underlie palatable food cravings and anxiety induced by high-fat diet withdrawal. Int J Obes. 2013;37(9):1183–91.
123. Sharma S, Fulton S. Diet-induced obesity promotes depressive-like behaviour that is associated with neural adaptations in brain reward circuitry. Int J Obes. 2013;37(3):382–9.

124. Kalyan-Masih P, Vega-Torres JD, Miles C, Haddad E, Rainsbury S, Baghchechi M, et al. Western high-fat diet consumption during adolescence increases susceptibility to traumatic stress while selectively disrupting hippocampal and ventricular volumes. eNeuro. 2016;3(5):1–10.
125. Wise RA, Koob GF. The development and maintenance of drug addiction. Neuropsychopharmacology. 2014;39(2):254–62.
126. Bocarsly ME, Berner LA, Hoebel BG, Avena NM. Rats that binge eat fat-rich food do not show somatic signs or anxiety associated with opiate-like withdrawal: implications for nutrient-specific food addiction behaviors. Physiol Behav. 2011;104(5):865–72.
127. Martin K, Woo J, Timmins V, Collins J, Islam A, Newton D, et al. Binge eating and emotional eating behaviors among adolescents and young adults with bipolar disorder. J Affect Disord. 2016;195:88–95.
128. Gibson EL. The psychobiology of comfort eating: implications for neuropharmacological interventions. Behav Pharmacol. 2012;23(5–6):442–60.
129. Wiss DA, Brewerton TD. Adverse childhood experiences and adult obesity: a systematic review of plausible mechanisms and Meta-analysis of cross-sectional studies. Physiol Behav. 2020;223:112964.
130. Kober H, Boswell RG. Potential psychological & neural mechanisms in binge eating disorder: implications for treatment. Clin Psychol Rev. 2018;60:32–44.
131. Koob GF. The dark side of emotion: the addiction perspective. Eur J Pharmacol. 2015;753:73–87.
132. Fischer S, Breithaupt L, Wonderlich J, Westwater ML, Crosby RD, Engel SG, et al. Impact of the neural correlates of stress and cue reactivity on stress related binge eating in the natural environment. J Psychiatr Res. 2017;92:15–23.
133. Daubenmier J, Lustig RH, Hecht FM, Kristeller J, Woolley J, Adam T, et al. A new biomarker of hedonic eating? A preliminary investigation of cortisol and nausea responses to acute opioid blockade. Appetite. 2014;74:92–100.
134. Donofry SD, Stillman CM, Erickson KI. A review of the relationship between eating behavior, obesity and functional brain network organization. Soc Cogn Affect Neurosci. 2020;15(10):1157–81.
135. Volkow ND, Wang GJ, Tomasi D, Baler RD. Obesity and addiction: neurobiological overlaps. Obes Rev. 2013;14(1):2–18.
136. Jentsch JD, Pennington ZT. Reward, interrupted: Inhibitory control and its relevance to addictions. Neuropharmacology. 2014;76(Pt B):479–86.
137. Hsu JS, Wang PW, Ko CH, Hsieh TJ, Chen CY, Yen JY. Altered brain correlates of response inhibition and error processing in females with obesity and sweet food addiction: a functional magnetic imaging study. Obes Res Clin Pract. 2017;11(6):677–86.
138. Batterink L, Yokum S, Stice E. Body mass correlates inversely with inhibitory control in response to food among adolescent girls: an fMRI study. NeuroImage. 2010;52(4):1696–703.
139. Ifland JR, Preuss HG, Marcus MT, Rourke KM, Taylor WC, Burau K, et al. Refined food addiction: a classic substance use disorder. Med Hypotheses. 2009;72(5):518–26.
140. Hardee JE, Phaneuf C, Cope L, Zucker R, Gearhardt A, Heitzeg M. Neural correlates of inhibitory control in youth with symptoms of food addiction. Appetite. 2020;148:104578.
141. Bechara A. Decision making, impulse control and loss of willpower to resist drugs: a neurocognitive perspective. Nat Neurosci. 2005;8(11):1458–63.
142. Clasen MM, Riley AL, Davidson TL. Hippocampal-dependent inhibitory learning and memory processes in the control of eating and drug taking. Curr Pharm Des. 2020;26(20):2334–52.
143. Martins-Silva T, Vaz JDS, Hutz MH, Salatino-Oliveira A, Genro JP, Hartwig FP, et al. Assessing causality in the association between attention-deficit/hyperactivity disorder and obesity: a Mendelian randomization study. Int J Obes. 2019;43(12):2500–8.
144. Koob GF. Neurobiology of opioid addiction: opponent process, hyperkatifeia, and negative reinforcement. Biol Psychiatry. 2020;87(1):44–53.
145. Koob GF, Powell P, White A. Addiction as a coping response: hyperkatifeia, deaths of despair, and COVID-19. Am J Psychiatry. 2020;177(11):1031–7.
146. Trifilieff P, Martinez D. Blunted dopamine release as a biomarker for vulnerability for substance use disorders. Biol Psychiatry. 2014;76(1):4–5.
147. Trifilieff P, Martinez D. Imaging addiction: D2 receptors and dopamine signaling in the striatum as biomarkers for impulsivity. Neuropharmacology. 2014;76(Pt B):498–509.
148. Courtney KE, Infante MA, Bordyug M, Simmons AN, Tapert SF. Prospective associations between BOLD markers of response inhibition and the transition to frequent binge drinking. Alcohol Clin Exp Res. 2020;44(2):463–9.
149. DelParigi A, Chen K, Salbe AD, Hill JO, Wing RR, Reiman EM, et al. Successful dieters have increased neural activity in cortical areas involved in the control of behavior. Int J Obes. 2007;31(3):440–8.
150. Goldman RL, Canterberry M, Borckardt JJ, Madan A, Byrne TK, George MS, et al. Executive control circuitry differentiates degree of success in weight loss following gastric-bypass surgery. Obesity. 2013;21(11):2189–96.
151. van der Zwaal EM, de Weijer BA, van de Giessen EM, Janssen I, Berends FJ, van de Laar A, et al. Striatal dopamine D2/3 receptor availability increases after long-term bariatric surgery-induced weight loss. Eur Neuropsychopharmacol. 2016;26(7):1190–200.
152. Baboumian S, Pantazatos SP, Kothari S, McGinty J, Holst J, Geliebter A. Functional magnetic resonance imaging (fMRI) of neural responses to visual and auditory food stimuli pre and post roux-en-Y gastric bypass (RYGB) and sleeve gastrectomy (SG). Neuroscience. 2019;409:290–8.

Additional Biological Mechanisms of Hedonic Eating

9

9.1 Interactions Between the Homeostatic System and Hedonic System

9.1.1 Anatomy

As was mentioned in Chap. 1 (Fig. 1.1), the lateral hypothalamus is the primary structure that bridges, or allows for communication between, the homeostatic feeding system and the hedonic eating system [1–3]. This structure has projections to and receives input from medial hypothalamus (the primary brain-based hub of the homeostatic feeding system) and brain areas such as the prefrontal cortex (PFC), amygdala, ventral and dorsal striatum, hippocampus, and insula [2]. For example, the lateral hypothalamus projects to the nucleus accumbens (NAc) (which resides in the ventral striatum; Fig. 7.2) [4] via neurons containing melanin-concentrating hormone (MCH), which stimulate feeding [5]. In addition, the NAc can disinhibit lateral hypothalamus neurons through GABAergic projections [5].

Appetite-regulating hormones, like leptin and ghrelin, are also able to directly influence the reward system and, as a result, hedonic eating behavior [5, 6]. Ghrelin receptors are dense in the ventral tegmental area (VTA), NAc, and amygdala and are expressed on DA neuron cell bodies, in particular [5–7]. Leptin receptors also exist on VTA DA neurons [8, 9].

9.1.2 Appetite-Regulating Neuropeptides Modulate Hedonic Eating

Appetite-regulating neuropeptides or hormones (Chap. 1) regulate homeostatic eating, but can also influence hedonic eating behavior or eating for pleasure or reward [5]. Recall that leptin and insulin are generally anorexigenic, or appetite-reducing, (except when obesity or diabetes are present is associated with resistance to leptin and insulin, blocking their functional effects on appetite). Recall, also, that ghrelin, agouti-related protein (AgRP), MCH, and orexins generally stimulate appetite (Chap. 1). Interestingly, these hormones also have effects on food craving and on hedonic eating behaviors, as well, with a similar directionality.

In terms of leptin, in rat studies, central administration of high levels of leptin reduces food intake [10] via effects on mesolimbic DA function: binding of leptin to receptors in the lateral hypothalamus (recall leptin receptors are present at high densities in the hypothalamus, Chap. 1) reduces extracellular DA in the NAc, attenuating brain reward signalling [5, 11]. It also affects firing in MCH-containing neurons that project from the lateral hypothalamus to the NAc [5, 6, 8, 12]. Furthermore, leptin acts through the opioid system, reversing μ-opioid receptor stimulated sugar feeding [13]. Leptin also acts more peripherally to reduce palatability of food by inhibiting

C. E. Wilcox, *Food Addiction, Obesity, and Disorders of Overeating*,
https://doi.org/10.1007/978-3-030-83078-6_9

responses of sweet-sensitive taste cells in the tongue [5]. Neuroimaging studies also show that leptin has effects on brain structures that mediate reward-based eating (Chaps. 7 and 8). For example, in one study, leptin deficiency was associated with greater NAc activation to food cue pictures, with the degree of deficiency positively correlated with valence ratings of food pictures in both the fasted and fed state [3]. After 1 week of leptin treatment, this activation correlated with valence ratings of food pictures in only the fasted state indicating that leptin was necessary to suppress the incentive value of food in the sated state or the state in which an animal might be eating beyond homeostatic needs [3]. In other work, higher leptin levels (often seen in obesity) predicted blunted ventromedial PFC and rostral anterior cingulate (ACC) activation to high-fat food images and to glucose and fructose intake in adolescents, as well [6, 14, 15].

Binding of ghrelin to receptors on neurons in the mesolimbic system (e.g., the VTA and NAc) has also been found in animal studies to cause an increase in the reward value of food [16] and to increase food intake [5, 7, 17–19], particularly sugary food intake [5]. Ghrelin also increases preferential intake of palatable food over standard chow [5, 20]. Ghrelin likely has this effect on feeding, in part, by facilitating DA release in the striatum [5, 16], and, in rats, the increase in motivation to consume sucrose induced by ghrelin is dependent on the amount of DA released into the NAc from neurons with cell bodies in the VTA, whereas ghrelin-induced increase in chow intake is not DA dependent [21]. Opioid signaling is also necessary to modulate the effects of ghrelin on food reward and intake [5]; ghrelin likely increases opioid activity in the VTA which facilitates DA release into NAc to augment reward-seeking behavior. As is seen with leptin, neuroimaging studies also show that ghrelin acts to stimulate reward circuitry in humans [3, 6, 8, 12]. One example of such a study showed greater activation to food cue following ghrelin administration compared with placebo, in the amygdala (bilaterally), right hippocampus, anterior and mid-dorsal insula, left orbitofrontal cortex (OFC), and left caudate nucleus. Furthermore, activation in amygdala and left OFC correlated with self-reported hunger [3, 12]. Another study found that, in healthy volunteers and in individuals with hyperphagic major depressive disorders, higher ghrelin levels were correlated with greater neural response to food pictures and food cravings [7].

Finally, chronically high levels of peripheral insulin and insulin resistance, as is observed in many individuals with obesity and certainly in those with type 2 diabetes, may promote rather than suppress food craving (in a healthy person, it should reduce appetite) and increase brain activation in DA-rich reward regions such as the VTA, NAc, and dorsal striatum [6, 22]. Higher insulin levels in response to eating predicted greater weight gain at a future 6-month follow-up assessment in one study [6, 23]. Furthermore, higher activity in the insula and dorsal striatum correlated with higher insulin levels, insulin resistance, and food craving when participants were placed in their favorite food contexts via imagined exposure [6, 22]. Disruption of insulin regulation (both increases during fasting and slow postprandial response) could lead to poor control of appetite and satiety, via effects on reward function [21].

AgRP, MCH, and orexins can also directly affect DA neuron firing influencing hedonic eating in a variety of ways, details about which can be accessed in these cited references [1, 11].

9.1.3 Appetite-Regulating Neuropeptides Moderate Drug and Alcohol Use

Further support for the overlap of neural systems that drive hedonic eating and substance use comes from evidence that many of these neuropeptides can influence addictive substance use and that substance use and SUD can affect, and be affected by, these anorexigenic and orexigenic peptide hormones [21, 24]. It is increasingly recognized that the hypothalamus is involved not only in the regulation of food and water intake but also in drug-seeking and other reward-based behaviors and that hunger and satiety states influence SUD behavior [5]. For example, food deprivation has been found to lower the threshold for activation of reward pathways increasing sensitivity to both drugs of abuse and food, potentially increasing consumption of, and reinforcement of future consumption of, both drugs and highly palatable (HP) food—which includes high-sugar, high-fat, high-salt, and/or highly processed foods [10, 21, 25]. Nutritional depletion will also encourage drug-seeking and alcohol-drinking in animals which is mediated by DA mechanisms [21].

A growing body of research implicates leptin in contributing to the development and maintenance of SUD [9, 11, 26]. Recall that leptin dampens the sensitivity of the reward system via reductions in DA function. In rat studies, central administration of high levels of leptin reduced heroin relapse [21, 24], and intra-VTA leptin reduced heroin seeking [26]. Leptin also blocks conditioned place preference for cocaine via attenuation of DA release [5]. Leptin also increases during abstinence from alcohol and smokers in some but not all studies [9] which could contribute to difficulty experiencing natural rewards via its reward-dampening effects.

A growing body of research implicates ghrelin in SUD as well [26, 27], including alcohol use disorder (AUD) [28]. Ghrelin, through binding to VTA receptors and facilitating DA release into the NAc [17, 18, 27], increases the rewarding and locomotor effects of cocaine, facilitates cocaine conditioned place preference, induces craving for alcohol, and increases alcohol consumption and other alcohol-seeking behaviors [5, 21, 28]. Likewise, ghrelin antagonists reduce alcohol intake [21] and heroin seeking in food-restricted rats [26]. Conversely, alcohol suppresses ghrelin production, and subjects with AUD have been shown to have significantly lower ghrelin levels than controls in most research studies in humans [21]; that said, ghrelin levels appear to rise in AUD during early abstinence (which is theorized to contribute to early relapse) and rebound after 30 days. At any rate, the role of ghrelin in AUD development and maintenance is likely complex, and despite prior study, there is no data to support the efficacy of ghrelin antagonism in AUD [21].

Finally, disruption of insulin regulation by drugs of abuse is theorized to cause increased drug and alcohol craving and poor control of appetite and satiety [21]. Drug use may cause these disruptions by increasing insulin levels during fasting and by slowing the postprandial response of insulin, with consequent adverse effects on glycaemia [21].

9.2 Stress, Hedonic Eating, and the Reward System

9.2.1 The Anatomy of the Stress Response

The physiological responses to acute stress manifest via two interacting neural pathways. The first is the hypothalamic-pituitary-adrenal (HPA) axis. Corticotropin-releasing hormone (CRH) is released from the paraventricular nucleus of the hypothalamus in response to stress, stimulating secretion of adreno-corticotrophin hormone from the anterior pituitary, which subsequently stimulates the secretion of glucocorticoids (cortisol or corticosterone) from the adrenal glands, which then feed back to the hypothalamus to modulate CRH release [6]. The second pathway that is involved in the stress response is the autonomic nervous system, which is coordinated by the sympathetic and the parasympathetic pathways, and moderates the fight or flight versus relaxation response and involves noradrenaline and acetylcholine, respectively [6]. The central nucleus of the amygdala (CeA) is also activated by cortisol and noradrenaline. A brain structure called the locus coeruleus produces and releases noradrenaline into the CeA under stress, triggering the subjective experience of anxiety and dysphoria, as well as other stress-related behaviors, and activity in the CeA feeds back to the hypothalamus to further modulate the stress response [29, 30].

9.2.2 Acute and Chronic Stress Promote Hedonic Eating

Both in humans and in animal models, acute stress promotes increased desire and craving (or evidence thereof, in animals) for high-calorie, high-sugar, and high-fat foods (think "comfort foods") and causes preferential selection, intake, and bingeing on these HP foods [6, 21, 31–33]. High levels of stress also promote weight gain and abdominal fat deposition [6, 32, 33] as well as susceptibility to developing eating disorder-like behavior, although the highest levels of acute stress will reduce feeding [6, 34]. Stress also triggers substance use via similar mechanisms [35, 36].

The stress response and its associated elevation in cortisol causes increased desire for HP foods [32, 33], and one way that they promote pleasure-related eating is via direct effects on the reward system. In particular, acute stress and cortisol release potentiates DA transmission and impacts reward seeking and food intake in laboratory animals [6]. Neuroimaging studies have also indicated an increase in dopamine transporter (DAT) density in PTSD, which may reflect a higher DA turnover among trauma survivors [37, 38]. Both an increase in the number of traumatic events early in life and an increase in levels of perceived stress were associated with a higher ventral striatal DA response to amphetamine [38, 39]. This evidence supports the biological embedding hypothesis which links early life adversity to addictive behaviors via hypersensitivity to reward [38].

Another way that stress promotes eating is through negative reinforcement learning or negative conditioning. Recall that hunger and food restriction causes a stress response. This makes evolutionary sense since the stress response promotes glucose mobilization increasing gluconeogenesis and glucose blood levels for immediate use [6]. Reducing blood glucose to mild hypoglycemic levels relative to normal euglycemic levels increases plasma cortisol [6], and women who engage in more restrained eating have higher cortisol levels [40]. This elevated cortisol is also correlated with increased craving for HP foods and brain activation of reward-motivational (striatal) and emotion-stress (limbic) regions in response to high-fat and high-sugar versus low-fat and non-food pictures [6, 41]. The withdrawal state from drugs or food is also marked by alterations similar to stress in terms of glucocorticoids and HPA axis function (and an increased intensity of HPA axis occurs over time with increased number and intensity of experienced withdrawal, leading to the vicious cycle of addiction [6]) (Chaps. 7 and 8). On the other hand, when HP foods are consumed in response to stress, people and animals experience reduced stress-associated dysphoria and negative affect. This reduction in negative affect is accompanied by a dampening of the stress-induced HPA axis and sympathetic nervous system responses [6]. Ultimately, if this process is repeated, it leads to conditioning, and the behavior reinforces itself, leading to a heightened incentive salience of HP foods and increased motivation to procure these foods and consume them, whenever similar dysphoric experiences present themselves [6]. This pattern also occurs with substances of abuse [35, 36].

Studies show that either due to the priming of the DA system or the negative reinforcement-induced positive feedback loop, stress can lead to progressively more and more weight gain for some people. Individuals with higher BMIs demonstrate stronger associations between experiences of psychological stress and future weight gain [6]. Stress may have more powerful effects in overweight individuals than lean individuals, as one study showed that it potentiates craving for desserts and snacks and leads to greater HP food intake in satiated overweight individuals relative to lean individuals [34]. One study showed that higher chronic stress, and associated insulin and cortisol responses, predicted greater weight gain at a future 6-month follow-up assessment [6, 23].

The stress response also affects neuropeptide function, which may further affect appetitive behavioral responses. For example, cortisol increases insulin levels, which may lead to worsening insulin resistance over time [6]. Stress-induced increases in cortisol also increase ghrelin in the periphery [28] which may in turn promote HP food seeking [6], and it also may even play a role in alcohol-seeking induced by stress [28].

It's important to mention, though, that chronic stress is usually associated with a different HPA axis profile than acute stress, with reduced cortisol levels and blunted HPA axis function. This state is often called "neuroendocrine tolerance." The HPA axis is usually stimulated by rewarding experiences, and this stimulation and associated elevated cortisol is believed to contribute to the pleasure experienced with use of drugs of abuse and HP foods, as we have mentioned. However, chronic stress and overuse of substances or HP food induces downregulation in cortisol release [6], which worsens tolerance and enhances blunting in DA and opioid function (reviewed in Chaps. 7 and 8) [6]. Indeed, blunted HPA axis responses to reward and low levels of morning cortisol are seen in higher BMI groups compared to normal BMI groups [6, 22, 42–44]. Chronic stress also promotes insulin resistance, and high levels of insulin, in turn, downregulate HPA axis responses and increase basal sympathetic tone even further [6]. Chronically elevated cortisol leads to a blunted leptin (and its associated satiety) response as well contributes further to increased desire for HP foods over healthier options, and the accumulation of abdominal fat [32, 33].

9.3 Genetics

Genetics likely play an important role in the risk for development of FA or hedonic eating tendencies [11, 45]. In a large twin study from the Netherlands, genetic factors explained 48% of the variance in high sugar consumption (52% of the variance was explained by unique environmental factors) [38, 46]. This is similar in magnitude to the heritability of SUD [35]. Future work is likely to find overlap in the genetic underpinnings of FA and SUD [47] as evidenced by the fact, for example, that FA are more likely to have a family history of mental health problems and addiction histories [38, 48].

Genome-wide association studies (GWAS) have not revealed much about the genetic underpinnings for hedonic eating or FA so far, however [38]. A genome-wide analysis in women with European ancestry showed two loci significantly related to FA at the genome-wide level (17q21.31 and 11q13.4) [49, 50], but the loci did not have any obvious functional roles in eating behavior. In another genome-wide investigation of FA, scores on the modified YFAS were significantly associated with signaling in the mitogen-activated protein kinase pathway, which has been identified as a possible drug addiction pathway in other works [40, 49].

Alterations in genes encoding components of the DA system influence SUD risk, and similar genetic variants could also be found to be important in FA risk, as well [51]. Indeed, higher loadings on the genetic DA multi-locus profile [40, 52] have been observed in FA, and the relationship between the genetic scores and FA were mediated by reward-driven eating. Furthermore, in drosophila, manipulating DA systems can cause inheritable overfeeding [53] although GWAS haven't implicated the DA system in any robust way [50]. In another study, a polymorphism in one of the DA transporters (e.g., SLC6A3, DAT1) has been implicated in FA [47, 54, 55]. Furthermore, differential genetically predicted gene expression of prefrontal type 4 dopamine receptor (D4) was found to be related to susceptibility to childhood emotional eating in response to positive environment [51, 56].

Genes encoding the type 2 dopamine receptor (D2) also are important in the risk for developing disorders associated with overeating and SUD [38, 47, 55, 57, 58]. This is not surprising given that obese individuals and individuals with SUD show low D2 receptor density on PET scans (although another mechanism by which this association might occur is through downregulation of these receptors with repeated use of HP food or substances during the development of tolerance) (Chaps. 7 and 8). In a Newfoundland population, the major allele A of rs2511521 located in the D2 receptor is significantly associated with FA [50]. The Taq1A allele polymorphism is an especially promising candidate: this allele can cause a

30–40% reduction in striatal D2 receptors and is also more prevalent in individuals with drug use disorders and obese individuals [3, 59, 60]. Other studies support the importance of this polymorphism in the genetic basis of overeating. For example, in Asian American college students, the A1 allele (versus A2 allele) was associated with greater carbohydrate craving, but not fat craving [50, 61]. Recall also that low D2 receptor density may contribute to FA via three mechanisms: impulsivity, the "reward deficiency syndrome," and emotional eating (Chaps. 7 and 8). Studies show that impulsivity and the "reward deficiency syndrome" may also be more prevalent in those with the A1 allele: obese compared with lean individuals showed a blunted striatal response to milkshake receipt, and this effect was amplified in those with the A1 allele [3, 59], and presence of that allele was found to be independently related to higher impulsivity, low reward sensitivity, and low grey matter volume in the anterior cingulate cortex (ACC) (a brain area mediating executive control) [60]. That a genetically-based low reward sensitivitywould lead to overeating is admittedly counerintuitive since heightened reward sensitivity is generally linked with addictive behavior (the better a substance or food feels, the more likely one is to return to it), but it is possible that an especially low reward sensitivity may also be a predictor, as evidenced by studies showing that reduced fat taste perception leads to greater fat consumption [50], for example. Further work is needed to confirm this, but it might be a situation where the genetic risk for development of an SUD or FA is heightened at both ends of the reward-sensitivity spectrum.

Genetic polymorphisms which are also linked to either SUD, reward sensitivity, or impulsivity have been found to increase risk for disordered eating and may be found to play a role in hedonic eating. Several genetic studies have linked polymorphisms at 5HTTLPR (in the promotor region for the that encodes for a serotonin transporter) to greater severity of SUD, as well as to higher levels of impulsivity among individuals with bulimia, with associated aberrations of serotonergic functioning being exacerbated by early life adversity [38]. Variants in the μ-opioid receptor gene (OPRM1) have been the focus of study for several decades as candidates for increasing opioid and alcohol use disorder etiology and predicting treatment-response, and early work shows variants in this gene may also play an important role in disordered eating [47]. Genetic factors may even influence the risk for inflammatory processes in the brain and gut that lead to diet-induced obesity either through more rapid fat absorption, via effects on neurotensin levels (which is a neuropeptide that interacts with the DA receptor), or via effects on the hypothalamus and resistance to leptin and insulin's effects [16, 54, 62]. Studies in humans also show that specific alleles for the CB1 receptor (implicated in both homeostatic feeding and hedonic eating via reward sensitivity) are more common in men and women with higher body fat content [5, 16]. Finally, polymorphisms in the gene encoding the CD36 receptor have been found to be associated with increased risk of obesity, and it may prove to play a role in FA as it also has been found to influence fat preference [50].

Sweet preference is a heritable trait that might prove useful to research more in the search for shared genetic underpinnings for FA and SUD. For one, genetic factors explain 50% of the variation in both sugar consumption and substance consumption (environment the other 50%) suggesting similar biological underpinnings [21]. Furthermore, in one study, men with a genetic link to AUD were also found to have a greater sweet preference than men with AUD without a genetic link [21]. Similarly, several studies of animal models that have preferences for both sweetness and alcohol have concluded that these preferences suggest strong and overlapping genetic determinants, as well [21].

9.4 In Utero Exposure

Prenatal exposure to excessive HP food intake and/or drug and alcohol use may also impact the risk for FA and SUD behaviors through effects on fetal neural reward and impulse control pathways [63]. For example, rats born to mothers fed with a palatable "junk food" diet of HP foods during gestation show an amplified preference for HP foods over healthy chow and eat beyond caloric need [63]. Prenatal exposure to high-calorie or HP diets also generates altered opioid and DA signaling in the offspring, such as increased sensitivity of μ-opioid receptor and amplified activity of DAT [63]. Furthermore, excessive exposure also leads to increased cocaine and amphetamine sensitivity as well as reduced basal dopamine levels in the VTA and striatum [16, 64]. In humans, observational studies show associations between maternal gestational diabetes and excessive weight gain during pregnancy and child adiposity in the first years of life, including weight gain promoting changes in infant eating behaviors and food preferences. The risk of obesity and effects on food preference linger through adolescence and into adulthood [63].

Similarly, prenatal exposure to substance use may also have implications for the development of disordered eating and excess weight across the lifespan, in addition to causing heightened risk of SUD-promoting behaviors in the offspring [63]. Based on studies in animal models, alcohol, cocaine, morphine, marijuana, and nicotine exposure in utero appear to cause, in the offspring, similar brain changes and alterations in neural reward circuitry as HP food exposure does and increases risk of related behaviors including weight gain and obesity [63]. In human studies, a meta-analysis concluded that prenatal exposure to maternal cigarette smoking was a consistent risk factor for overweight and obesity from ages 3 to 33 [63]. Observational studies have also identified prenatal exposure to maternal alcohol use as a risk factor for overweight and obesity in youth ages 2–19 [63].

9.5 Neuroinflammation

There is a growing literature implicating inflammation, and particularly inflammation occurring in the brain, as a common mechanism underlying obesity, eating disorders associated with binge eating, and SUD [29, 30, 65].

Studies have shown that excess intake of palatable foods, especially high-fat foods, is associated with increased inflammation in a variety of body systems and increased levels of numerous cytokines [2, 65, 66]. Adipose tissue cytokines and adipokines (e.g., adiponectin, TNF alpha, IL-6, IL-8) can also induce or reduce inflammation, with some being pro-inflammatory and diabetogenic (TNF alpha, IL-6 IL-8) and others anti-inflammatory and insulin-mimetic (I-10 adiponectin) [66], and greater body weight will also lead to more systemic and neural inflammation by adversely affecting the balance in these systems. Ghrelin, glucagon-like peptide 1 (GLP-1), and gastric inhibitory peptide (GIP) affect the immune system in various ways, too [66–68].

Neuroinflammation, in turn, influences feeding. One way it does so is via its effects in the hypothalamus [2, 65, 66]. Parts of this brain structure are not protected by the blood-brain barrier making it more accessible to inflammatory processes, and it has been shown that inflammation in the hypothalamus (especially via cytokines like TNF alpha and NF-kB) causes obesity. High-fat diets lead to changes in the hypothalamus such as reactive gliosis, neuronal injury, synaptic plasticity changes, and neurodegeneration, as well as reduced insulin sensitivity and leptin resistance, all of which ultimately causes more overeating and weight gain [2, 62, 69, 70].

Other brain regions that are fully protected by the blood-brain barrier (and which likely play important roles in regulating hedonic eating and food intake) also undergo neuroinflammatory responses after excessive intake of high-fat diet and from obesity. For example, studies show that continuous high-fat diets cause microglial activation in the PFC [71, 72], important since deficient function in this brain region can lead to deficits in attention, executive function, and impulse control [73, 74]. Obesity has been shown to increase microglial activation in the hippocampus as well [2], a state which is also associated with heightened negative affect and memory problems, both of which could lead to excessive drug and HP food-seeking via mechanisms we've already discussed at length (Chaps. 7 and 8). Long-term misuse of such HP food has also been linked to chronic neuroimmune maladaptation that may predispose individuals to neurodegenerative conditions such as Alzheimer's disease [16] and could affect weight loss abilities through adverse cognitive effects.

Neuroinflammation may also increase appetitive drive and food-seeking behavior through effects on reward sensitivity [75, 76]. For example, microglial activation in the VTA has been implicated in the pathophysiology of SUD: cocaine causes microglial activation in the VTA which then primes VTA DA neurons, leading to heightened DA release upon further drug exposure in NAc [75–78]. Notably, both +naloxone and +naltrexone [which are microglial inhibitors acting via the type 4 Toll-like receptor (TLR-4)] reverse both the DA release and cocaine reward and reinforcement behavior [75–78]. Although it is not known with certainty whether HP food causes microglial activation in the VTA, it seems likely given the known effects of high-fat diets on other brain regions. If shown true in future research, this would be another possible mechanism by which neuroinflammatory processes cause a vicious cycle of addiction.

Several other important factors can also increase inflammation and initiate the aforementioned cascades which could culminate in a habit of reward seeking and overeating. Psychological stress, as seen with early life adversity and childhood trauma studies, also causes systemic and neuroinflammation which could subsequently lead to heightened risk for impaired PFC function and reduced executive control, negative affect and anxiety, and a primed reward system, all of which could contribute to heightened risk for development of SUD or FA (Chaps. 7 and 8) [38, 79]. Oxidative stress and changes in the gut-brain-microbiome also interact with and affect neuroinflammatory processes [80].

Excitingly, there is a growing literature on the therapeutic use of anti-inflammatory medicines and/or diets for both SUD and obesity treatment. Some medicines which have been studied but not yet found to be highly effective include minocycline and phosphodiesterase inhibitors like ibudilast: although they reduce microglial activation and showed promise in animal studies, they have not been found to be effective in clinical trials, yet, but very few human studies have been done, and more work is needed [81–85]. Topiramate, which is an efficacious treatment for AUD, obesity (when combined with phentermine), and binge eating disorder (Chaps. 2, 3, and 10) may actually be working through anti-inflammatory mechanisms: it reduces TNF-alpha and has been shown to be neuroprotective [86]. Finally, studies indicate that weight regain after weight loss shows inter-individual variability and is dependent on macronutrient intake, where protein and fiber seem to be protective against weight regain—greater protein and fiber intake are associated with reduced inflammation, better adipokine secretion ratios, and reduced cellular stress [87].

9.6 Oxidative Stress

Oxidative stress (OS) results from excessive production of reactive oxygen species and reduced elimination by protective mechanisms. This kind of stress is caused by nutritional imbalances, including excess sugar and fat intake, as well as by excess use of drugs of abuse (e.g., cocaine and opiates) [80]. Other known causes of oxidative stress include excessive dopamine stimulation, as well as chronic stress, and HPA axis activation [80], which are obviously closely related to obesity and SUD, as we have discussed in previous sections and chapters.

OS is implicated in the etiology of SUD and obesity and will likely be found to play a role in hedonic eating or FA [80]. Preventing weight regain after weight loss seems to depend on an adequate intake of protein and fiber, which probably is in part due to the fact that these macronutrients reduce reactive oxygen species formation and levels in the blood [80].

There are several mechanisms by which OS may increase risk for and severity of SUD, disordered eating, and FA. For one, OS can lead to inflammation which then can then cause increased addictive behavior through mechanisms we have discussed in the previous section on inflammation

[80]. OS can also increase DA stimulation, which further promotes conditioning and habit formation [88]. Third, OS reduces executive function and could thereby contribute to impulsivity and loss of control [80]. Finally, OS can cause blunting of HPA axis and can reduce serotonin receptor expression, both of which can contribute to addictive behavior through mechanisms discussed in other previous sections in this chapter [88].

9.7 Gut Microbiome and Gut-Brain Axis

Increasing research into the gut-brain axis points to the importance of the gut microbiome in brain health, and vice versa (besides the nervous system, the gut is the most innervated organ in the body) [89]. Animal studies implicate the relevance of the gut microbiome profile in driving obesity and FA-like behavior [89–91], conclusions which are supported by associative studies in humans showing that there are distinct brain-gut-microbiome profiles in obese women and women with FA compared to controls [92], although cause and effect are not clear. However, that fecal transplant experiments in mice and humans are capable of transferring obese, and lean phenotypes from one individual to the next indicate that the gut microbiome is at least in part a causal factor for overeating behavior [66]. Recently, gut microbiota has been increasingly implicated in alcohol and other SUD as well [93, 94].

How the microbiome affects the risk and severity of these disorders is unknown but may be in part due to effects on the absorptive capacity of the gut [62, 66, 95]. Furthermore, derangements in microbiota induce inflammation through activation of pattern recognition receptors such as toll-like receptors [66], and, as we have discussed, inflammation can affect addictive behavior via several posited mechanisms. Inflammation triggered by high-fat or high-sugar diets can also cause local inflammation that leads to even greater absorption of fat and sugar, and larger, faster changes in glucose levels with HP food consumption, which can lead to even more intense conditioning effects from HP foods (Chap. 8) [96]. Impulsiveness has even been linked to gut microbiome, with one study showing that reduced microbial alpha diversity affected self-regulation [91].

9.8 Adrenergic System

The adrenergic system is important in the stress response, in inhibitory control, and in reward system sensitivity, and imbalances in this system might contribute to overeating and addictive behavior. Alpha-1 antagonists such as prazosin and doxazosin are used frequently to treat hyperarousal and nightmares in post-traumatic stress disorder, and growing evidence in humans and animals shows this category of medication may also be beneficial in reducing substance use (alcohol, opioids, stimulant), although the mechanism by which they work for SUD treatment is still unclear [97–100]. In preliminary work, prazosin has been found to also reduce binge eating in animal models [101], indicating potential promise for this relatively safe category of medicines for FA treatment; however, although they are generally safe, they are yet to be tested in human populations with overeating behaviors.

9.9 Sleep and Circadian Rhythm

Impaired sleep or insomnia is an important treatment target for patients with SUD and obesity since it clearly contributes to poorer treatment outcomes and heightened risk for relapse for both categories of disorder. Insomnia is associated with higher anxiety and depressed mood, it can reduce impulse control, memory, and executive functions, and it can increase craving and sensitivity to drug and food cues (Chaps. 2 and 8) [102–106]. Sleep debt makes the brain hypersensitive to food cues and increases appetite [107] even in people who aren't aware they need sleep. Daily feeding times, and time-linked appetitive drive, are controlled by the circadian clock in the suprachiasmatic nucleus, which has close connections with the hypothalamus and brain regions in hedonic eating pathways. Disruptions of the circadian clock (e.g., social jet-lag, shift work) lead to eating and metabolic disorders as well regardless of whether or not there is actual sleep debt [1]. Neurotransmitters and hormones that are believed to play important roles in both sleep and feeding behavior include the orexins, ghrelin, serotonin, and histamine [108].

9.10 Serotonin System

The serotonergic system plays an important role in regulating feeding behavior in general and hedonic eating in particular, likely via its positive effects on mood and impulse control [109]. As a general rule, higher serotonin levels appear to reduce feeding behavior. Higher serotonin is also associated with lower depression levels, less frequent or intense suicidal thoughts and behaviors, and reduced anxiety [109]. Serotonin also plays a role in global impulse control [38, 109]. For example, lower cerebrospinal fluid levels of 5-HT and metabolites have been reported [109] in both BED and trait impulsivity.

Agonists at the 5HT2C receptor like lorcaserin (a medication that was FDA approved for obesity treatment but taken off the market due to heightened cancer risk) (Chaps. 2 and 10) increase satiety and reduce food intake in animal models and human studies and promote weight loss, via binding to receptors in the arcuate nucleus of the hypothalamus, which leads to increased pro-opiomelanocortin production (an anorexigenic neuropeptide) (Chap. 1) [109, 110]. Interestingly, though, agonists at this receptor also reduce substance use, especially nicotine use, and they reduce hedonic eating (one study demonstrated a reduction in binge-like eating of a high-fat diet but did not affect feeding induced by deprivation [109, 110]) which indicates that it is also acting via extra-hypothalamic mechanisms as well. Mechanistic studies using electrophysiological and chemo-genetic techniques indicate that its anti-bingeing actions may be attributable to an excitatory effect on 5-HT2C receptors localized to midbrain DA neurons, which has a net effect of reducing mesolimbic DA tone, and thereby reducing reward [38, 109, 111].

9.11 Endocannabinoid System

Cannabinoids act at every point of the regulatory network that controls energy homeostasis by decreasing satiety signals and increasing orexigenic signals; they also act within the hedonic system to control pleasure-related eating [16, 29, 30, 112]. Cannabinoid type 1 receptor (CB1) receptors are located both peripherally and centrally [in the central nervous system (CNS)], and stimulation of this receptor influences preferences for fat and sugary food. Administration of agonists at the CB1 receptor, such as delta-9THC or 2-arachidonylglyceral, causes a shift towards higher-fat and sweet-fat diet preferences and stimulates food intake [5]. Blockade at the CB1 receptor, on the other hand, attenuates reinstatement of responding for Ensure by cues and causes lower levels of fat preference (with little effect on general feeding) among mice [5, 50]. CB1 antagonism also reduces drug seeking in many animal models [67, 68] and human studies (Chaps. 1 and 10). Cannabinoid type 2 (CB2) receptors are primarily located peripherally (not in the CNS), and CB2 agonists have the opposite effect, promoting weight loss [112, 113].

CB1 receptors are found throughout the cortex, including in the VTA, NAc, PFC, and hypothalamus as well as peripherally. CB1 agonists influence feeding and food choice by acting in the reward network. For one, CB1 agonists increase DA release in the NAc, stimulating VTA DA neurons [5]. Focal infusion of compounds like delta-9-THC into the NAc stimulates food intake [5]. A mouse model lacking CB1 receptors failed to develop FA behavior, which was due to the fact that the absence of this receptor also blocked excitatory glutamate transmission from the medial PFC to the NAc [114]. The CB1 receptor plays a role in synaptic plasticity and therefore in conditioning—by blocking glutamate and DA function in key brain regions and receptors, it might reduce the initiation and perpetuation of conditioning effects of HP food and possibly drugs of abuse, as well [113]. Endocannabinoids also play a role in mood, and CB1 agonists reduce stress-induced palatable food seeking [113]. Human studies support its important functional effects on reward-based eating as well: CB1 antagonists in humans reduced orbitofrontal cortex and ventral striatal activation to chocolate [3].

CB1 and CB2 both also influence eating via effects on the homeostatic system. For example, studies have shown that CB1 agonists block insulin release to a spike in sugar, blunt GLP-1 release, and increase ghrelin release all of which would theoretically increase appetite (or reduce the appetite suppressing effect of eating sugar) [115]. Antagonists at CB1 receptors might also promote weight loss via peripheral effects: CB1 receptors exist in adipose tissue, liver, and skeletal muscle, and agonists at peripheral CB1 receptors promote lipogenesis and energy storage [5, 62, 112, 113]. For this reason, peripherally restricted CB1 receptor inverse agonists are also now being explored for obesity treatment. These would potentially be beneficial in that they would have less centrally acting side effects, like depression (which was a major problem with rimonabant, a CB1 central antagonist once under study for obesity treatment), but might still increase metabolic rate and cause weight loss via peripheral mechanisms partially reducing circulating leptin levels to reverse leptin resistance [67, 68]. CB2 agonists also promote weight loss via thermogenesis, apparently transforming white adipose tissue towards beige or brown adipocytes, the latter two of which are better for weight loss; beige adipocytes have the potential to still become brown, and brown adipocytes are protective against obesity and associated with greater thermogenesis (Chap. 1) [112]. Also stimulation of CB2 receptors reduces inflammation and likely has anti-obesity effects via this mechanism as well [112].

Finally, and interestingly, highly palatable food and drugs also activate cannabinoid pathways [21]. Increased intake of highly palatable calorically dense foods heightens the activation of CB1 receptors in this region which could have a feed-forward effect but might lead to downregulation long-term [5].

9.12 Functional Connectivity

Functional connectivity is a metric derived from functional MRI or PET data that reflects the degree to which different brain regions act in synchrony with one another. Higher functional connectivity indicates that the regions are more "in sync" with one another or are more likely to activate at the same time, and therefore high connectivity between regions indicates that the structures likely exist in a network with one another. Alterations in functional connectivity in SUD are related to SUD diagnosis and SUD severity, and, in some cases, can predict treatment outcome. Altered connectivity is both caused by and contributes to problematic behavior around substance use [116].

Similar functional connectivity patterns exist in the brains of people with obesity and SUD in clusters of regions involved in executive control [executive control network (ECN)], emotional processing and introspection [default mode network (DMN)], and reward valuation and attention [salience network (SN)] [116, 117]. Specifically, obesity and SUD are both associated with reduced connectivity in the executive control network (ECN) and heightened connectivity in the salience (SN) and default mode networks (DMN) [116, 118]. People with FA also show heightened connectivity between the reward regions of the brain (striatum) and DMN, which has also been seen in SUD [40, 50, 116, 119, 120], and this heightened connectivity was, interestingly, greater in the fasted compared to fed state in one study. Other studies have been done in small samples, with some interesting findings. One study showed that greater self-control over eating was associated with negative functional connectivity between the dorsal ACC and the right anterior insula (within-SN connectivity) during a decision-making task. Authors suggested this indicated a "greater response conflict" during decision-making—the insula receives sensory signals from the body, and the dorsal ACC is a structure with more of a behavioral control function [40]. Another study reported increased connectivity between the hypothalamus and dopamine-rich regions of the ventral and dorsal striatum and insula in healthy individuals in response to a high-glucose drink [6, 121] suggesting that this palatable reward-stimulating drink increases functional coherence between the homeostatic and reward systems.

9.13 Conclusions

In summary, regulation of hedonic feeding behavior is complex and multifactorial. For one, the homeostatic systems and hedonic systems of feeding influence one another. Furthermore, there are numerous other systems and mechanisms at play. The etiology of FA is also likely very complex and affected broadly by numerous body systems and states and factors. Despite that there is a theme that runs through the last several chapters which is notable: it is striking how many commonalities there are between the biological underpinnings of hedonic eating and substance use and the development of FA and SUD.

References

1. Mendoza J. Food intake and addictive-like eating behaviors: time to think about the circadian clock(s). Neurosci Biobehav Rev. 2018;106:122–32.
2. Lin Z, Qu S. Legend of weight loss: a crosstalk between the bariatric surgery and the brain. Obes Surg. 2020;30(5):1988–2002.
3. Schlogl H, Horstmann A, Villringer A, Stumvoll M. Functional neuroimaging in obesity and the potential for development of novel treatments. Lancet Diabetes Endocrinol. 2016;4(8):695–705.
4. Bond CW, Trinko R, Foscue E, Furman K, Groman SM, Taylor JR, et al. Medial nucleus accumbens projections to the ventral tegmental area control food consumption. J Neurosci. 2020;40(24):4727–38.
5. Blanco-Gandia MC, Minarro J, Rodriguez-Arias M. Common neural mechanisms of palatable food intake and drug abuse: knowledge obtained with animal models. Curr Pharm Des. 2020;26(20):2372–84.
6. Sinha R. Role of addiction and stress neurobiology on food intake and obesity. Biol Psychol. 2018;131:5–13.
7. Cerit H, Christensen K, Moondra P, Klibanski A, Goldstein JM, Holsen LM. Divergent associations between ghrelin and neural responsivity to palatable food in hyperphagic and hypophagic depression. J Affect Disord. 2019;242:29–38.
8. DiLeone RJ. The influence of leptin on the dopamine system and implications for ingestive behavior. Int J Obes. 2009;33(Suppl 2):S25–9.
9. Aguiar-Nemer AS, Toffolo MC, da Silva CJ, Laranjeira R, Silva-Fonseca VA. Leptin influence in craving and relapse of alcoholics and smokers. J Clin Med Res. 2013;5(3):164–7.
10. Carr KD. Chronic food restriction: enhancing effects on drug reward and striatal cell signaling. Physiol Behav. 2007;91(5):459–72.
11. Onaolapo AY, Onaolapo OJ. Food additives, food and the concept of 'food addiction': is stimulation of the brain reward circuit by food sufficient to trigger addiction? Pathophysiology. 2018;25(4):263–76.
12. Malik S, McGlone F, Bedrossian D, Dagher A. Ghrelin modulates brain activity in areas that control appetitive behavior. Cell Metab. 2008;7(5):400–9.
13. Figlewicz DP, MacDonald Naleid A, Sipols AJ. Modulation of food reward by adiposity signals. Physiol Behav. 2007;91(5):473–8.
14. Jastreboff AM, Lacadie C, Seo D, Kubat J, Van Name MA, Giannini C, et al. Leptin is associated with exaggerated brain reward and emotion responses to food images in adolescent obesity. Diabetes Care. 2014;37(11):3061–8.
15. Jastreboff AM, Sinha R, Arora J, Giannini C, Kubat J, Malik S, et al. Altered brain response to drinking glucose and fructose in obese adolescents. Diabetes. 2016;65(7):1929–39.
16. Morin JP, Rodriguez-Duran LF, Guzman-Ramos K, Perez-Cruz C, Ferreira G, Diaz-Cintra S, et al. Palatable hyper-caloric foods impact on neuronal plasticity. Front Behav Neurosci. 2017;11:19.
17. Jerlhag E. Systemic administration of ghrelin induces conditioned place preference and stimulates accumbal dopamine. Addict Biol. 2008;13(3–4):358–63.
18. Wellman PJ, Clifford PS, Rodriguez JA. Ghrelin and ghrelin receptor modulation of psychostimulant action. Front Neurosci. 2013;7:171.
19. Naef L, Pitman KA, Borgland SL. Mesolimbic dopamine and its neuromodulators in obesity and binge eating. CNS Spectr. 2015;20(6):574–83.
20. Egecioglu E, Skibicka KP, Hansson C, Alvarez-Crespo M, Friberg PA, Jerlhag E, et al. Hedonic and incentive signals for body weight control. Rev Endocr Metab Disord. 2011;12(3):141–51.
21. Jeynes KD, Gibson EL. The importance of nutrition in aiding recovery from substance use disorders: a review. Drug Alcohol Depend. 2017;179:229–39.
22. Jastreboff AM, Sinha R, Lacadie C, Small DM, Sherwin RS, Potenza MN. Neural correlates of stress- and food cue-induced food craving in obesity: association with insulin levels. Diabetes Care. 2013;36(2):394–402.
23. Chao A, Grilo CM, White MA, Sinha R. Food cravings, food intake, and weight status in a community-based sample. Eat Behav. 2014;15(3):478–82.

24. Mysels DJ, Sullivan MA. The relationship between opioid and sugar intake: review of evidence and clinical applications. J Opioid Manag. 2010;6(6):445–52.
25. Volkow ND, Wang GJ, Fowler JS, Tomasi D, Baler R. Food and drug reward: overlapping circuits in human obesity and addiction. Curr Top Behav Neurosci. 2012;11:1–24.
26. D'Cunha TM, Chisholm A, Hryhorczuk C, Fulton S, Shalev U. A role for leptin and ghrelin in the augmentation of heroin seeking induced by chronic food restriction. Psychopharmacology. 2020;237(3):787–800.
27. Revitsky AR, Klein LC. Role of ghrelin in drug abuse and reward-relevant behaviors: a burgeoning field and gaps in the literature. Curr Drug Abuse Rev. 2013;6(3):231–44.
28. Morris LS, Voon V, Leggio L. Stress, motivation, and the gut-brain axis: a focus on the ghrelin system and alcohol use disorder. Alcohol Clin Exp Res. 2018; https://doi.org/10.1111/acer.13781.
29. Koob GF. Neurobiology of opioid addiction: opponent process, hyperkatifeia, and negative reinforcement. Biol Psychiatry. 2020;87(1):44–53.
30. Koob GF, Powell P, White A. Addiction as a coping response: hyperkatifeia, deaths of despair, and COVID-19. Am J Psychiatry. 2020;177(11):1031–7.
31. Boggiano MM, Chandler PC, Viana JB, Oswald KD, Maldonado CR, Wauford PK. Combined dieting and stress evoke exaggerated responses to opioids in binge-eating rats. Behav Neurosci. 2005;119(5):1207–14.
32. Torres SJ, Nowson CA. Relationship between stress, eating behavior, and obesity. Nutrition. 2007;23(11–12):887–94.
33. Kinasz KR, Ross DA Cooper JJ. Eat to live or live to eat? The neurobiology of appetite regulation. Biol Psychiatry. 2017;81(9):e73–e5.
34. Novelle MG, Dieguez C. Food addiction and binge eating: lessons learned from animal models. Nutrients. 2018;10(1):71.
35. Galanter M, Kleber HD, editors. Textbook of substance abuse treatment. 4th ed. Washington DC/ London: American Psychiatric Publishing Inc; 2008.
36. Sinha R. Chronic stress, drug use, and vulnerability to addiction. Ann N Y Acad Sci. 2008;1141:105–30.
37. Hoexter MQ, Fadel G, Felicio AC, Calzavara MB, Batista IR, Reis MA, et al. Higher striatal dopamine transporter density in PTSD: an in vivo SPECT study with [(99m)Tc]TRODAT-1. Psychopharmacology. 2012;224(2):337–45.
38. Wiss D, Brewerton T. Separating the signal from the noise: how psychiatric diagnoses can help discern food addiction from dietary restraint. Nutrients. 2020;12(10):2937.
39. Oswald LM, Wand GS, Kuwabara H, Wong DF, Zhu S, Brasic JR. History of childhood adversity is positively associated with ventral striatal dopamine responses to amphetamine. Psychopharmacology. 2014;231(12):2417–33.
40. Gordon EL, Ariel-Donges AH, Bauman V, Merlo LJ. What is the evidence for "food addiction?" a systematic review. Nutrients. 2018;10(4):477.
41. Page KA, Seo D, Belfort-DeAguiar R, Lacadie C, Dzuira J, Naik S, et al. Circulating glucose levels modulate neural control of desire for high-calorie foods in humans. J Clin Invest. 2011;121(10):4161–9.
42. Appelhans BM, Pagoto SL, Peters EN, Spring BJ. HPA axis response to stress predicts short-term snack intake in obese women. Appetite. 2010;54(1):217–20.
43. Packard AE, Egan AE, Ulrich-Lai YM. HPA axis interactions with behavioral systems. Compr Physiol. 2016;6(4):1897–934.
44. Tyrka AR, Walters OC, Price LH, Anderson GM, Carpenter LL. Altered response to neuroendocrine challenge linked to indices of the metabolic syndrome in healthy adults. Horm Metab Res. 2012;44(7):543–9.
45. Eskander N, Chakrapani S, Ghani MR. The risk of substance use among adolescents and adults with eating disorders. Cureus. 2020;12(9):e10309.
46. Treur JL, Boomsma DI, Ligthart L, Willemsen G, Vink JM. Heritability of high sugar consumption through drinks and the genetic correlation with substance use. Am J Clin Nutr. 2016;104(4):1144–50.
47. Hauck C, Cook B, Ellrott T. Food addiction, eating addiction and eating disorders. Proc Nutr Soc. 2020;79(1):103–12.
48. Wenzel KR, Weinstock J, McGrath AB. The clinical significance of food addiction. J Addict Med. 2020;14(5):e153–e9.
49. Cornelis MC, Flint A, Field AE, Kraft P, Han J, Rimm EB, et al. A genome-wide investigation of food addiction. Obesity. 2016;24(6):1336–41.
50. Sarkar S, Kochhar KP, Khan NA. Fat addiction: psychological and physiological trajectory. Nutrients. 2019;11(11):2785.
51. Botticelli L, Micioni Di Bonaventura E, Del Bello F, Giorgioni G, Piergentili A, Romano A, et al. Underlying susceptibility to eating disorders and drug abuse: genetic and pharmacological aspects of dopamine D4 receptors. Nutrients. 2020;12(8):2288.
52. Davis C, Loxton NJ, Levitan RD, Kaplan AS, Carter JC, Kennedy JL. 'Food addiction' and its association with a dopaminergic multilocus genetic profile. Physiol Behav. 2013;118:63–9.
53. Moulin TC, Ferro F, Berkins S, Hoyer A, Williams MJ, Schioth HB. Transient administration of dopaminergic precursor causes inheritable overfeeding behavior in young Drosophila melanogaster adults. Brain Sci. 2020;10(8):487.
54. Heber D, Carpenter CL. Addictive genes and the relationship to obesity and inflammation. Mol Neurobiol. 2011;44(2):160–5.
55. Davis C, Zai C, Levitan RD, Kaplan AS, Carter JC, Reid-Westoby C, et al. Opiates, overeating and obesity: a psychogenetic analysis. Int J Obes. 2011;35(10):1347–54.

56. Barth B, Bizarro L, Miguel PM, Dube L, Levitan R, O'Donnell K, et al. Genetically predicted gene expression of prefrontal DRD4 gene and the differential susceptibility to childhood emotional eating in response to positive environment. Appetite. 2020;148:104594.
57. Blum K, Oscar-Berman M, Barh D, Giordano J, Gold M. Dopamine genetics and function in food and substance abuse. J Genet Syndr Gene Ther. 2013;4(121):1000121.
58. Blum K, Thanos PK, Wang GJ, Febo M, Demetrovics Z, Modestino EJ, et al. The food and drug addiction epidemic: targeting dopamine homeostasis. Curr Pharm Des. 2018;23(39):6050–61.
59. Stice E, Spoor S, Bohon C, Small DM. Relation between obesity and blunted striatal response to food is moderated by TaqIA A1 allele. Science. 2008;322(5900):449–52.
60. Adams RC, Sedgmond J, Maizey L, Chambers CD, Lawrence NS. Food addiction: implications for the diagnosis and treatment of overeating. Nutrients. 2019;11(9):2086.
61. Yeh J, Trang A, Henning SM, Wilhalme H, Carpenter C, Heber D, et al. Food cravings, food addiction, and a dopamine-resistant (DRD2 A1) receptor polymorphism in Asian American college students. Asia Pac J Clin Nutr. 2016;25(2):424–9.
62. O'Rourke RW. The pathophysiology of obesity and obesity-related disease. In: The ASMBS textbook of bariatric surgery. Springer. https://link.springer.com/chapter/10.1007/978-3-030-27021-6_2?s...internal_7078_20200917&mkt-key=42010A0550671EEAA2988DEEB95A0F3A; 2019.
63. Schiestl ET, Rios JM, Parnarouskis L, Cummings JR, Gearhardt AN. A narrative review of highly processed food addiction across the lifespan. Prog Neuro-Psychopharmacol Biol Psychiatry. 2021;106:110152.
64. Peleg-Raibstein D, Sarker G, Litwan K, Kramer SD, Ametamey SM, Schibli R, et al. Enhanced sensitivity to drugs of abuse and palatable foods following maternal overnutrition. Transl Psychiatry. 2016;6(10):e911.
65. Thaler JP, Yi CX, Schur EA, Guyenet SJ, Hwang BH, Dietrich MO, et al. Obesity is associated with hypothalamic injury in rodents and humans. J Clin Invest. 2012;122(1):153–62.
66. O'Rourke RW. The pathophysiology of obesity and obesity-related disease. In: Nguyen N, Brethauer SA, Morton JM, Ponce J, Rosenthal RJ, editors. The ASMBS textbook of bariatric surgery. Cham: Springer; 2020.
67. Zhao S, Zhu Y, Schultz RD, Li N, He Z, Zhang Z, et al. Partial leptin reduction as an insulin sensitization and weight loss strategy. Cell Metab. 2019;30(4):706–19. e6
68. Hankir MK, Seyfried F. Partial leptin reduction: an emerging weight loss paradigm. Trends Endocrinol Metab. 2020;31(6):395–7.
69. Li J, Tang Y, Cai D. IKKbeta/NF-kappaB disrupts adult hypothalamic neural stem cells to mediate a neurodegenerative mechanism of dietary obesity and pre-diabetes. Nat Cell Biol. 2012;14(10):999–1012.
70. Chun SK, Jo YH. Loss of leptin receptors on hypothalamic POMC neurons alters synaptic inhibition. J Neurophysiol. 2010;104(5):2321–8.
71. Tramullas M, Finger BC, Dinan TG, Cryan JF. Obesity takes its toll on visceral pain: high-fat diet induces toll-like receptor 4-dependent visceral hypersensitivity. PLoS One. 2016;11(5):e0155367.
72. Guillemot-Legris O, Muccioli GG. Obesity-induced neuroinflammation: beyond the hypothalamus. Trends Neurosci. 2017;40(4):237–53.
73. Crews FT, Sarkar DK, Qin L, Zou J, Boyadjieva N, Vetreno RP. Neuroimmune function and the consequences of alcohol exposure. Alcohol Res. 2015;37(2):331–41. 44–51
74. Aurelian L, Warnock KT, Balan I, Puche A, June H. TLR4 signaling in VTA dopaminergic neurons regulates impulsivity through tyrosine hydroxylase modulation. Transl Psychiatry. 2016;6:e815.
75. Northcutt AL, Hutchinson MR, Wang X, Baratta MV, Hiranita T, Cochran TA, et al. DAT isn't all that: cocaine reward and reinforcement require toll-like receptor 4 signaling. Mol Psychiatry. 2015;20(12):1525–37.
76. Watkins LR, Wang X, Mustafa S, Hutchinson MR. In vivo veritas: (+)-Naltrexone's actions define translational importance: a letter in response to Skolnick et al. 'Translational potential of naloxone and naltrexone as TLR4 antagonists'. Trends Pharmacol Sci. 2014;35(9):432–3.
77. Bachtell R, Hutchinson MR, Wang X, Rice KC, Maier SF, Watkins LR. Targeting the toll of drug abuse: the translational potential of toll-like receptor 4. CNS Neurol Disord Drug Targets. 2015;14(6):692–9.
78. Warden A, Erickson E, Robinson G, Harris RA, Mayfield RD. The neuroimmune transcriptome and alcohol dependence: potential for targeted therapies. Pharmacogenomics. 2016;17(18):2081–96.
79. Ziobrowski HN, Buka SL, Austin SB, Sullivan AJ, Horton NJ, Simone M, et al. Using latent class analysis to empirically classify maltreatment according to the developmental timing, duration, and co-occurrence of abuse types. Child Abuse Negl. 2020;107:104574.
80. Tobore TO. Towards a comprehensive theory of obesity and a healthy diet: the causal role of oxidative stress in food addiction and obesity. Behav Brain Res. 2020;384:112560.
81. Heinzerling KG, Swanson AN, Kim S, Cederblom L, Moe A, Ling W, et al. Randomized, double-blind, placebo-controlled trial of modafinil for the treatment of methamphetamine dependence. Drug Alcohol Depend. 2010;109(1–3):20–9.
82. Ray LA, Bujarski S, Shoptaw S, Roche DJ, Heinzerling K, Miotto K. Development of the neuroimmune modulator ibudilast for the treatment

of alcoholism: a randomized, placebo-controlled, human laboratory trial. Neuropsychopharmacology. 2017;42(9):1776–88.
83. Crews FT, Lawrimore CJ, Walter TJ, Coleman LG Jr. The role of neuroimmune signaling in alcoholism. Neuropharmacology. 2017;122:56–73.
84. Ray LA, Roche DJ, Heinzerling K, Shoptaw S. Opportunities for the development of neuroimmune therapies in addiction. Int Rev Neurobiol. 2014;118:381–401.
85. Syapin PJ, Martinez JM, Curtis DC, Marquardt PC, Allison CL, Groot JA, et al. Effective reduction in high ethanol drinking by semisynthetic tetracycline derivatives. Alcohol Clin Exp Res. 2016;40(12):2482–90.
86. Su W, Xie M, Li Y, Gong X, Li J. Topiramate reverses physiological and behavioral alterations by postoperative cognitive dysfunction in rat model through inhibiting TNF signaling pathway. NeuroMolecular Med. 2020;22(2):227–38.
87. Sethi Dalai S, Sinha A, Gearhardt AN. Low carbohydrate ketogenic therapy as a metabolic treatment for binge eating and ultraprocessed food addiction. Curr Opin Endocrinol Diabetes Obes. 2020;27(5):275–82.
88. Gibson AS, Keefe KA, Furlong TM. Accelerated habitual learning resulting from L-dopa exposure in rats is prevented by N-acetylcysteine. Pharmacol Biochem Behav. 2020;198:173033.
89. De Lorenzo A, Romano L, Di Renzo L, Di Lorenzo N, Cenname G, Gualtieri P. Obesity: a preventable, treatable, but relapsing disease. Nutrition. 2020;71:110615.
90. Gupta A, Osadchiy V, Mayer EA. Brain-gut-microbiome interactions in obesity and food addiction. Nat Rev Gastroenterol Hepatol. 2020;17(11):655–72.
91. Peterson VL, Richards JB, Meyer PJ, Cabrera-Rubio R, Tripi JA, King CP, et al. Sex-dependent associations between addiction-related behaviors and the microbiome in outbred rats. EBioMedicine. 2020;55:102769.
92. Dong TS, Mayer EA, Osadchiy V, Chang C, Katzka W, Lagishetty V, et al. A distinct brain-gut-microbiome profile exists for females with obesity and food addiction. Obesity. 2020;28(8):1477–86.
93. Qin C, Hu J, Wan Y, Cai M, Wang Z, Peng Z, et al. Narrative review on potential role of gut microbiota in certain substance addiction. Prog Neuro-Psychopharmacol Biol Psychiatry. 2021;106:110093.
94. Wang SC, Chen YC, Chen SJ, Lee CH, Cheng CM. Alcohol addiction, gut microbiota, and alcoholism treatment: a review. Int J Mol Sci. 2020;21(17):6413.
95. Perrault L. Genetic contribution and pathophysiology of obesity. In: Pi-Sunyer FX, Martin KA, editors. UpToDate. Wolters Kluwer; 2018. Available from: www.uptodate.com.
96. Jamar G, Ribeiro DA Pisani LP. High-fat or high-sugar diets as trigger inflammation in the microbiota-gut-brain axis. Crit Rev Food Sci Nutr. 2021;61(5):836–54.
97. Wilcox CE, Tonigan JS, Bogenschutz MP, Clifford J, Bigelow R, Simpson T. A randomized, placebo-controlled, clinical trial of prazosin for the treatment of alcohol use disorder. J Addict Med. 2018;12(5):339–45.
98. Raskind MA, Peskind ER, Kanter ED, Petrie EC, Radant A, Thompson CE, et al. Reduction of nightmares and other PTSD symptoms in combat veterans by prazosin: a placebo-controlled study. Am J Psychiatry. 2003;160(2):371–3.
99. Rasmussen DD, Alexander LL, Raskind MA, Froehlich JC. The alpha1-adrenergic receptor antagonist, prazosin, reduces alcohol drinking in alcohol-preferring (P) rats. Alcohol Clin Exp Res. 2009;33(2):264–72.
100. Greenwell TN, Walker BM, Cottone P, Zorrilla EP, Koob GF. The alpha1 adrenergic receptor antagonist prazosin reduces heroin self-administration in rats with extended access to heroin administration. Pharmacol Biochem Behav. 2009;91(3):295–302.
101. Hicks C, Sabino V, Cottone P. The alpha-1 adrenergic receptor antagonist prazosin reduces binge-like eating in rats. Nutrients. 2020;12(6):1569.
102. Hasler BP, Soehner AM, Clark DB. Circadian rhythms and risk for substance use disorders in adolescence. Curr Opin Psychiatry. 2014;27(6):460–6.
103. Brower KJ. Insomnia, alcoholism and relapse. Sleep Med Rev. 2003;7(6):523–39.
104. Lin CY, Cheung P, Imani V, Griffiths MD, Pakpour AH. The mediating effects of eating disorder, food addiction, and insomnia in the association between psychological distress and being overweight among Iranian adolescents. Nutrients. 2020;12(5):1371.
105. Meyer RE. Craving: what can be done to bring the insights of neuroscience, behavioral science and clinical science into synchrony. Addiction. 2000;95(8s2):219–27.
106. Greer SM, Goldstein AN, Walker MP. The impact of sleep deprivation on food desire in the human brain. Nat Commun. 2013;4:2259.
107. Katsunuma R, Oba K, Kitamura S, Motomura Y, Terasawa Y, Nakazaki K, et al. Unrecognized sleep loss accumulated in daily life can promote brain hyperreactivity to food cue. Sleep. 2017;40(10) https://doi.org/10.1093/sleep/zsx137.
108. Karasu SR. Gravity of weight: the daunting science of weight control. Washington, DC: American Psychiatric Publishing Incorporated; 2010.
109. Higgins GA, Zeeb FD, Fletcher PJ. Role of impulsivity and reward in the anti-obesity actions of 5-HT2C receptor agonists. J Psychopharmacol. 2017;31(11):1403–18.
110. Xu P, He Y, Cao X, Valencia-Torres L, Yan X, Saito K, et al. Activation of serotonin 2C receptors in dopamine neurons inhibits binge-like eating in mice. Biol Psychiatry. 2017;81(9):737–47.
111. Howell LL, Cunningham KA. Serotonin 5-HT2 receptor interactions with dopamine function:

implications for therapeutics in cocaine use disorder. Pharmacol Rev. 2015;67(1):176–97.

112. Rossi F, Punzo F, Umano GR, Argenziano M, Del Giudice E. Role of cannabinoids in obesity. Int J Mol Sci. 2018;19(9):2690.
113. Coccurello R, Maccarrone M. Hedonic eating and the "delicious circle": from lipid-derived mediators to brain dopamine and back. Front Neurosci. 2018;12:271.
114. Domingo-Rodriguez L, Ruiz de Azua I, Dominguez E, Senabre E, Serra I, Kummer S, et al. A specific prelimbic-nucleus accumbens pathway controls resilience versus vulnerability to food addiction. Nat Commun. 2020;11(1):782.
115. Farokhnia M, McDiarmid GR, Newmeyer MN, Munjal V, Abulseoud OA, Huestis MA, et al. Effects of oral, smoked, and vaporized cannabis on endocrine pathways related to appetite and metabolism: a randomized, double-blind, placebo-controlled, human laboratory study. Transl Psychiatry. 2020;10(1):71.
116. Wilcox CE, Abbott CC, Calhoun VD. Alterations in resting-state functional connectivity in substance use disorders and treatment implications. Prog Neuro-Psychopharmacol Biol Psychiatry. 2018;91:79–93.
117. Peng-Li D, Sorensen TA, Li Y, He Q. Systematically lower structural brain connectivity in individuals with elevated food addiction symptoms. Appetite. 2020;155:104850.
118. Donofry SD, Stillman CM, Erickson KI. A review of the relationship between eating behavior, obesity and functional brain network organization. Soc Cogn Affect Neurosci. 2020;15(10):1157–81.
119. Contreras-Rodriguez O, Burrows T, Pursey KM, Stanwell P, Parkes L, Soriano-Mas C, et al. Food addiction linked to changes in ventral striatum functional connectivity between fasting and satiety. Appetite. 2019;133:18–23.
120. Contreras-Rodriguez O, Martin-Perez C, Vilar-Lopez R, Verdejo-Garcia A. Ventral and dorsal striatum networks in obesity: link to food craving and weight gain. Biol Psychiatry. 2017;81(9):789–96.
121. Page KA, Sinha R, Sherwin RS. Differential effects of fructose and glucose on cerebral blood flow–reply. JAMA. 2013;309(17):1769.

10 Treatment-Related Evidence that Food Addiction Is a Valid Construct

10.1 Pharmacotherapy-Related Evidence

10.1.1 Stimulants

Several stimulant medications are currently FDA-approved for the treatment of BED (lisdexamfetamine) and obesity (topiramate/phentermine, bupropion/naltrexone), and these medicines reduce binging and promote weight loss [1–10]. Over the last several decades, several other medicines in the stimulant class have been tested, were found to be effective, and were FDA-approved for weight loss, but subsequently were taken off the market for adverse effects (e.g., fenfluramine/phentermine, sibutramine, lorcaserin) [8, 11]. Older FDA-approved stimulants, such as diethylpropion, benzphetamine, and phendimetrazine, are rarely used because they are only FDA-approved for short-term use, thus limiting their efficacy [2]. Atomoxetine, another medication in the stimulant class, is utilized off-label for binge eating reduction when individuals have comorbid attention-deficit hyperactivity disorders (ADHD) (atomoxetine), and tesofensine is in the stimulant class and being studied [1, 12].

Stimulant medications also have and continue to be studied for the treatment of SUD, especially cocaine and methamphetamine use disorders, and although the results are mixed, stimulants are also occasionally used to treat illicit stimulant use disorders in clinical practice [13, 14]. There is even promising data for the use of stimulants in combination with topiramate for cocaine and methamphetamine use disorders [15, 16]. That said, none of the stimulants approved for the treatment of obesity or BED have yet been found to be effective in stimulant use disorders. Bupropion, though, is a mainstay of treatment for nicotine use disorder and is FDA-approved for smoking cessation [13].

All stimulants inhibit reuptake of norepinephrine and dopamine, thereby causing increases in dopamine and norepinephrine in the synapse [8]. As centrally acting sympathomimetic agents, stimulants are directly anorexigenic and suppress appetite [8]; any drug that increases norepinephrine in the brain causes hypophagia, weight loss, and, in some cases, increased energy expenditure [1, 17, 18]. However, another mechanism by which stimulants work in both SUD and obesity/binge-based eating disorders (ED) is by reducing impulsivity [19] and improving dorsolateral prefrontal cortex (DLPFC) and cognitive function [17, 19–22]. If this mechanism is a primary reason for their efficacy, as data suggests, it would indicate a possible mechanism by which it works in both SUD and disorders of overeating. Indeed, bupropion, lisdexamfetamine, and atomoxetine are mainstays of treatment for attention deficit hyperactivity disorder (ADHD), a condition characterized by impulsivity, and lisdexamfetamine is FDA approved for ADHD as well as BED treatment [16, 19, 20].

C. E. Wilcox, *Food Addiction, Obesity, and Disorders of Overeating*,
https://doi.org/10.1007/978-3-030-83078-6_10

Research is needed to test long-term outcomes of lisdexamfetamine and other stimulant medications in people with FA. It may prove important to consider the presence of ADHD when conceptualizing FA phenotypes in the context of medication choices as has been done in early work in cocaine use disorders, where researchers have found that people with comorbid ADHD have more clinical improvement on a stimulant than those without [14]. One might surmise that FA would predict a better response to treatment with stimulants in people with BED or obesity too, since FA, like ADHD, is characterized by high levels of impulsivity. Surprisingly, though, one study found that a stimulant was *not* effective in adults who screened positive for FA on the Yale Food Addiction Scale (YFAS) compared with controls [23–25], which was theorized to be due to the fact that the stimulant oversensitized the reward system. A priming mechanism may also explain why, despite extensive study, stimulants for the treatment of stimulant use disorder have been found to be only marginally effective. Further work to investigate for whom stimulants are most helpful, and for whom stimulants are most harmful, in reducing overeating is needed.

10.1.2 Opioid Antagonists

Opioid blockers have been studied for the treatment of BED and bulimia, but demonstrate mixed efficacy in human research when used alone [26]. Indeed, some studies indicate bupropion alone may work just as well for weight loss as the combination naltrexone-bupropion medication [2, 9]. Animal studies have shown that μ-opioid receptor antagonists reduce hedonic eating behavior and associated brain pathway function.

Naltrexone is both FDA approved for and used as a first-line treatment for alcohol use disorder (AUD) and opioid use disorder (OUD) [13, 27, 28]. Naltrexone may reduce SUD and overeating behaviors via similar biological mechanisms. As discussed in detail in Chap. 8, μ-opioid receptor agonists have hedonic properties; therefore antagonists block hedonic effects. Dopamine contributes to the hedonic experience of drug and food consumption and plays an important role in conditioning [29, 30]. Antagonists at μ-opioid receptors will reduce dopamine release in the nucleus accumbens (NAc) in response to drug use and palatable food ingestion [28, 29, 31]. In this way naltrexone likely works for both SUD and binge eating/obesity by reducing the pleasure experienced with consumption (mediated by dopamine and opioids), the perpetuation of conditioning effects (mediated by dopamine and glutamate), and the ability of environmental drug or food cues to trigger craving (mediated by opioids and dopamine) [19, 28, 29, 31].

Several human studies support that naltrexone and opioid antagonists act via these mechanisms in obesity and binge eating. GSK1521498, an experimental μ-opioid receptor antagonist reduced hedonic preferences for high-calorie foods and reduced calorie intake in binge-eating obese subjects [32–34]. It also reduced brain activation to high-calorie food images in the pallidum/putamen, a brain region recognized as central to motivational and hedonic components of reward-seeking behavior [33, 34].

In AUD and OUD, naltrexone blocks both craving and cue-induced brain activation as well [13, 27, 28, 35] and reduces use and conditioning by blocking the "high" associated with drug use [13, 27]. A growing body of work also indicates that naltrexone may be useful in improving global impulse control, although this effect may be limited to μ- agonist-triggered impulsivity (e.g., impulsivity after consuming something pleasurable) rather than general impulsivity [19, 36]. One study showed that 4 weeks of combined naltrexone/bupropion not only caused decreased activation in the hypothalamus in response to food cues, supporting the possibility that the treatment has some beneficial effects on homeostatic appetitive mechanisms, but also increased activation in the anterior cingulate cortex (ACC), superior frontal cortex, superior parietal cortex, insula, and hippocampus, the latter findings of which might indicate beneficial effects on impulse control [37–39]. Whether increased cortical response might have been due to bupropion rather than naltrexone is not known. Naltrexone might also improve impulse control and cause restoration of prefrontal functioning in AUD, though, in support of this possibility [40].

10.1.3 Topiramate and Zonisamide

Topiramate, which has been extensively studied, and zonisamide, another promising medication in the same class with fewer side effects, are both effective in BED, reducing binge eating and promoting weight loss compared to placebo. When used in combination with phentermine, topiramate is approved for obesity treatment by the FDA [1, 7, 8, 41]. Zonisamide reduces binge eating and weight, as well, but effects on weight may be more pronounced than on binge eating [41], particularly when used in combination with bupropion [42]. Both drugs not only have direct appetite suppressant effects, but they also have effects on hedonic eating pathways as discussed below [1, 7, 8, 41].

Topiramate, and to a lesser degree zonisamide, have been studied in a wide variety of SUD. Topiramate is highly effective in AUD and possibly effective in stimulant use disorder especially when used in combination with a stimulant [13, 14, 43–45]. Topiramate has also been shown to reduce impulsivity in individuals with AUD [46].

The exact mechanism of effect of these two anticonvulsant medications on eating and substance use behavior is not entirely clear, since the drugs affect many neurotransmitter systems. They have GABA agonist activity, glutamate AMPA antagonist effects, block voltage-dependent sodium channels, and inhibit carbonic anhydrase activity, all of which could affect reward and impulse control circuits [8, 41, 44, 47]. Furthermore, there is growing evidence that topiramate may reduce neuroinflammation and have other neuroprotective effects [48]. Via GABA agonist activity, they may cause reduction in withdrawal symptoms and anxiety; via blockade of AMPA glutamate receptors, they may block ability of drug or food cues to trigger craving (Chap. 8); via dopamine and glutamate, they may reduce reinforcing effects and hedonic properties [41]; and via glutamate and neuroinflammation, they may reduce global impulsivity [44, 46].

10.1.4 GLP-1 Agonists

GLP-1 agonists such as liraglutide, semaglutide, and exenatide are indicated for the treatment of type 1 diabetes and obesity, reducing insulin resistance and enhancing weight loss [1, 2, 10, 49–51]. It is not known whether they reduce binge eating in BED, but this is an area of active study [10]. This class of medicines is also being studied in SUD based on promising results in animal models indicating potential efficacy [52], although whether they work in human populations is still unknown.

These agents have a primary effect on appetite and weight by directly affecting hypothalamic homeostatic circuitry [1, 37, 53, 54]. Recall, GLP-1 is a hormone released by the gut that works on homeostatic feeding circuits by binding to receptors in the hypothalamus, directly stimulating proopiomelanocortin release and the activity of other hypothalamic anorexigenic neurons, and intestinal vagal afferents to activate neurons in the nucleus tractus solitarius [1, 37, 53, 54]. Exenatide, a GLP-1 agonist, increased connectivity between the hypothalamus and other brain regions in neuroimaging studies, and in those whose connectivity was not altered, no anorectic effect was seen [37, 53]. However, other work indicates that GLP-1 agonists also act directly on reward networks, prompting the study of its role in SUD. For example, animal data shows that GLP-1 activates the reward system including the ventral tegmental area (VTA) and the NAc [1, 55]. Specifically, infusion of a GLP-1 agonist into the VTA and NAc reduced motivated behavior for sucrose in animals [55, 56]. In humans, liraglutide decreased the activation in insula and putamen in response to highly versus less desirable food images and decreased insular activation to a meal [37, 39, 50], indicating reductions in reward system reactivity. Finally GLP-1 agonists may enhance hippocampal functioning, indicating promise for improvement in memory and cognitive systems important for self-control [51], but whether these medicines also affect impulse control circuits is still only speculative.

10.1.5 Other Medications to Note

Selective serotonin reuptake inhibitors (SSRIs) are not FDA approved for BED treatment, but most treatment recommendations for BED suggest SSRIs be first-line, if pharmacotherapy is used [7, 19]. They are not very effective for SUD behavior reduction or weight loss, in obesity, although they are clearly very useful in the case of a comorbid anxiety or depressive disorder [13]. SSRIs have widespread benefits on mood, cognition, feeding, satiety, appetite, and impulsivity and reduce "yo-yo dieting" [19]. However, they might not specifically be useful for FA.

Alpha-1 adrenergic antagonists (prazosin and doxazosin), which are being more frequently studied in AUD and stimulant use disorder [57, 58], have also been found to reduce binge eating in animal models [59]. Mechanisms that could explain the cross-diagnostic benefit include reductions in irritability, improvement in sleep and hyperarousal [this class of medicines is utilized frequently for this purpose in post-traumatic stress disorder (PTSD)], and reductions in craving and cue reactivity [57, 58, 60].

Lorcaserin is an agonist at 5-HT2C receptors. This medication was well-studied for the treatment of obesity and finally FDA approved after being found to reduce caloric intake and promote weight loss [1, 2, 34, 39, 61]. Further research indicated it was also beneficial in nicotine use disorder and helped promote smoking cessation [34, 61, 62]. However, this medicine was recently taken off the market for concerns of increased cancer risk [11]. In animal models, 5HT2C receptor agonists reduce feeding behavior and operant responding for food in such a way that suggests that this class of medications works directly on reward circuitry [34, 61]. For example, it blocks conditioned responding, self-administration, and conditioned place preference behaviors maintained by several drugs of abuse including cocaine, nicotine, ethanol, and opioids [34, 61]. In humans, meta-chlorophenylpiperazine (mCPP), another 5HT2c agonist, was found to reduce reward eating (palatable cookie snack) but did not affect eating when hungry (pasta meal) [34, 39, 63, 64]. It also blocked food cue-induced activation in parietal and visual cortex, amygdala, insula, DLPFC, and ACC [34, 39, 63], and changes in the brain activation in reward areas were correlated with weight loss effects [34, 64]. Moreover, greater baseline activation of the amygdala was found to be associated with increased efficacy, suggesting that lorcaserin or 5HT2C drugs might be of particular benefit to emotional eaters, which might also imply a mechanism by which they reduce substance use in SUD [34, 64].

As reviewed in Chap. 9, and as discussed in Murphy et al., CB1 agonists stimulate the reward system [65]. Rimonabant, a CB1 antagonist was one drug designed to block this effect, and which had potential for both SUD and obseity, but it was taken off the market because it was associated with depression side effects [37, 65].

10.2 Bariatric Surgery

Bariatric surgeries are the most effective treatments for obesity in terms of weight loss and maintenance, and they cause reductions in caloric intake, changes in food preferences from high to low energy foods, reduction in binge eating, and reduction in FA symptoms [39]. Of course, it is also the most invasive set of treatments available and they come with several surgically related risks, as discussed in Chaps. 2 and 4. Bariatric surgery likely exerts its effects through many of the same mechanisms as do effective treatments for SUD, e.g., by restoring the balance between the reward and inhibitory control systems. That said, there are many studies that show addiction transfer can (but does not always) occur post bariatric surgery (reviewed in Chap. 6), which would not be expected to occur if surgery caused resolution of all reward circuitry imbalances. In addition, this is certainly not an intervention under study for the treatment of SUD. That said, the fact that it reverses brain changes also seen and believed to underlie SUD behavior reinforces the validity of the FA construct.

For one, bypass surgery may dampen appetite for sweet foods by interfering with postprandial striatal dopamine release, as evidenced in a rodent study [66, 67]. Reduced dopamine release to eating could subsequently lead to reductions in the conditioning effect and the power of cues such as visual or taste cues to trigger craving.

Moreover, studies with gastric bypass patients have demonstrated increased D2 receptor availability following weight loss [68, 69]. Recall from Chap. 10 that people with SUD and who suffer from overeating disorders have D2 receptor downregulation in the striatum, which is believed to contribute to impaired impulse control and "reward deficiency" to natural rewards [68–71]. Bariatric surgery seems to reverse this deficit.

Furthermore, bariatric surgery also shows pronounced effects on brain activity. First, it can alter neural activity in brain regions related to taste perception and reward in humans [66, 72]. Multiple fMRI and other imaging studies show decreased activation after surgery in the reward network and other brain regions to food cues (fusiform gyrus, parahippocampal gyrus, medial prefrontal cortex, inferior frontal gyrus, insula, and striatum) and increased activation in inhibitory control regions (i.e., DLPFC) [39, 68, 71, 73–77]. Activation in the hypothalamus and OFC in response to glucose ingestion was also reduced to levels similar to those of lean controls 8 months post-surgery [37, 78]. Studies in rats have similarly shown reduced neural activity in regions related to taste perception and reward [66, 72]. Again, these studies indicate that bariatric surgery restores the brain to more normal states. These brain changes are also associated with lower reports of cravings and less hunger and less behavioral disinhibition [39, 73]. Relatedly, reductions in visual attentional bias towards food cues after obesity surgery using an eye-tracking paradigm have been observed [79].

In fact, it appears that the surgeries may be directly affecting hedonic and inhibitory control-mediating brain circuits, rather than the brain circuits simply changing as a consequence of weight loss. For example, one group compared the fMRI data from 16 behavioral dieters and 15 patients after obesity surgery with similar weight loss amounts of about 10% and found that the behavioral dieters showed increased responses to food cues in the medial prefrontal cortex when compared to patients with obesity surgery [39, 80]. Another study compared a weight loss behavioral intervention with bariatric surgery and found that the surgical patients demonstrated increased DLPFC and decreased memory network (parahippocampal gyrus) activation to high energy diet versus low energy diet, whereas those with behavior intervention and no surgery showed the opposite effects in these brain regions [39, 77]. Furthermore, patients who are less successful at losing weight after surgery were shown to have reduced activation of the areas of the brain involved in inhibition but no significant change in the reward areas compared with their more successful weight loss counterparts [39, 81]. These brain changes are associated with improved global cognitive function [66].

Functional connectivity studies have also shown reversal of some typical deficits seen in both overeaters and individuals with SUD (Chap. 9), namely, reductions in heightened DMN connectivity and restoration of impaired connectivity in and between brain regions involved in executive control [39, 82].

Finally, one mechanism by which these surgeries restore reward and inhibitory control brain networks may be via effects on the gut microbiome. For example, a recent study demonstrated that improvement in loss of control around feeding was associated with changes in the brain-gut-microbiome axis in obese women [83]. As discussed in Chap. 9, there is a growing appreciation of the role of the brain-gut-microbiome axis in regulating behavior and impulse control in both SUD and overeating.

10.3 Conclusion

Treatments for disorders of overeating (BED and obesity) overlap with treatment for SUDs and target similar brain regions and mechanisms affected by both. Unfortunately, pharmacological treatment for both still requires substantial research given the limited effectiveness of the current available treatments.

References

1. Coulter AA, Rebello CJ, Greenway FL. Centrally acting agents for obesity: past, present, and future. Drugs. 2018;78:1113–32.
2. Gadde KM, Atkins KD. The limits and challenges of antiobesity pharmacotherapy. Expert Opin Pharmacother. 2020;21:1319–28.
3. Davis H, Attia E. Pharmacotherapy of eating disorders. Curr Opin Psychiatry. 2017;30:452–7.
4. Hudson JI, McElroy SL, Ferreira-Cornwell MC, Radewonuk J, Gasior M. Efficacy of lisdexamfetamine in adults with moderate to severe binge-eating disorder: a randomized clinical trial. JAMA Psychiat. 2017;74:903–10.
5. Gadde KM, Allison DB, Ryan DH, Peterson CA, Troupin B, Schwiers ML, et al. Effects of low-dose, controlled-release, phentermine plus topiramate combination on weight and associated comorbidities in overweight and obese adults (CONQUER): a randomised, placebo-controlled, phase 3 trial. Lancet. 2011;377:1341–52.
6. Carbone EA, Caroleo M, Rania M, Calabrò G, Staltari FA, de Filippis R, et al. An open-label trial on the efficacy and tolerability of naltrexone/bupropion SR for treating altered eating behaviours and weight loss in binge eating disorder. Eat Weight Disord. 2021;26:779–88.
7. Wilcox CE. Binge eating disorder. CMEtoGo.com. American Physician Institute; 2019.
8. Vardanyan GS, Harutyunyan HS, Aghajanov MI, Vardanyan RS. Neurochemical regulators of food behavior for pharmacological treatment of obesity: current status and future prospects. Future Med Chem. 2020;12:1865–84.
9. Greenway FL, Fujioka K, Plodkowski RA, Mudaliar S, Guttadauria M, Erickson J, et al. Effect of naltrexone plus bupropion on weight loss in overweight and obese adults (COR-I): a multicentre, randomised, double-blind, placebo-controlled, phase 3 trial. Lancet. 2010;376:595–605.
10. Chao AM, Wadden TA, Walsh OA, Gruber KA, Alamuddin N, Berkowitz RI, et al. Effects of liraglutide and behavioral weight loss on food cravings, eating behaviors, and eating disorder psychopathology. Obesity. 2019;27:2005–10.
11. FDA requests the withdrawal of the weight-loss drug Belviq, Belviq XR (lorcaserin) from the market [Internet]. U.S. Food & Drug Administration. 2020 [cited 2021 Apr 23]. Available from: https://www.fda.gov/drugs/drug-safety-and-availability/fda-requests-withdrawal-weight-loss-drug-belviq-belviq-xr-lorcaserin-market
12. Gadde KM, Yonish GM, Wagner HR 2nd, Foust MS, Allison DB. Atomoxetine for weight reduction in obese women: a preliminary randomised controlled trial. Int J Obes. 2006;30:1138–42.
13. Wilcox CE, Bogenschutz MB. Psychopharmacologies for alcohol and drug use disorders. In: McCrady BS, Epstein EE, editors. Addictions: a comprehensive guidebook. 2nd ed. New York: Oxford University Press; 2013. p. 526–50.
14. Blevins D, Choi CJ, Pavlicova M, Martinez D, Mariani JJ, Grabowski J, et al. Impulsiveness as a moderator of amphetamine treatment response for cocaine use disorder among ADHD patients. Drug Alcohol Depend. 2020;213:108082.
15. Mariani JJ, Pavlicova M, Bisaga A, Nunes EV, Brooks DJ, Levin FR. Extended-release mixed amphetamine salts and topiramate for cocaine dependence: a randomized controlled trial. Biol Psychiatry. 2012;72:950–6.
16. Levin FR, Mariani JJ, Pavlicova M, Choi CJ, Mahony AL, Brooks DJ, et al. Extended release mixed amphetamine salts and topiramate for cocaine dependence: a randomized clinical replication trial with frequent users. Drug Alcohol Depend. 2020;206:107700.
17. Wiss D, Brewerton T. Separating the signal from the noise: how psychiatric diagnoses can help discern food addiction from dietary restraint. Nutrients. 2020;12:2937. https://doi.org/10.3390/nu12102937.
18. Jeffers A, Benotsch EG, Koester S. Misuse of prescription stimulants for weight loss, psychosocial variables, and eating disordered behaviors. Appetite. 2013;65:8–13.
19. Hutson PH, Balodis IM, Potenza MN. Binge-eating disorder: clinical and therapeutic advances. Pharmacol Ther. 2018;182:15–27.
20. McElroy SL, Hudson JI, Mitchell JE, Wilfley D, Ferreira-Cornwell MC, Gao J, et al. Efficacy and safety of lisdexamfetamine for treatment of adults with moderate to severe binge-eating disorder: a randomized clinical trial. JAMA Psychiat. 2015;72:235–46.
21. Brady KT, Gray KM, Tolliver BK. Cognitive enhancers in the treatment of substance use disorders: clinical evidence. Pharmacol Biochem Behav. 2011;99:285–94.
22. Spencer RC, Devilbiss DM, Berridge CW. The cognition-enhancing effects of psychostimulants involve direct action in the prefrontal cortex. Biol Psychiatry. 2015;77:940–50.
23. Joos L, Goudriaan AE, Schmaal L, Fransen E, van den Brink W, Sabbe BGC, et al. Effect of modafinil on impulsivity and relapse in alcohol dependent patients: a randomized, placebo-controlled trial. Eur Neuropsychopharmacol. 2013;23:948–55.
24. Davis C, Levitan RD, Kaplan AS, Kennedy JL, Carter JC. Food cravings, appetite, and snack-food consumption in response to a psychomotor stimulant drug: the moderating effect of "food-addiction". Front Psychol. 2014;5:403.
25. Gordon EL, Ariel-Donges AH, Bauman V, Merlo LJ. What is the evidence for "food addiction?" A systematic review. Nutrients. 2018;10(4):477.
26. Valbrun LP, Zvonarev V. The opioid system and food intake: use of opiate antagonists in treatment of binge

eating disorder and abnormal eating behavior. J Clin Med Res. 2020;12:41–63.
27. Anton RF, O'Malley SS, Ciraulo DA, Cisler RA, Couper D, Donovan DM, et al. Combined pharmacotherapies and behavioral interventions for alcohol dependence: the COMBINE study: a randomized controlled trial. JAMA. 2006;295:2003–17.
28. Myrick H, Anton RF, Li X, Henderson S, Randall PK, Voronin K. Effect of naltrexone and ondansetron on alcohol cue-induced activation of the ventral striatum in alcohol-dependent people. Arch Gen Psychiatry. 2008;65:466–75.
29. Morales I, Berridge KC. "Liking" and "wanting" in eating and food reward: brain mechanisms and clinical implications. Physiol Behav. 2020;227:113152.
30. Berridge KC, Robinson TE, Aldridge JW. Dissecting components of reward: "liking", "wanting", and learning. Curr Opin Pharmacol. 2009;9:65–73.
31. Giraudo SQ, Billington CJ, Levine AS. Effects of the opioid antagonist naltrexone on feeding induced by DAMGO in the central nucleus of the amygdala and in the paraventricular nucleus in the rat. Brain Res. 1998;782:18–23.
32. Ziauddeen H, Chamberlain SR, Nathan PJ, Koch A, Maltby K, Bush M, et al. Effects of the mu-opioid receptor antagonist GSK1521498 on hedonic and consummatory eating behaviour: a proof of mechanism study in binge-eating obese subjects. Mol Psychiatry. 2013;18:1287–93.
33. Cambridge VC, Ziauddeen H, Nathan PJ, Subramaniam N, Dodds C, Chamberlain SR, et al. Neural and behavioral effects of a novel mu opioid receptor antagonist in binge-eating obese people. Biol Psychiatry. 2013;73:887–94.
34. Higgins GA, Zeeb FD, Fletcher PJ. Role of impulsivity and reward in the anti-obesity actions of 5-HT2C receptor agonists. J Psychopharmacol. 2017;31:1403–18.
35. Mann K, Vollstädt-Klein S, Reinhard I, Leménager T, Fauth-Bühler M, Hermann D, et al. Predicting naltrexone response in alcohol-dependent patients: the contribution of functional magnetic resonance imaging. Alcohol Clin Exp Res. 2014;38:2754–62.
36. Pattij T, Schetters D, Janssen MCW, Wiskerke J, Schoffelmeer ANM. Acute effects of morphine on distinct forms of impulsive behavior in rats. Psychopharmacology. 2009;205:489–502.
37. Schlögl H, Horstmann A, Villringer A, Stumvoll M. Functional neuroimaging in obesity and the potential for development of novel treatments. Lancet Diabetes Endocrinol. 2016;4:695–705.
38. Wang G-J, Tomasi D, Volkow ND, Wang R, Telang F, Caparelli EC, et al. Effect of combined naltrexone and bupropion therapy on the brain's reactivity to food cues. Int J Obes. 2014;38:682–8.
39. Lin Z, Qu S. Legend of weight loss: a crosstalk between the bariatric surgery and the brain. Obes Surg. 2020;30:1988–2002.
40. Boettiger CA, Kelley EA, Mitchell JM, D'Esposito M, Fields HL. Now or later? An fMRI study of the effects of endogenous opioid blockade on a decision-making network. Pharmacol Biochem Behav. 2009;93:291–9.
41. McElroy SL, Kotwal R, Guerdjikova AI, Welge JA, Nelson EB, Lake KA, et al. Zonisamide in the treatment of binge eating disorder with obesity: a randomized controlled trial. J Clin Psychiatry. 2006;67:1897–906.
42. Srivastava G, Apovian C. Future pharmacotherapy for obesity: new anti-obesity drugs on the horizon. Curr Obes Rep. 2018;7:147–61.
43. Johnson BA, Rosenthal N, Capece JA, Wiegand F, Mao L, Beyers K, et al. Topiramate for treating alcohol dependence: a randomized controlled trial. JAMA. 2007;298:1641–51.
44. Johnson BA, Ait-Daoud N. Topiramate in the new generation of drugs: efficacy in the treatment of alcoholic patients. Curr Pharm Des. 2010;16:2103–12.
45. Rubio G, López-Muñoz F, Ferre F, Martínez-Gras I, Ponce G, Pascual JM, et al. Effects of zonisamide in the treatment of alcohol dependence. Clin Neuropharmacol. 2010;33:250–3.
46. Rubio G, Martínez-Gras I, Manzanares J. Modulation of impulsivity by topiramate: implications for the treatment of alcohol dependence. J Clin Psychopharmacol. 2009;29:584–9.
47. Rawls SM, Thomas T, Adeola M, Patil T, Raymondi N, Poles A, et al. Topiramate antagonizes NMDA- and AMPA-induced seizure-like activity in planarians. Pharmacol Biochem Behav. 2009;93:363–7.
48. Su W, Xie M, Li Y, Gong X, Li J. Topiramate reverses physiological and behavioral alterations by postoperative cognitive dysfunction in rat model through inhibiting TNF signaling pathway. NeuroMolecular Med. 2020;22:227–38.
49. Khalil H, Ellwood L, Lord H, Fernandez R. Pharmacological treatment for obesity in adults. An umbrella review. Ann Pharmacother. 2020;54:691–705.
50. Farr OM, Sofopoulos M, Tsoukas MA, Dincer F, Thakkar B, Sahin-Efe A, et al. GLP-1 receptors exist in the parietal cortex, hypothalamus and medulla of human brains and the GLP-1 analogue liraglutide alters brain activity related to highly desirable food cues in individuals with diabetes: a crossover, randomised, placebo-controlled trial. Diabetologia. 2016;59:954–65.
51. Clasen MM, Riley AL, Davidson TL. Hippocampal-dependent inhibitory learning and memory processes in the control of eating and drug taking. Curr Pharm Des. 2020;26:2334–52.
52. Hernandez NS, Schmidt HD. Central GLP-1 receptors: novel molecular targets for cocaine use disorder. Physiol Behav. 2019;206:93–105.
53. Schlögl H, Kabisch S, Horstmann A, Lohmann G, Müller K, Lepsien J, et al. Exenatide-induced reduction in energy intake is associated with increase in hypothalamic connectivity. Diabetes Care. 2013;36:1933–40.
54. De Silva A, Salem V, Long CJ, Makwana A, Newbould RD, Rabiner EA, et al. The gut hormones PYY 3-36

and GLP-1 7-36 amide reduce food intake and modulate brain activity in appetite centers in humans. Cell Metab. 2011;14:700–6.
55. van Bloemendaal L, Ten Kulve JS, la Fleur SE, Ijzerman RG, Diamant M. Effects of glucagon-like peptide 1 on appetite and body weight: focus on the CNS. J Endocrinol. 2014;221:T1–16.
56. Dickson SL, Shirazi RH, Hansson C, Bergquist F, Nissbrandt H, Skibicka KP. The glucagon-like peptide 1 (GLP-1) analogue, exendin-4, decreases the rewarding value of food: a new role for mesolimbic GLP-1 receptors. J Neurosci. 2012;32:4812–20.
57. Wilcox CE, Tonigan JS, Bogenschutz MP, Clifford J, Bigelow R, Simpson T. A randomized, placebo-controlled, clinical trial of prazosin for the treatment of alcohol use disorder. J Addict Med. 2018;12:339–45.
58. Sinha R. Prazosin for the treatment of alcohol use disorders. Am J Psychiatry. 2018;175(12):1159–60.
59. Hicks C, Sabino V, Cottone P. The Alpha-1 adrenergic receptor antagonist prazosin reduces binge-like eating in rats. Nutrients. 2020;12(6):1569. https://doi.org/10.3390/nu12061569.
60. Wilcox CE, Pommy J, Adinoff BA, Bigelow RC, Mayer AR. Prazosin decreases striatal BOLD response to conditioned threat stimulus in alcohol use disorder. Recent Dev Alcohol. 2015;26:102162.
61. Higgins GA, Sellers EM, Fletcher PJ. From obesity to substance abuse: therapeutic opportunities for 5-HT2C receptor agonists. Trends Pharmacol Sci. 2013;34:560–70.
62. Shanahan WR, Rose JE, Glicklich A, Stubbe S, Sanchez-Kam M. Lorcaserin for smoking cessation and associated weight gain: a randomized 12-week clinical trial. Nicotine Tob Res. 2017;19:944–51.
63. Thomas JM, Dourish CT, Tomlinson J, Hassan-Smith Z, Hansen PC, Higgs S. The 5-HT2C receptor agonist meta-chlorophenylpiperazine (mCPP) reduces palatable food consumption and BOLD fMRI responses to food images in healthy female volunteers. Psychopharmacology. 2018;235:257–67.
64. Farr OM, Upadhyay J, Gavrieli A, Camp M, Spyrou N, Kaye H, et al. Lorcaserin administration decreases activation of brain centers in response to food cues and these emotion- and salience-related changes correlate with weight loss effects: a 4-week-long randomized, placebo-controlled, double-blind clinical trial. Diabetes. 2016;65:2943–53.
65. Murphy T, Le Foll B. Targeting the endocannabinoid CB1 receptor to treat body weight disorders: a preclinical and clinical review of the therapeutic potential of past and present CB1 drugs. Biomolecules. 2020;10(6):855. https://doi.org/10.3390/biom10060855.
66. Morin J-P, Rodríguez-Durán LF, Guzmán-Ramos K, Perez-Cruz C, Ferreira G, Diaz-Cintra S, et al. Palatable hyper-caloric foods impact on neuronal plasticity. Front Behav Neurosci. 2017;11:19.
67. Han W, Tellez LA, Niu J, Medina S, Ferreira TL, Zhang X, et al. Striatal dopamine links gastrointestinal rerouting to altered sweet appetite. Cell Metab. 2016;23:103–12.
68. Adams RC, Sedgmond J, Maizey L, Chambers CD, Lawrence NS. Food addiction: implications for the diagnosis and treatment of overeating. Nutrients. 2019;11(9):2086. https://doi.org/10.3390/nu11092086.
69. van der Zwaal EM, de Weijer BA, van de Giessen EM, Janssen I, Berends FJ, van de Laar A, et al. Striatal dopamine D2/3 receptor availability increases after long-term bariatric surgery-induced weight loss. Eur Neuropsychopharmacol. 2016;26:1190–200.
70. Steele KE, Prokopowicz GP, Schweitzer MA, Magunsuon TH, Lidor AO, Kuwabawa H, et al. Alterations of central dopamine receptors before and after gastric bypass surgery. Obes Surg. 2010;20:369–74.
71. Ochner CN, Kwok Y, Conceição E, Pantazatos SP, Puma LM, Carnell S, et al. Selective reduction in neural responses to high calorie foods following gastric bypass surgery. Ann Surg. 2011;253:502–7.
72. Thanos PK, Michaelides M, Subrize M, Miller ML, Bellezza R, Cooney RN, et al. Roux-en-Y gastric bypass alters brain activity in regions that underlie reward and taste perception. PLoS One. 2015;10:e0125570.
73. Bruce JM, Hancock L, Bruce A, Lepping RJ, Martin L, Lundgren JD, et al. Changes in brain activation to food pictures after adjustable gastric banding. Surg Obes Relat Dis. 2012;8:602–8.
74. Frank S, Wilms B, Veit R, Ernst B, Thurnheer M, Kullmann S, et al. Altered brain activity in severely obese women may recover after Roux-en Y gastric bypass surgery. Int J Obes. 2014;38:341–8.
75. Behary P, Miras AD. Food preferences and underlying mechanisms after bariatric surgery. Proc Nutr Soc. 2015;74:419–25.
76. Hansen TT, Jakobsen TA, Nielsen MS, Sjödin A, Le Roux CW, Schmidt JB. Hedonic changes in food choices following Roux-en-Y gastric bypass. Obes Surg. 2016;26:1946–55.
77. Baboumian S, Pantazatos SP, Kothari S, McGinty J, Holst J, Geliebter A. Functional magnetic resonance imaging (fMRI) of neural responses to visual and auditory food stimuli pre and post Roux-en-Y Gastric bypass (RYGB) and sleeve gastrectomy (SG). Neuroscience. 2019;409:290–8.
78. van de Sande-Lee S, Pereira FRS, Cintra DE, Fernandes PT, Cardoso AR, Garlipp CR, et al. Partial reversibility of hypothalamic dysfunction and changes in brain activity after body mass reduction in obese subjects. Diabetes. 2011;60:1699–704.
79. Schäfer L, Schmidt R, Müller SM, Dietrich A, Hilbert A. Changes in visual attention towards food cues after obesity surgery: an eye-tracking study. J Psychiatr Res. 2020;129:214–21.
80. Bruce AS, Bruce JM, Ness AR, Lepping RJ, Malley S, Hancock L, et al. A comparison of functional brain

changes associated with surgical versus behavioral weight loss. Obesity. 2014;22:337–43.

81. Goldman RL, Canterberry M, Borckardt JJ, Madan A, Byrne TK, George MS, et al. Executive control circuitry differentiates degree of success in weight loss following gastric-bypass surgery. Obesity. 2013;21:2189–96.
82. Li G, Ji G, Hu Y, Xu M, Jin Q, Liu L, et al. Bariatric surgery in obese patients reduced resting connectivity of brain regions involved with self-referential processing. Hum Brain Mapp. 2018;39:4755–65.
83. Dong TS, Gupta A, Jacobs JP, Lagishetty V, Gallagher E, Bhatt RR, et al. Improvement in uncontrolled eating behavior after laparoscopic sleeve gastrectomy is associated with alterations in the brain-gut-microbiome axis in obese women. Nutrients. 2020;12(10):2924. https://doi.org/10.3390/nu12102924.

11 Highly Palatable Foods Are Addictive

11.1 Problematic and "Addictive" Foods

The construct of FA is usually discussed with specific relevance to high-fat (particularly high in trans-fat or saturated fat) [1, 2], high-sugar [3, 4], high-salt, highly processed, highly refined, high-glycemic index foods [3, 5–8] and foods containing high-fructose corn syrup [3, 4]. These kinds of foods are also more generally palatable [4, 5, 7, 9–11] and have an innate capacity to promote their own overconsumption [12–15]. However, one single macronutrient isn't likely to blame. Indeed, many of the foods listed on the Yale Food Addiction Scale (YFAS; e.g., chocolate, ice cream, French fries, pizza, cookies, chips, cake, sodas, breakfast cereal, potato chips) are also not found in nature but "processed," meaning extra sugars, refined carbohydrates such as white flour, and fats are added to maximize palatability [3–5, 7, 16, 17]. Foods that are "addictive" (meaning foods that are consumed in ways that are harmful and consumption is continued, despite significant consequences [18]) often contain high amounts of both sweet and fat, the combination being more commonly associated with addictive symptoms than sugar alone [4, 19]. But "whole foods" can also sometimes be addictive too: in humans, nuts (typically considered a whole food, without added sugars) were rated more addictive on average than granola bars (typically processed, with added sugars and fats) [4, 16, 17]. Highly processed foods were also self-reported as being uniquely related to symptoms of FA [16, 17].

That said, as a general rule, foods that are naturally occurring and minimally processed such as fruits, vegetables, lean meats, and brown rice are reported by participants to rarely induce addictive-like eating [4, 16, 17]. Foods that are high in dietary protein and high in fiber with whole grains tend also to increase satiety and limit weight gain [12, 20–22], with a high-fiber (pectin) diet leading to increased levels of the satiety hormones GLP-1 and PYY and weight loss in obese rats accustomed to a high-fat diet [23]. Protein and fiber may also promote weight loss via beneficial effects on inflammatory processes, adipokine secretion, cellular stress, and extracellular matrix remodeling [24].

11.2 Association Between HP Food Intake and Addiction in Animal Models

As reviewed in detail in Chap. 8, highly palatable (HP) food consumption can clearly cause obesity and disordered eating behaviors in animal models [12, 25–27]. HP foods induce obesity in rodents who would not otherwise have become obese, and the weight gain persists and increases even after they are switched back to normal chow [12]. Rats given intermittent access to sugar dis-

C. E. Wilcox, *Food Addiction, Obesity, and Disorders of Overeating*,
https://doi.org/10.1007/978-3-030-83078-6_11

play a repertoire of behaviors and brain modifications (bingeing, craving, and cross-sensitization) that are characteristic of rats that voluntarily self-administer addictive drugs [25, 28]. High-fat diets have a more immediate effect than high-sugar diets, higher-fat diets stimulating an even greater acute desire to overconsume, and induce shorter latency between meals [28]. By contrast, there has been no evidence for addictive-like symptoms to develop in relation to rodent chow alone [4, 27].

11.3 Association Between HP Food Intake and Weight Gain/Disordered Eating in Humans

In the general population, fast foods such as potato chips, processed meats and sugar-sweetened beverages all predicted long-term weight gain in large prospective cohorts of US men and women [29, 30]. Higher food craving for these HP foods, in particular, was observed in a community sample, and higher food craving was significantly associated with greater intake of these foods, and those with higher body mass index (BMI) reported greater levels of craving for these foods [31].

In terms of FA in particular, in a qualitative study using a semi-structured interview of people with binge eating disorder (BED) probing for *Diagnostic and Statistical Manual of Mental Disorders* (DSM V) substance use disorder (SUD) symptoms, participants noticed that only highly processed foods triggered symptoms such as consuming more than intended, persistent desire but unsuccessful attempts to cut down, continued use despite persistent physical or psychological problems and cravings [17]. In other work, highly processed foods are implicated in symptoms such as compulsive need to have them around, high levels of craving, and feeling addicted. This is characterized by preoccupation and loss of control and is triggered by situational cues such as negative affect and being home alone in other qualitative studies in women [19, 32–34]. Subjects with high FA scores report a high consumption of saturated fat, as well [1, 2].

11.4 Why Are HP Foods More Associated with Addictive Eating Patterns?

11.4.1 Innate Preferences

Three tastes have been described with regard to innate food preferences: sugar, fat or lipids, and umami (the taste of glutamate, which adds a savory flavor to food) [12]. Sugar, in particular, is easily detected by the sweet taste receptors in the oral cavity, and it elicits a strong taste or flavor preference in many animals [12]. Several studies have also reported that foods that are high in protein are less innately liked than low-protein foods [12, 35, 36].

Highly processed foods are modified by the food industry to match common innate preferences to maximize palatability [5, 12]. The combination of fat and sugar in highly processed foods doesn't occur generally in naturally occurring foods, which may give these foods an additive rewarding effect in the gut and brain [12, 17, 37].

11.4.2 Conditioning from Rapid Post-oral Glucose Rise

Interestingly, most flavor preferences are learned; however conditioning (see Chaps. 7 and 8) [12, 38, 39] can happen for fat and sugar and their combination and can be especially enhanced by the post-oral actions of sugars (e.g., the rise in blood glucose after consumption) [12, 40]. Recall that a food's addictive potential is dependent on the rate of its absorption and metabolism (Chap. 8), which speaks to the effects of conditioning mediated by the post-oral rise in glucose [16, 41, 42]. Indeed, absorbed foods that contain sucrose or fructose but that also have high fiber contents (e.g., fruit) may not be prone to causing brain changes that lead to conditioning and binge use or overconsumption because the fiber limits rapid absorption [43]. Related to this is the glucostatic theory which theorizes that the intensity of sugar spikes after eating and the glycemic index of foods drive food intake [24, 44–46].

11.4.3 Stimulation of Reward System by HP Foods

Consumption of diets high in sugar, fat, or both stimulate the brain reward system in ways that are similar to drugs of abuse and thereby stimulate excessive eating [12, 47]. Neurochemically, as we have discussed in Chap. 8, this includes dopamine and opioid release in the nucleus accumbens (NAc), basolateral amygdala, and cortical areas [1, 12, 26, 48, 49]. Compared to less palatable foods, foods higher in sugar have more powerful effects on the reward system. In one study participants consumed 5 g of a commercially available chocolate with increasing amounts of sugar (90% cocoa, 85% cocoa, 70% cocoa, and milk chocolate) with the higher sugar content leading to higher scores on the excitement subscale, higher well-being, and greater euphoria [50, 51]. Several studies have also reported that foods that are high in protein are less liked than low-protein foods [12, 35, 36]. There is clear evidence that the composition of a high sugar diet can also affect the subsequent intake of drugs of abuse [26, 28, 52]: for example, sugar-dependent rats have been shown to exhibit increased alcohol intake, indicating priming of the reward system and increased reward sensitivity due to prior sugar exposure [28, 53].

11.4.4 Effects on Inflammatory Processes, Oxidative Stress and Gut Microbiome

Highly processed foods, as opposed to healthier foods (such as those high in antioxidants), impact appetitive behavior via effects on neurohormonal and inflammatory signaling pathways as well [9, 11]. Oxidative stress caused by consumption of pro-oxidant foods can lead to gut dysbiosis, resistance to leptin and insulin, increases in ghrelin, disordered sleep, and chronic inflammation [11].

11.4.5 Cessation Leads to Withdrawal

As discussed in Chap. 8, and as has been demonstrated in numerous studies, excessive consumption of sugar followed by sudden cessation leads to measurable withdrawal symptoms in animals, with increased anxiety, a heightened stress response, and elevated palatable food seeking during discontinuation [54]. The evidence for withdrawal from high-fat diets in animals is less compelling [54]. As discussed in Chap. 6, and as has been demonstrated in numerous studies, food withdrawal occurs in human populations as well. High-fat sweet and high-fat savory foods may be more likely than low-fat sugary foods to cause tolerance and withdrawal in human populations, which differs slightly from animals [4, 19]. In addition, cessation of highly processed foods are especially likely to precipitate withdrawal as has been validated in the development of the " Highly Processed Food Withdrawal Scale" for clinical use [3, 17, 55–58].

11.4.6 Adverse Effects on Mood and Anxiety

Depression and anxiety occur at higher rates in obesity, eating disorders (ED), and FA (Chap. 6). This is likely a bidirectional relationship: depressed or anxious individuals may turn to highly palatable foods to alleviate negative affect and then the short-term mood enhancing effect of the palatable food fuels addictive behavior via negative reinforcement.

HP foods have adverse long term effects on mood via several other mechanisms as well [9]. Overweight and obesity can increase negative mood due to stigma and physical limitations [9], for one. Furthermore, deficits in antioxidants and micronutrients in an unbalanced diet can cause mood deterioration [11, 59], with pro-inflammatory foods and low-fiber foods appearing to be especially problematic [9, 60, 61].

Indeed, HP foods, which are most enjoyable initially, cause more long-term mood troubles than other kinds of food. For example, a Spanish cohort of graduate students initially free of depression (n = 14,907) was followed for a median 10.3 years in one study. Participants with the highest consumption of ultra-processed foods had the highest risk of developing depression over time, particularly among those with low levels of physical activity [9, 62]. Another large French cohort of adults followed for a mean of 5.4 years demonstrated a positive association between ultra-processed food and the risk of incident depression [9, 63]. Furthermore, anxiety disorders show a dose–response association with worsening diet quality, such that higher levels of processed foods are associated with greater anxiety [9]. The role of gastrointestinal microbiota has also received attention as a potential mediator linking poor diet quality to anxiety and mood symptoms [9, 64, 65]. A randomized controlled trial (RCT) showed that dietary support (nutrition counseling by a dietitian) for 12 weeks can improve depression symptoms [9, 66]. Compelling evidence for beneficial mood effects exists for the Mediterranean diet, known for its anti-inflammatory properties, which appears to have an antidepressant [67] and anxiolytic effect [9, 68].

11.4.7 Reduction in Executive Function

In animal models and humans, high-fat diets and the obese state are associated with and likely cause impulsivity and deterioration in executive function (reviewed in Chap. 8), which contributes to loss of control of food intake [9–11, 41, 69, 70]. High-fat foods cause several other cognitive impairments, including memory deficits [41, 71–74], as does nutritional deficiency when not consuming a balanced diet [11] although tere may be some cognitive and cardiac benefits of mono-unsaturated fatty acid and controlled amounts of saturated fat intake with some additional measureable benefits in synaptic connectivity, and membrane stability [1, 75]. But more work to find out the ideal amounts and kinds of fat to consume for optimal brain health is needed.

11.4.8 Reduction in Satiety Due to Changes in Homeostatic Feeding

In Chap. 1 we discussed the hormonal and hypothalamic mechanisms underlying homeostatic feeding. These systems can be affected by HP foods to cause impaired satiety mechanisms. Highly palatable foods interfere with post-ingestive satiety processes and reduce the effectiveness with which intestinal and post-absorptive satiation signals suppress food intake [12, 76]. In particular, high-sucrose and high-carbohydrate foods can cause blood sugar and insulin spikes (whereas high-fat foods do not) which is believed to cause lower satiety [24, 44].

Exposure to sucrose and glucose causes animals to modify their feeding behavior with binge-like consumption, "eating when not physically hungry", and feeding beyond the daily energy requirements, thereby contributing to weight gain and obesity [12, 77].

Trans-fat may lead to greater short-term consumption than polyunsaturated fat, as the latter is more rapid than the former to trigger satiety [1]. Chronic exposure to foods high in fat raise the body's adiposity and satiation threshold via effects on insulin and leptin and ghrelin, such that higher degrees of change in levels of these hormone are required to adequately suppress feeding [12, 14]. Interestingly, neurons sensitive to fat in the hypothalamus (arcuate and ventromedial nucleus of the hypothalamus, primarily) when chronically stimulated become less sensitive (downregulate) over time in response to long-chain fatty acids, but not to polyunsaturated fatty acids, partially explaining the beneficial effects of the latter over the former [78].

By contrast, foods high in dietary protein tend to increase the perception of satiety [12, 20, 79]. A high-protein diet can induce several weight-loss benefiting changes (Chap. 2) including increased release of gut-derived, anorexigenic proteins glucagon-like peptide-1, cholecystokinin, and peptide-tyrosine-tyrosine and reduced release of orexigenic hormone ghrelin [80]. These effects increase satiety signaling and eventually reduce food intake [80].

11.4.9 Individual Variability

That said, not all people have equal degrees of susceptibility to develop "addiction" to these foods [59, 81]. Sugars, fats, and highly processed foods affect human and animal behavior in those at risk for developing obesity differently than in those not at risk [12, 16, 25, 27, 81–83]. People with high reward sensitivity show a higher preference for sweet and fat foods as well as increased alcohol consumption, binge eating and other addictive behaviors compared to those with low reward sensitivity, for example [59, 84].

11.4.10 Feeding Patterns Influence Food Addiction

The way a substance or food is consumed may alter the way in which the reward system responds and the degree of conditioning that ensues [25, 28, 53, 85]. Research in animal models has mainly focused on two models of feeding in studies of overeating: the continuous access model and the limited access model [28]. The continuous access model (wherein animals have ad libitum access to HP food) leads to obesity and metabolic syndrome, while the limited access model (intermittent access to HP food) leads to binge eating and progressive increases in intake in fat and sugar over time [28].

Continuous access produces long-term decreases in striatal dopamine concentrations and dopamine-transporter density [28, 86–89]. By contrast, intermittent access produces a persistently activated dopaminergic system as escalation occurs, more similar to changes seen in SUD, leading animals that would otherwise be satiated to overeat for pleasure and reward [8, 28, 54, 90, 91]. Rats that binge either on sugar or fat also exhibit enhanced locomotor sensitization to cocaine and amphetamine, stronger continued place preference, and more quickly develop cocaine self-administration, whereas these behaviors do not seem to occur after exposure to continuously administered diets [28].

The continuous access models may apply more to obesity, in a general sense, whereas the intermittent and limited access model may more accurately mirror BED and FA. If this is true, this would indicate that treatment of FA needs to include a stabilization component (which we will discuss more in Chap. 13) – e.g., frequently stopping and starting or engaging in semi-starvation will only make things worse. It also is in line with traditional eating disorder treatment models that argue that cessation of binging is the most important element for mental health, even if that means letting go of short-term goals to lose weight [92]. That said, continuous exposure to these foods encourages obesity too, which is not conducive to physical health and wellness. Success will likely depend on finding an appropriate balance between restricting consumption of certain foods while still allowing enough "healthy" food, in FA food plans.

11.5 State Effects of Hunger/Food Restriction on Reward Circuitry and Brain Function

Satiety, and related homeostatic indicators, affects the degree of pleasure experienced, the degree of reward, and the brain's response to food [59]. When someone is hungry or food-deprived, food is pleasurable [28], and activity in DA reward systems have heightened response to palatable, energy-rich food, which could lead to increasing consumption of HP food later on, due to conditioning effects [28, 59, 90, 93]. By contrast, food is unpleasant after satiation [28]. Food restriction also enhances the positive effects of μ-opioid agonism on binge eating behavior [59, 94]. Indeed, food deprivation lowers the threshold for activation of reward pathways in a general sense, increasing sensitivity to drugs of abuse as well as food [59, 93] potentially further reinforcing consumption of either [59].

Variance in brain activity to food from satiated to fasting states may have clinical relevance. For example, FA symptoms are associated with activation in the ventral striatum, amygdala, anterior insula, and medial and lateral orbitofrontal cortex (OFC) to high-calorie versus low-calorie foods, but only in a fasted session [95]. Increased intra-individual variability in the NAc's response to highly palatable food between fasting and fed states correlated with higher BMI, as well as higher variance in food intake and glucose levels [96, 97].

Sensitivity to food cues also increases during food restriction which may feed into greater craving and attentional bias for food cues [98]. Increased activation in reward-related brain regions to food cues [putamen, caudate, reward and motivation; OFC, reward; anterior cingulate cortex (ACC), visual cortex, ventromedial prefrontal cortex (vmPFC), attention; precentral gyrus, motivation; hippocampus, memory] were found to be greater during calorie-deficient states, and brain reward systems are also more biased towards high-calorie foods when calorie deficient [59, 95, 99]. Fasting for hours correlated positively with activation in regions implicated in attention (ACC), reward (putamen, OFC), and motivation (precentral gyrus) in response to food cues [100, 101]. Negative energy balance for 2 weeks (weight loss ≥1 kg) resulted in increased activation in attention (ACC, vmPFC, superior visual cortex) and reward (caudate) regions in response to food cues [100, 101]. Finally, mild food restriction resulted in increased HP food craving, activation of striatal and emotional regions in response to HP food pictures, and increases in plasma cortisol [29, 102]. Relatedly, increased food cue reactivity was observed on a liquid-only diet compared to a calorie-matched solid diet in the ACC, the left insular cortex, the bilateral NAc, the primary motor cortex, the OFC, and the bilateral dorsolateral prefrontal cortex (DLPFC) [101, 108].

Although short-term deprivation increases reward sensitivity and cravings for avoided foods, long-term restriction and weight loss results in reduction of food cravings that can facilitate extinction of conditioned responses [9, 109]. Indeed, several studies in patients who lost weight through dieting (Chap. 8) or bariatric surgery also show reduced conditioned responses (e.g., cue reactivity) over time (Chap. 10). Moreover, a healthy diet and weight loss can restore objective measures of cognitive functioning and PFC recruitment (Chaps. 8 and 10).

11.6 Artificial Sweeteners and Sugar Substitutes

Polyols (mannitol, sorbitol, isomalt, lactitol, maltitol, polydextrose, and xylitol) are nutritive and high in fiber and have very low-calorie content [12, 105]. When consumed in large quantities, they have laxative effects. Polyols don't appear to cause addiction in animal studies, and some of them have been found to increase satiety and reduce energy intake [12, 105]. Effects on satiety may be mediated in part by their high fiber content, as well as induction of GLP1 and peptide YY release, reduced ghrelin release, and delays in gastric emptying [12].

Non-nutritive sweeteners (NNS) (acesulfame-K, aspartame, neo-tame, saccharin, sucralose, and stevia) have no effect on blood sugar [12, 106]. NNS in an energy-animal increases hunger in some studies, but not others, and, if given with food/calories, increases in hunger are minimal [12]. Furthermore, animals prefer NNS over water, but nutritive sugar over NNS, indicating that NNS don't induce the same type or degree of reward as sugar. Human studies don't indicate strong effects on appetite or satiety of NNS [12, 106].

Several imaging studies support their safety in terms of addictive potential. The ingestion of sucrose as opposed to sucralose causes greater activation in "higher gustatory areas" including the orbitofrontal cortex, insula and amygdala, and reward areas like striatum and anterior cingulate cortex, but both sucrose and sucralose cause similar activation in primary taste pathways [107]. This is likely due to the fact that although they both stimulate sweet sensory pathways, the post-ingestion component of glucose consumption, i.e., the blood sugar rise that leads to conditioning, does not occur with sucralose. It is posited that these differences reflect greater dopamine release in reward areas to sucrose compared to sucralose [12, 41, 107, 108]. Sucralose also doesn't cause the same hypothalamic signal depression that is seen in response to sucrose [12, 109].

Therefore, it can be said that polyols and NNS do not elicit the same effects on appetite, satiety, conditioned preferences, or the brain reward circuit as is observed with sugars. Also, they are not likely to potentiate the effects of other foods or lead to conditioning although more research is needed.

11.7 What Should Be Considered Addictive Food?

The use of glycemic index, protein, and fat content in weight loss diets has produced varied results, and no single approach has been found to work better for weight loss or maintenance (Chap. 2). However, there are a few clear messages across human and animal neuroscience studies, observational studies, randomized controlled trials, and epidemiological analyses that can inform nutritional recommendations for people with FA (see Table 11.1). One message is that although excessive consumption of simple sugars and fats has adverse effects, data suggests a more definitive adverse role for simple sugars than for fats in obesity, ED, and FA [24]. Second, foods high in protein, fiber, and micronutrients are helpful for satiety and cardiometabolic health. Third, carbohydrates, when consumed as fruit or whole grains such as oats and barley, are associated with decreased cardiometabolic risk factors and weight [46, 110], whereas sugary foods such as sugar sweetened beverages, sweetened breakfast cereals and desserts, and foods high in refined white flour are likely best to avoid [45, 111]. Fourth, data from human studies suggests that the combination of sugar and fat is more commonly associated with addictive symptoms than sugar or fat alone [4, 19]. Finally, and perhaps most importantly, highly processed and highly refined foods, and foods designed to maximize palatability, are wise to avoid almost completely [45, 111].

Table 11.1 Foods that have been associated with FA, binge eating and obesity ("foods to avoid"), and foods that are less associated with these conditions ("foods to encourage") [7, 11, 34, 35]. See also https://www.drfuhrman.com/

Foods to avoid	Examples
High fat	Steak, bacon, hamburgers, cheeseburgers, pizza, and French fries
High fat/high sugar	Ice cream, chocolate, doughnuts, cookies, cake, candy
High-fructose corn syrup/high sugar	Candy, soda pop, lemonade, sports drinks, and energy drinks
High salt	Chips, pretzels, and crackers
Highly processed/refined	Baked goods, candy, packaged snack foods
High glycemic index	White bread, high sugar cereal, white rice
Inflammatory (pro-oxidant)	Deep fried foods, red/processed meats, sugary sodas, margarine/butter, white rice, pizza/pasta
Foods to encourage	Examples
Fruits	Antioxidant-rich: grapes, plum, pineapple, lemon, date, kiwi, clementine, grapefruit, pomegranates, cherries, blueberries
Vegetables	Antioxidant-rich: broccoli, peppers, asparagus, chard, kale, cabbage, brussels sprouts, eggplant, tomatoes, onions
Lean meats	Chicken, eggs, seafood
Whole grains	Brown rice
High fiber	Fruits, vegetables, legumes, nuts
High protein	Lean meats, lentils, beans

11.8 Conclusion

There is still controversy about whether some natural foods, such as sugar, are truly addictive and whether all highly processed foods should be considered addictive for all people [17, 112]. Despite this controversy, the vast majority of data indicates that FA exists and that it is more like a substance use disorder than a behavioral disorder, with certain food components having clear toxic effects on brain function, behavior, and physical health; alternate nosology to reflect the above findings might be considered, i.e., instead of food addiction, "refined food use disorder," "highly palatable food use disorder," or simply "food use disorder" [4, 43, 113–115].

References

1. Sarkar S, Kochhar KP, Khan NA. Fat addiction: psychological and physiological trajectory. Nutrients. 2019;11:2785. https://doi.org/10.3390/nu11112785.
2. Pursey KM, Collins CE, Stanwell P, Burrows TL. Foods and dietary profiles associated with "food addiction" in young adults. Addict Behav Rep. 2015;2:41–8.
3. Ifland JR, Preuss HG, Marcus MT, Rourke KM, Taylor WC, Burau K, et al. Refined food addiction: a classic substance use disorder. Med Hypotheses. 2009;72:518–26.
4. Gordon EL, Ariel-Donges AH, Bauman V, Merlo LJ. What is the evidence for "food addiction?" a systematic review. Nutrients. 2018;10(4):477. https://doi.org/10.3390/nu10040477.
5. Gearhardt AN, Davis C, Kuschner R, Brownell KD. The addiction potential of hyperpalatable foods. Curr Drug Abuse Rev. 2011;4:140–5.
6. Pretlow RA. Addiction to highly pleasurable food as a cause of the childhood obesity epidemic: a qualitative Internet study. Eat Disord. 2011;19:295–307.
7. Gearhardt AN, Corbin WR, Brownell KD. Development of the Yale Food Addiction Scale Version 2.0. Psychol Addict Behav. 2016;30:113–21.
8. Adams RC, Sedgmond J, Maizey L, Chambers CD, Lawrence NS. Food addiction: implications for the diagnosis and treatment of overeating. Nutrients. 2019;11:2086. https://doi.org/10.3390/nu11092086.
9. Wiss D, Brewerton T. Separating the signal from the noise: how psychiatric diagnoses can help discern food addiction from dietary restraint. Nutrients. 2020;12:2937. https://doi.org/10.3390/nu12102937.
10. Small DM, DiFeliceantonio AG. Processed foods and food reward. Science. 2019;363:346–7.
11. Tobore TO. Towards a comprehensive theory of obesity and a healthy diet: the causal role of oxidative stress in food addiction and obesity. Behav Brain Res. 2020;384:112560.
12. Onaolapo AY, Onaolapo OJ. Food additives, food and the concept of "food addiction": is stimulation of the brain reward circuit by food sufficient to trigger addiction? Pathophysiology. 2018;25:263–76.
13. Berthoud H-R. Metabolic and hedonic drives in the neural control of appetite: who is the boss? Curr Opin Neurobiol. 2011;21:888–96.
14. Ryan KK, Woods SC, Seeley RJ. Central nervous system mechanisms linking the consumption of palatable high-fat diets to the defense of greater adiposity. Cell Metab. 2012;15:137–49.
15. Egecioglu E, Skibicka KP, Hansson C, Alvarez-Crespo M, Friberg PA, Jerlhag E, et al. Hedonic and incentive signals for body weight control. Rev Endocr Metab Disord. 2011;12:141–51.
16. Schulte EM, Avena NM, Gearhardt AN. Which foods may be addictive? The roles of processing, fat content, and glycemic load. PLoS One. 2015;10:e0117959.
17. Schulte EM, Wadden TA, Allison KC. An evaluation of food addiction as a distinct psychiatric disorder. Int J Eat Disord. 2020;53:1610–22.
18. ASAM Definition of Addiction [Internet]. American Society of Addiction Medicine. 2019 [cited 2021 May 2]. Available from: https://www.asam.org/Quality-Science/definition-of-addiction
19. Markus CR, Rogers PJ, Brouns F, Schepers R. Eating dependence and weight gain; no human evidence for a "sugar-addiction" model of overweight. Appetite. 2017;114:64–72.
20. Luhovyy BL, Akhavan T, Anderson GH. Whey proteins in the regulation of food intake and satiety. J Am Coll Nutr. 2007;26:704S–12S.
21. Sivertsen HK, Ueland O, Westad F. Development of satiating and palatable high-protein meat products by using experimental design in food technology. Food Nutr Res. 2010;54 https://doi.org/10.3402/fnr.v54i0.5114.
22. Larsen TM, Dalskov S-M, van Baak M, Jebb SA, Papadaki A, Pfeiffer AFH, et al. Diets with high or low protein content and glycemic index for weight-loss maintenance. N Engl J Med. 2010;363:2102–13.
23. Adam CL, Gratz SW, Peinado DI, Thomson LM, Garden KE, Williams PA, et al. Effects of dietary fibre (pectin) and/or increased protein (casein or pea) on satiety, body weight, adiposity and caecal fermentation in high fat diet-induced obese rats. PLoS One. 2016;11:e0155871.
24. San-Cristobal R, Navas-Carretero S, Martínez-González MÁ, Ordovas JM, Martínez JA. Contribution of macronutrients to obesity: implications for precision nutrition. Nat Rev Endocrinol. 2020;16:305–20.
25. Avena NM, Rada P, Hoebel BG. Evidence for sugar addiction: behavioral and neurochemical effects of intermittent, excessive sugar intake. Neurosci Biobehav Rev. 2008;32:20–39.
26. Avena NM, Gold JA, Kroll C, Gold MS. Further developments in the neurobiology of food and addiction: update on the state of the science. Nutrition. 2012;28:341–3.

27. Johnson PM, Kenny PJ. Dopamine D2 receptors in addiction-like reward dysfunction and compulsive eating in obese rats. Nat Neurosci. 2010;13:635–41.
28. Blanco-Gandía MC, Miñarro J, Rodríguez-Arias M. Common neural mechanisms of palatable food intake and drug abuse: knowledge obtained with animal models. Curr Pharm Des. 2020;26:2372–84.
29. Sinha R. Role of addiction and stress neurobiology on food intake and obesity. Biol Psychol. 2018;131:5–13.
30. Mozaffarian D, Hao T, Rimm EB, Willett WC, Hu FB. Changes in diet and lifestyle and long-term weight gain in women and men. N Engl J Med. 2011;364:2392–404.
31. Chao A, Grilo CM, White MA, Sinha R. Food cravings, food intake, and weight status in a community-based sample. Eat Behav. 2014;15:478–82.
32. Malika NM, Hayman LW Jr, Miller AL, Lee HJ, Lumeng JC. Low-income women's conceptualizations of food craving and food addiction. Eat Behav. 2015;18:25–9.
33. Paterson C, Lacroix E, von Ranson KM. Conceptualizing addictive-like eating: a qualitative analysis. Appetite. 2019;141:104326.
34. Atkinson FS, Foster-Powell K, Brand-Miller JC. International tables of glycemic index and glycemic load values: 2008. Diabetes Care. 2008;31:2281–3.
35. Fuhrman J. Smart Nutrition, Superior Health [Internet]. [cited 2021 May 9]. Available from: https://www.drfuhrman.com/
36. Bachmanov AA, Bosak NP, Floriano WB, Inoue M, Li X, Lin C, et al. Genetics of sweet taste preferences. Flavour Fragr J. 2011;26:286–94.
37. Johnson J, Vickers Z. Factors influencing sensory-specific satiety. Appetite. 1992;19:15–31.
38. DiFeliceantonio AG, Small DM. Dopamine and diet-induced obesity. Nat Neurosci. 2019;22(1):1–2.
39. Yamamoto T, Ueji K. Brain mechanisms of flavor learning. Front Syst Neurosci. 2011;5:76.
40. Sclafani A, Ackroff K. Role of gut nutrient sensing in stimulating appetite and conditioning food preferences. Am J Physiol Regul Integr Comp Physiol. 2012;302:R1119–33.
41. Myers KP, Sclafani A. Conditioned enhancement of flavor evaluation reinforced by intragastric glucose. II. Taste reactivity analysis. Physiol Behav. 2001;74:495–505.
42. Morin J-P, Rodríguez-Durán LF, Guzmán-Ramos K, Perez-Cruz C, Ferreira G, Diaz-Cintra S, et al. Palatable hyper-caloric foods impact on neuronal plasticity. Front Behav Neurosci. 2017;11:19.
43. Criscitelli K, Avena NM. The neurobiological and behavioral overlaps of nicotine and food addiction. Prev Med. 2016;92:82–9.
44. Lustig RH, Schmidt LA, Brindis CD. Public health: the toxic truth about sugar. Nature. 2012;482:27–9.
45. Sethi Dalai S, Sinha A, Gearhardt AN. Low carbohydrate ketogenic therapy as a metabolic treatment for binge eating and ultraprocessed food addiction. Curr Opin Endocrinol Diabetes Obes. 2020;27:275–82.
46. Sievenpiper JL. Low-carbohydrate diets and cardiometabolic health: the importance of carbohydrate quality over quantity. Nutr Rev. 2020;78:69–77.
47. Wang W, Li J, Chen X, Yu M, Pan Q, Guo L. Whole grain food diet slightly reduces cardiovascular risks in obese/overweight adults: a systematic review and meta-analysis. BMC Cardiovasc Disord. 2020;20:82.
48. Liang N-C, Hajnal A, Norgren R. Sham feeding corn oil increases accumbens dopamine in the rat. Am J Physiol Regul Integr Comp Physiol. 2006;291:R1236–9.
49. Adachi S-I, Endo Y, Mizushige T, Tsuzuki S, Matsumura S, Inoue K, et al. Increased levels of extracellular dopamine in the nucleus accumbens and amygdala of rats by ingesting a low concentration of a long-chain Fatty Acid. Biosci Biotechnol Biochem. 2013;77:2175–80.
50. Dela Cruz JAD, Coke T, Bodnar RJ. Simultaneous detection of c-Fos activation from mesolimbic and mesocortical dopamine reward sites following naive sugar and fat ingestion in rats. J Vis Exp. 2016;2016:53897. https://doi.org/10.3791/53897.
51. Casperson SL, Lanza L, Albajri E, Nasser JA. Increasing chocolate's sugar content enhances its psychoactive effects and intake. Nutrients. 2019;11:596. https://doi.org/10.3390/nu11030596.
52. Carter A, Hardman CA, Burrows T. Food addiction and eating addiction: scientific advances and their clinical, social and policy implications. Nutrients. 2020;12:1485. https://doi.org/10.3390/nu12051485.
53. Blanco-Gandía MC, Cantacorps L, Aracil-Fernández A, Montagud-Romero S, Aguilar MA, Manzanares J, et al. Effects of bingeing on fat during adolescence on the reinforcing effects of cocaine in adult male mice. Neuropharmacology. 2017;113:31–44.
54. Blanco-Gandía MC, Ledesma JC, Aracil-Fernández A, Navarrete F, Montagud-Romero S, Aguilar MA, et al. The rewarding effects of ethanol are modulated by binge eating of a high-fat diet during adolescence. Neuropharmacology. 2017;121:219–30.
55. Gearhardt AN, Corbin WR, Brownell KD. Preliminary validation of the Yale Food Addiction Scale. Appetite. 2009;52:430–6.
56. Avena NM, Rada P, Hoebel BG. Sugar and fat bingeing have notable differences in addictive-like behavior. J Nutr. 2009;139:623–8.
57. Schulte EM, Smeal JK, Lewis J, Gearhardt AN. Development of the highly processed food withdrawal scale. Appetite. 2018;131:148–54.
58. Parnarouskis L, Schulte EM, Lumeng JC, Gearhardt AN. Development of the highly processed food withdrawal scale for children. Appetite. 2020;147:104553.
59. Jeynes KD, Gibson EL. The importance of nutrition in aiding recovery from substance use disorders: a review. Drug Alcohol Depend. 2017;179:229–39.

60. Gearhardt AN, Corbin WR, Brownell KD. Food addiction: an examination of the diagnostic criteria for dependence. J Addict Med. 2009;3:1–7.
61. Xu H, Li S, Song X, Li Z, Zhang D. Exploration of the association between dietary fiber intake and depressive symptoms in adults. Nutrition. 2018;54:48–53.
62. Adjibade M, Andreeva VA, Lemogne C, Touvier M, Shivappa N, Hébert JR, et al. The inflammatory potential of the diet is associated with depressive symptoms in different subgroups of the general population. J Nutr. 2017;147:879–87.
63. Gómez-Donoso C, Sánchez-Villegas A, Martínez-González MA, Gea A, et al. Ultra-processed food consumption and the incidence of depression in a Mediterranean cohort: the SUN Project. Eur J Nutr. 2020;59:1093–103.
64. Adjibade M, Julia C, Allès B, Touvier M, Lemogne C, Srour B, et al. Prospective association between ultra-processed food consumption and incident depressive symptoms in the French NutriNet-Santé cohort. BMC Med. 2019;17:78.
65. Cryan JF, O'Riordan KJ, Cowan CSM, Sandhu KV, Bastiaanssen TFS, Boehme M, et al. The microbiota-gut-brain axis. Physiol Rev. 2019;99:1877–2013.
66. Noonan S, Zaveri M, Macaninch E, Martyn K. Food & mood: a review of supplementary prebiotic and probiotic interventions in the treatment of anxiety and depression in adults. BMJ Nutr Prev Health. 2020;3:351–62.
67. Jacka FN, O'Neil A, Opie R, Itsiopoulos C, Cotton S, Mohebbi M, et al. A randomised controlled trial of dietary improvement for adults with major depression (the "SMILES" trial). BMC Med. 2017;15:23.
68. Lassale C, Batty GD, Baghdadli A, Jacka F, Sánchez-Villegas A, Kivimäki M, et al. Correction: healthy dietary indices and risk of depressive outcomes: a systematic review and meta-analysis of observational studies. Mol Psychiatry. 2019;24:1094.
69. Sadeghi O, Keshteli AH, Afshar H, Esmaillzadeh A, Adibi P. Adherence to Mediterranean dietary pattern is inversely associated with depression, anxiety and psychological distress. Nutr Neurosci. 2021;24:248–59.
70. Wiss DA, Criscitelli K, Gold M, Avena N. Preclinical evidence for the addiction potential of highly palatable foods: current developments related to maternal influence. Appetite. 2017;115:19–27.
71. Martins-Silva T, Vaz JDS, Hutz MH, Salatino-Oliveira A, Genro JP, Hartwig FP, et al. Assessing causality in the association between attention-deficit/hyperactivity disorder and obesity: a Mendelian randomization study. Int J Obes. 2019;43:2500–8.
72. Clasen MM, Riley AL, Davidson TL. Hippocampal-dependent inhibitory learning and memory processes in the control of eating and drug taking. Curr Pharm Des. 2020;26:2334–52.
73. Webber L, Divajeva D, Marsh T, McPherson K, Brown M, Galea G, et al. The future burden of obesity-related diseases in the 53 WHO European-Region countries and the impact of effective interventions: a modelling study. BMJ Open. 2014;4:e004787.
74. Xu B-L, Wang R, Ma L-N, Dong W, Zhao Z-W, Zhang J-S, et al. Effects of caloric intake on learning and memory function in juvenile C57BL/6J mice. Biomed Res Int. 2015;2015:759803.
75. Kalyan-Masih P, Vega-Torres JD, Miles C, Haddad E, Rainsbury S, Baghchechi M, et al. Western high-fat diet consumption during adolescence increases susceptibility to traumatic stress while selectively disrupting hippocampal and ventricular volumes. eNeuro. 2016;3 https://doi.org/10.1523/ENEURO.0125-16.2016.
76. Power R, Prado-Cabrero A, Mulcahy R, Howard A, Nolan JM. The role of nutrition for the aging population: implications for cognition and Alzheimer's disease. Annu Rev Food Sci Technol. 2019;10:619–39.
77. Sclafani A. Gut-brain nutrient signaling. Appetition vs satiation. Appetite. 2013;71:454–8.
78. Kenny PJ. Reward mechanisms in obesity: new insights and future directions. Neuron. 2011;69:664–79.
79. O'Rourke RW. The pathophysiology of obesity and obesity-related disease. In: Nguyen NT, Brethauer SA, Morton JM, Ponce J, Rosenthal RJ, editors. The ASMBS textbook of bariatric surgery. Cham: Springer International Publishing; 2020. p. 15–36.
80. Schoeller DA, Buchholz AC. Energetics of obesity and weight control: does diet composition matter? J Am Diet Assoc. 2005;105:S24–8.
81. Moon J, Koh G. Clinical evidence and mechanisms of high-protein diet-induced weight loss. J Obes Metab Syndr. 2020;29:166–73.
82. Davis C, Curtis C, Levitan RD, Carter JC, Kaplan AS, Kennedy JL. Evidence that "food addiction" is a valid phenotype of obesity. Appetite. 2011;57:711–7.
83. Avena NM, Bocarsly ME, Hoebel BG. Animal models of sugar and fat bingeing: relationship to food addiction and increased body weight. Methods Mol Biol. 2012;829:351–65.
84. Borengasser SJ, Kang P, Faske J, Gomez-Acevedo H, Blackburn ML, Badger TM, et al. High fat diet and in utero exposure to maternal obesity disrupts circadian rhythm and leads to metabolic programming of liver in rat offspring. PLoS One. 2014;9:e84209.
85. Davis C. A narrative review of binge eating and addictive behaviors: shared associations with seasonality and personality factors. Front Psych. 2013;4:183.
86. Blanco-Gandía MC, Aracil-Fernández A, Montagud-Romero S, Aguilar MA, Manzanares J, Miñarro J, et al. Changes in gene expression and sensitivity of cocaine reward produced by a continuous fat diet. Psychopharmacology. 2017;234:2337–52.
87. Kelley AE, Schiltz CA, Landry CF. Neural systems recruited by drug- and food-related cues: studies of gene activation in corticolimbic regions. Physiol Behav. 2005;86:11–4.

88. Rada P, Avena NM, Hoebel BG. Daily bingeing on sugar repeatedly releases dopamine in the accumbens shell. Neuroscience. 2005;134:737–44.
89. Narayanaswami V, Thompson AC, Cassis LA, Bardo MT, Dwoskin LP. Diet-induced obesity: dopamine transporter function, impulsivity and motivation. Int J Obes. 2013;37:1095–103.
90. Davis C, Patte K, Levitan R, Reid C, Tweed S, Curtis C. From motivation to behaviour: a model of reward sensitivity, overeating, and food preferences in the risk profile for obesity. Appetite. 2007;48:12–9.
91. Valdivia S, Cornejo MP, Reynaldo M, De Francesco PN, Perello M. Escalation in high fat intake in a binge eating model differentially engages dopamine neurons of the ventral tegmental area and requires ghrelin signaling. Psychoneuroendocrinology. 2015;60:206–16.
92. Colantuoni C, Schwenker J, McCarthy J, Rada P, Ladenheim B, Cadet JL, et al. Excessive sugar intake alters binding to dopamine and mu-opioid receptors in the brain. Neuroreport. 2001;12:3549–52.
93. Fairburn CG, Cooper Z, Shafran R. Cognitive behaviour therapy for eating disorders: a "transdiagnostic" theory and treatment. Behav Res Ther. 2003;41:509–28.
94. Volkow ND, Wang GJ, Fowler JS, Tomasi D, Baler R. Food and drug reward: overlapping circuits in human obesity and addiction. Curr Top Behav Neurosci. 2012;11:1–24.
95. Boggiano MM, Chandler PC, Viana JB, Oswald KD, Maldonado CR, Wauford PK. Combined dieting and stress evoke exaggerated responses to opioids in binge-eating rats. Behav Neurosci. 2005;119:1207–14.
96. Goldstone AP, Prechtl de Hernandez CG, Beaver JD, Muhammed K, Croese C, Bell G, et al. Fasting biases brain reward systems towards high-calorie foods. Eur J Neurosci. 2009;30:1625–35.
97. Gordon EL, Lent MR, Merlo LJ. The effect of food composition and behavior on neurobiological response to food: a review of recent research. Curr Nutr Rep. 2020;9:75–82.
98. Kroemer NB, Sun X, Veldhuizen MG, Babbs AE, de Araujo IE, Small DM. Weighing the evidence: variance in brain responses to milkshake receipt is predictive of eating behavior. NeuroImage. 2016;128:273–83.
99. Schlögl H, Horstmann A, Villringer A, Stumvoll M. Functional neuroimaging in obesity and the potential for development of novel treatments. Lancet Diabetes Endocrinol. 2016;4:695–705.
100. Leidy HJ, Lepping RJ, Savage CR, Harris CT. Neural responses to visual food stimuli after a normal vs. higher protein breakfast in breakfast-skipping teens: a pilot fMRI study. Obesity. 2011;19:2019–25.
101. Lin Z, Qu S. Legend of weight loss: a crosstalk between the bariatric surgery and the brain. Obes Surg. 2020;30:1988–2002.
102. Stice E, Burger K, Yokum S. Caloric deprivation increases responsivity of attention and reward brain regions to intake, anticipated intake, and images of palatable foods. NeuroImage. 2013;67:322–30.
103. Page KA, Seo D, Belfort-DeAguiar R, Lacadie C, Dzuira J, Naik S, et al. Circulating glucose levels modulate neural control of desire for high-calorie foods in humans. J Clin Invest. 2011;121:4161–9.
104. Kahathuduwa CN, Davis T, O'Boyle M, Boyd LA, Chin S-H, Paniukov D, et al. Effects of 3-week total meal replacement vs. typical food-based diet on human brain functional magnetic resonance imaging food-cue reactivity and functional connectivity in people with obesity. Appetite. 2018;120:431–41.
105. Meule A. The psychology of food cravings: the role of food deprivation. Curr Nutr Rep. 2020;9:251–7.
106. Gee JM, Johnson IT. Dietary lactitol fermentation increases circulating peptide YY and glucagon-like peptide-1 in rats and humans. Nutrition. 2005;21:1036–43.
107. Fernstrom JD. Non-nutritive sweeteners and obesity. Annu Rev Food Sci Technol. 2015;6:119–36.
108. Frank GKW, Oberndorfer TA, Simmons AN, Paulus MP, Fudge JL, Yang TT, et al. Sucrose activates human taste pathways differently from artificial sweetener. NeuroImage. 2008;39:1559–69.
109. Haase L, Cerf-Ducastel B, Murphy C. Cortical activation in response to pure taste stimuli during the physiological states of hunger and satiety. NeuroImage. 2009;44:1008–21.
110. Smeets PAM, de Graaf C, Stafleu A, van Osch MJP, van der Grond J. Functional magnetic resonance imaging of human hypothalamic responses to sweet taste and calories. Am J Clin Nutr. 2005;82:1011–6.
111. Karl JP, Meydani M, Barnett JB, Vanegas SM, Goldin B, Kane A, et al. Substituting whole grains for refined grains in a 6-wk randomized trial favorably affects energy-balance metrics in healthy men and postmenopausal women. Am J Clin Nutr. 2017;105:589–99.
112. Hebebrand J, Albayrak O, Adan R, Antel J, Dieguez C, Jong J. "Eating addiction", rather than "food addiction", better captures addictive-like eating behavior. Neurosci Biobehav Rev. 2014;47:295–306.
113. Guise S. Mini habits for weight loss: stop dieting. Form new habits. Change your lifestyle without suffering. Selective Entertainment LLC; 2016.
114. Schulte EM, Potenza MN, Gearhardt AN. A commentary on the "eating addiction" versus "food addiction" perspectives on addictive-like food consumption. Appetite. 2017;115:9–15.
115. Ifland J, Preuss HG, Marcus MT, Rourke KM, Taylor W, Theresa WH. Clearing the confusion around processed food addiction. J Am Coll Nutr. 2015;34:240–3.

Part V

Assessment and Treatment of Food Addiction

12 Evaluation of Food Addiction: Importance, Epidemiology, Diagnosis, and Assessment

12.1 Importance of Assessing for Food Addiction

Because of the range of potential health problems associated with obesity and binge eating (Chaps. 2 and 3), the poor response to treatment for these disorders (Chap. 4), and the intense popularity of diet books in our culture, providers should go the extra step and consider an FA diagnosis to improve their ability to help people lose weight and reduce distress around food. Although more treatment studies are needed, addressing FA directly with FA-focused approaches may improve outcomes for our patients with obesity and eating disorders (ED).

One reason to identify FA is that people with FA often also need greater support, as evidenced by their higher levels of psychosocial impairment [1], higher general psychological distress and levels of mental health problems [2–6], reduced general quality of life [3, 5], reduced health-related quality of life, impaired self-esteem, and struggles with dating, socialization, and work [7, 8].

Identifying FA will also help providers be on the alert for more severe and potentially difficult to treat obese patients (a FA diagnosis predicts higher body mass index (BMI)) [4, 5, 9–11] and to identify people more likely to eat unhelpful foods or to have more problematic medical issues. For example, individuals with FA tend to have lower diet quality, with lower intake of fruits and vegetables and higher intakes of highly processed foods such as chips and chocolate, and higher fat and sugar consumption [4, 9, 10, 12]. They also tend to consume more high-fat, high-sugar, and caloric food during binge episodes, which may result in higher obesity and ED severity [5, 13]. Higher FA scores are also associated with higher risks of medical complications in patients with type 2 diabetes, including higher hemoglobin A1c levels, and higher risks of diabetic retinopathy, neuropathy, and nephropathy [13–20].

Recognizing and treating FA can also alert providers to the existence of an undiagnosed ED and/or a more severe ED picture. FA is associated with higher rates of ED, especially bulimia nervosa and binge eating disorder (BED) [3, 5, 10, 13, 15–23]. FA is also associated with more severe ED [24], with a higher frequency of binge episodes and greater eating psychopathology [5, 11, 12, 25, 26]. In addition to more frequent binging, individuals with YFAS-diagnosed FA and BED may have more intense cravings, elevated symptoms of depression, and higher MDD prevalence than individuals with BED alone [19, 27–29]. Furthermore, the association between YFAS diagnosis and frequency of binge eating episodes persists after controlling for ED psychopathology and depressive symptoms [19, 28, 30]. FA is also associated with higher shape and weight concern,

C. E. Wilcox, *Food Addiction, Obesity, and Disorders of Overeating*,
https://doi.org/10.1007/978-3-030-83078-6_12

eating concern, global eating disorder psychopathology, and food craving, even after correcting for BMI and binge eating episodes [11]. Identifying FA in people with EDs can also help alert providers to patients who might need more intensive treatment and a more comprehensive treatment team approach.

FA also likely indicates a greater risk of comorbid psychopathology in bariatric surgery patients. In a group of 131 adults seeking treatment for post sleeve gastrectomy surgery, the FA group experienced greater ED scores, depression scores, and nibbling picking and loss of control eating and lower functioning [31]. Diagnosing FA may help surgeons both to make pre-op decisions and/or make referrals for comorbidity treatment to enhance the potential for a good outcome for surgery.

Not surprisingly, FA diagnosis also predicts poor response to some of the standard existing treatments for obesity. Adhering to a diet is much more difficult, as implied in several of the diagnostic criteria for the disorders. For example, in preoperative cases of bariatric surgery, the initial dietary intervention is less effective in individuals with FA [5, 12] who lose less weight. These individuals may ultimately be better off with an abstinence-based approach during this time.

Furthermore, FA predicts outcome in ED treatment. In a sample of 49 individuals with bulimia and 29 with BED, although FA did not predict treatment outcome for the whole sample, it was associated with poorer prognosis in the BED group [26, 32]. Worse outcomes are also seen for patients with bulimia nervosa: for example, patients with higher FA severity at baseline were less likely to obtain abstinence from binge-purge behavior following treatment for bulimia [5, 32, 33]. Mediation studies also support the important role that FA plays in ED recovery: in one study, FA was found to be a mediator in the relationship between ED severity and treatment outcome [26] indicating that those with higher FA symptoms were less likely to respond to the standard ED treatment provided in that study. For these reasons, many experts believe that people with FA may need tailored ED treatment approaches [27, 32].

Finally FA has been found to predict weight loss outcomes post-bariatric surgery with less response to secondary problems like sugar control in type 2 diabetes [15–17] and less favorable weight loss outcomes and BMI post sleeve gastrectomy at year one [34, 35], although not all studies have shown poorer outcomes in those with FA [12]. Bariatric surgery likely improves FA symptoms (Chap. 10), but more work needs to be done to confirm this is true.

12.2 Epidemiology of FA

FA is common even in the general population. The frequency of FA in a general sample recruited from a MTurk worker pool in the United States was measured at 16% in the original YFAS 2.0 psychometric evaluation study [16]. Severe FA (i.e., six or more symptoms) was more common (11–12%) than moderate (2%) or mild (2%) FA. Obese participants also had a higher prevalence of FA (25%) than overweight (17%) or normal weight (8%) participants on the YFAS 2.0 [16].

The prevalence of FA in the United States in other studies ranges from 11% to 20% [12, 17, 32, 36–39]. A meta-analysis of 51 studies determined that the mean prevalence of FA worldwide is about the same as in the United States, at about 16% [3, 32]. Prevalence may vary greatly from country to country, however, and even within a country depending on the study. For example, in Taiwan, 13% of young adults met criteria for FA based on the YFAS in one study [40], whereas in another study in students in several Asian countries, FA prevalence was 6% overall (with 8% in South Korea, 5% in Japan, and 4% in Taiwan). In France and Germany, the general prevalence was 8% and 9%, respectively [36]. In Canada it was 5% [36]. In Italy it was 11% in a general population [36]. In summary, somewhere between 5% and 20% of the general population meets criteria for food addiction (in the last year) including the United States and other parts of the world.

Rates of FA are higher, and FA symptoms are more severe, in people with obesity compared to normal weight individuals [14, 41]. As was seen in the original YFAS 2.0 validation study, other studies have shown that about 25% of obese individuals can be classified as food addicted although rates can be as low as 7–17% in samples of people with obesity seeking weight loss [8, 15, 32, 38, 42–45] but reach up to 50% in extremely obese treatment-seeking samples [12, 17, 32, 39, 44, 46]. In another sample of patients with type 2 diabetes, 29% screened positive for FA [14].

Higher rates of FA are also seen in EDs, especially BED and bulimia nervosa, compared to the general population [3, 5, 10, 13, 15–23]. In a systematic review of studies on FA in non-clinical and clinical cohorts, BED was associated with the most severe FA symptoms of the ED subtypes [5, 18], and in BED in various other studies, rates of FA range from 42% to 92% depending on the population (treatment seekers tend to have higher rates of FA) [13, 19, 21–23, 28, 30, 38, 44, 47]. Furthermore, rates of FA in bulimia nervosa are typically around 80% [21, 22] but as low as 42% [16]. In one study of patients receiving ED treatment, the prevalence of FA in the entire ED population was 84% [24] with the highest rates in bulimia (98%), BED (93%), and anorexia binge-purge type (88%) and lowest in anorexia restrictive type (62%) [24]. In other work, in a sample of treatment seekers with either BED or bulimia, FA was diagnosed in 87% [26]. Some patients with anorexia might have higher FA rates too: one study showed that FA was seen at higher rates in bulimia than in anorexia but that in severely underweight people (especially with anorexia with a binge-purge type) FA becomes more prevalent again (in a "U-shaped" pattern when graphed) [32].

Rates of FA are also fairly high in surgical populations, as well, with one study finding that FA was positive in 41% of their sleeve gastrectomy patients and 48% reporting binge eating [34], with all of the FA patients also meeting criteria for binge eating. In another study in a sample of people 6 months post-op sleeve gastrectomy who also reported loss of control eating, only 18% met FA criteria [14].

FA occurs at higher rates in younger patients, but FA rates are lowest in adolescents [6, 14, 32] suggesting that FA develops slightly later in life. Female sex is positively associated with FA frequency and more severe FA, especially in those with obesity too [4, 5, 12, 14, 48]. Unlike obesity, rates of FA in the United States are elevated among individuals with higher incomes [32, 39]. Also, rates of FA are higher in clinical samples as compared to community samples [4, 12, 17].

12.3 YFAS: Scoring and Interpretation

Our first step towards identifying patients more likely to respond to interventions targeting mechanisms like reward hypersensitivity and loss of control should be to utilize the most ubiquitously utilized scale for the diagnosis of FA, the YFAS. Recall, the original YFAS is a self-report questionnaire that screens for the seven DSM-IV symptoms of substance dependence in relation to certain foods. The symptoms evaluated for include continued use despite negative consequences, withdrawal, and the persistent desire to cut down on certain foods but an inability to do so [49]. A diagnosis of FA is obtained on the original YFAS if three symptoms were endorsed above a certain severity threshold based on frequency, plus either clinically significant impairment or distress related to addictive-like eating behavior paralleling the DSM-IV criteria [49].

The YFAS 2.0 should be utilized currently (Table 12.1, reproduced with permission from [16]). It is based on the DSM-V instead of the older, fourth, version, and it assesses for all 11 of the criteria for a SUD applied to highly palatable food.

Box 12.1 describes the method for calculating the final YFAS 2.0 score and for determining whether or not someone meets criteria for food addiction. It is reproduced with permission from [16].

Table 12.1 Full Yale Food Addiction Scale Version 2.0

This survey asks about your eating habits in the past year. People sometimes have difficulty controlling how much they eat of certain foods such as:

- Sweets like ice cream, chocolate, doughnuts, cookies, cake, candy
- Starches like white bread, rolls, pasta, and rice
- Salty snacks like chips, pretzels, and crackers
- Fatty foods like steak, bacon, hamburgers, cheeseburgers, pizza, and French fries
- Sugary drinks like soda pop, lemonade, sports drinks, and energy drinks

When the following questions ask about "CERTAIN FOODS" please think of ANY foods or beverages similar to those listed in the food or beverage groups above or ANY OTHER foods you have had difficulty with in the past year

In the past 12 months:	Never	Less than monthly	Once a month	2–3 times a month	Once a week	2–3 times a week	4–6 times a week	Every day
1. When I started to eat certain foods, I ate much more than planned.	0	1	2	3	4	5	6	7
2. I continued to eat certain foods even though I was no longer hungry.	0	1	2	3	4	5	6	7
3. I ate to the point where I felt physically ill	0	1	2	3	4	5	6	7
4. I worried a lot about cutting down on certain types of food, but I ate them anyways.	0	1	2	3	4	5	6	7
5. I spent a lot of time feeling sluggish or tired from overeating.	0	1	2	3	4	5	6	7
6. I spent a lot of time eating certain foods throughout the day.	0	1	2	3	4	5	6	7
7. When certain foods were not available, I went out of my way to get them. For example, I went to the store to get certain foods even though I had other things to eat at home.	0	1	2	3	4	5	6	7
8. I ate certain foods so often or in such large amounts that I stopped doing other important things. These things may have been working or spending time with family or friends.	0	1	2	3	4	5	6	7
9. I had problems with my family or friends because of how much I overate.	0	1	2	3	4	5	6	7
10. I avoided work, school or social activities because I was afraid I would overeat there.	0	1	2	3	4	5	6	7
11. When I cut down on or stopped eating certain foods, I felt irritable, nervous or sad.	0	1	2	3	4	5	6	7
12. If I had physical symptoms because I hadn't eaten certain foods, I would eat those foods to feel better.	0	1	2	3	4	5	6	7
13. If I had emotional problems because I hadn't eaten certain foods, I would eat those foods to feel better.	0	1	2	3	4	5	6	7
14. When I cut down on or stopped eating certain foods, I had physical symptoms. For example, I had headaches or fatigue.	0	1	2	3	4	5	6	7
15. When I cut down or stopped eating certain foods, I had strong cravings for them.	0	1	2	3	4	5	6	7
16. My eating behavior caused me a lot of distress.	0	1	2	3	4	5	6	7
17. I had significant problems in my life because of food and eating. These may have been problems with my daily routine, work, school, friends, family, or health.	0	1	2	3	4	5	6	7

Table 12.1 (continued)

In the past 12 months:	Never	Less than monthly	Once a month	2–3 times a month	Once a week	2–3 times a week	4–6 times a week	Every day
18. I felt so bad about overeating that I didn't do other important things. These things may have been working or spending time with family or friends.	0	1	2	3	4	5	6	7
19. My overeating got in the way of me taking care of my family or doing household chores.	0	1	2	3	4	5	6	7
20. I avoided work, school or social functions because I could not eat certain foods there.	0	1	2	3	4	5	6	7
21. I avoided social situations because people wouldn't approve of how much I ate.	0	1	2	3	4	5	6	7
22. I kept eating in the same way even though my eating caused emotional problems.	0	1	2	3	4	5	6	7
23. I kept eating the same way even though my eating caused physical problems.	0	1	2	3	4	5	6	7
24. Eating the same amount of food did not give me as much enjoyment as it used to.	0	1	2	3	4	5	6	7
25. I really wanted to cut down on or stop eating certain kinds of foods, but I just couldn't.	0	1	2	3	4	5	6	7
26. I needed to eat more and more to get the feelings I wanted from eating. This included reducing negative emotions like sadness or increasing pleasure.	0	1	2	3	4	5	6	7
27. I didn't do well at work or school because I was eating too much.	0	1	2	3	4	5	6	7
28. I kept eating certain foods even though I knew it was physically dangerous. For example, I kept eating sweets even though I had diabetes. Or I kept eating fatty foods despite having heart disease.	0	1	2	3	4	5	6	7
29. I had such strong urges to eat certain foods that I couldn't think of anything else.	0	1	2	3	4	5	6	7
30. I had such intense cravings for certain foods that I felt like I had to eat them right away.	0	1	2	3	4	5	6	7
31. I tried to cut down on or not eat certain kinds of food, but I wasn't successful.	0	1	2	3	4	5	6	7
32. I tried and failed to cut down on or stop eating certain foods.	0	1	2	3	4	5	6	7
33. I was so distracted by eating that I could have been hurt (e.g., when driving a car, crossing the street, operating machinery).	0	1	2	3	4	5	6	7
34. I was so distracted by thinking about food that I could have been hurt (e.g., when driving a car, crossing the street, operating machinery).	0	1	2	3	4	5	6	7
35. My friends or family were worried about how much I overate.	0	1	2	3	4	5	6	7

This table is reproduced with permission from the following Ref. [16]

Box 12.1 YFAS 2.0 Scoring [16]

Scoring Instructions for the YFAS 2.0

Development of YFAS 2.0 Scoring Thresholds

All questions on the YFAS 2.0 are continuous. To reflect diagnostic thresholds, a cutoff for each question was established to allow for determination of a diagnosis and severity level. Questions on the YFAS 2.0 have eight frequency response options that range from "Never" to "Every Day." The threshold for the YFAS 2.0 symptom questions were determined by examining specificity for each response option based on receiver operator characteristic (ROC) curves. There is no existing gold standard for assessing "food addiction"; thus we created a multivariate latent variable that included constructs that are theoretically associated with addictive-like eating (e.g., BMI, binge eating frequency, TFEQ disinhibition, and TFEQ hunger). A confirmatory factor analysis of the multivariate latent variable suggested an excellent fit to a one-factor solution, χ^2 (2 df) = 1.53, $p = 0.47$, CFI = 1.00, RMSEA = 0.00 (95% CI; 0.000, 0.075), SRMR = 0.008, with standardized factor loadings ranging from 0.37 to 0.95. The latent variable was saved and imported into the data set for purposes of conducting ROC analyses. The highest quartile of the multivariate latent factor scores was used as the outcome indicator for the ROC curve analyses to identify YFAS 2.0 question thresholds. To reduce the likelihood of over-pathologizing normal eating behaviors, thresholds with specificity of 0.90 or greater were chosen as the cutoff for each question. Thresholds for these questions ranged from once a month to 4–6 times a week, although the threshold for the majority of YFAS 2.0 questions was once a week (eight questions) or 2–3 times a week (eight questions). To maintain consistency with the diagnostic scoring option of the original YFAS, the same thresholds used for the clinical significance questions (impairment or distress) were retained for the YFAS 2.0 (i.e., two to three times a week or more).

Each question falls under a DSM-V Substance-Related and Addictive Disorders (SRAD) symptom criterion or clinical impairment/distress:

1. Substance taken in larger amount and for longer period than intended
   Questions #1, #2, #3
2. Persistent desire or repeated unsuccessful attempts to quit
   Questions #4, #25, #31, #32
3. Much time/activity to obtain, use, recover
   Questions #5, #6, #7
4. Important social, occupational, or recreational activities given up or reduced
   Questions #8, #10, #18, #20
5. Use continues despite knowledge of adverse consequences (e.g., emotional problems, physical problems)
   Questions, #22, #23
6. Tolerance (marked increase in amount; marked decrease in effect)
   Questions #24, #26
7. Characteristic withdrawal symptoms; substance taken to relieve withdrawal
   Questions #11, #12, #13, #14, #15
8. Continued use despite social or interpersonal problems
   Questions #9, #21, #35
9. Failure to fulfill major role obligation (e.g., work, school, home)
   Questions #19, #27
10. Use in physically hazardous situations
    Question #28, #33, #34
11. Craving, or a strong desire or urge to use
    Questions #29, #30
12. Use causes clinically significant impairment or distress
    Questions #16, #17

Each question has a different threshold: 0 = threshold not met, 1 = threshold is met

1. Once a month: #9, #10, #19, #27, #33, #35
2. Two to three times a month: #8, #18, #20, #21, #34
3. Once a week: #3, #11, #13, #14, #22, #28, #29
4. Two to three times a week: #5, #12, #16, #17, #23, #24, #26, #30, #31, #32
5. Four to six times a week: #1, #2, #4, #6, #7, #15, #25

After computing the threshold for each question, sum up the questions under each criterion (e.g., Tolerance, Withdrawal, Clinical Significance, etc.). If the score for the symptom criterion is ≥1, then the criterion has been met and is scored as 1. If the score = 0, then the symptom criterion has not been met and is scored as 0.

Example:

- Tolerance: (#24 = 1) + (#26 = 0) = 1, Criterion Met
- Craving (#29 = 0) + (#30 = 0), Criterion Not Met
- Failure to fulfill role obligations (#19 = 1) + (#27 = 1), Criterion Met and scored as 1

For the symptom count scoring option, add up all of the scores for each of the 11 criterion (e.g., Tolerance, Withdrawal, Use Despite Negative Consequence). Do not add clinical significance to the score. This score should range from 0 to 11 (0 symptoms to 11 symptoms).

For the "diagnosis" scoring option, a participant can meet for mild, moderate, or severe food addiction. Both the symptom count score and the clinical significance criterion are used.

- No Food Addiction = 1 or fewer symptoms
- No Food Addiction = Does not meet criteria for clinical significance
- Mild Food Addiction = 2 or 3 symptoms and clinical significance
- Moderate Food Addiction = 4 or 5 symptoms and clinical significance
- Severe Food Addiction = 6 or more symptoms and clinical significance

For each question, be it a yes/no or continuous answer, there is a "cutoff," which, if met, indicates that the person meets the criteria [16]. Only one question above the cutoff out of several options is needed to meet a particular criterion. The continuous FA score is on a scale of 1–11 which is based on how many criteria they meet (possible score from 1 to 11). Like with the DSM-V for SUD, the cutoff of SUD is based on whether or not they meet two or more criteria (2–3 criteria = mild, 4–5 = moderate, 6 or more = severe). Looking closely at the answers to individual questions on the YFAS may also clue clinicians into the domains in which a person might be especially struggling/weak and which might need attention during treatment, such as reward sensitivity, attentional bias and other cognitive biases for food, craving, impulsivity, and other executive function deficits, emotion regulation difficulties, heightened tendencies towards stress and emotional distress, and negative urgency [5, 15, 50], as well as whether the person struggles primarily with reward-motivated or comfort-seeking eating.

Other self-report scales and questionnaires for assessment of FA are also available and have been validated, though they are less ubiquitously utilized in research studies. These questionnaires rely on features like craving and eating patterns and include Eating Behaviors Questionnaire, the Food Cravings Questionnaire, the Eating Behaviors Patterns Questionnaire, and the Power of Food Scale [12]. It has been suggested that assessing fat addiction separately might have important implications for interventions [12], and that developing a questionnaire to identify the subtypes of food that the individual is more drawn to may help the field, given fat and sugar may affect the reward circuits differently. The Highly Processed Food Withdrawal Scale [51, 52] is also useful for assessment of acute food withdrawal, which might significantly affect mood and decision-making. Finally, the TFEQ Restraint and Disinhibition scale [53] helps decide if someone is too focused on restraint to safely introduce the concept of an abstinence-based approach [32].

12.4 Other Important Assessment Considerations and Common Comorbidities

12.4.1 SUD

During assessments, providers should ask about whether or not the person has a prior history of or current diagnosis of a SUD or past or current substance misuse. Relatedly it's important to find out about any history of addiction transfer between food and substances of abuse or vice versa, and, if so, whether the SUD or the FA came first [32]. If either were the case, it might indicate the person has an underlying propensity for FA which might lower the threshold for considering an FA diagnosis and an FA-based treatment approach. Prior or current SUD or an addiction transfer history would also indicate that caution should be utilized if there is a reason to consider prescription of a stimulant-like medication, which is sometimes indicated in obesity treatment, for example (Chaps. 2 and 14). If a medication with heightened addiction risk is deemed worthy of prescribing after careful assessment of the risk-benefit ratios, frequent urine drug screens, checking patient profiles on pharmacy board prescription monitoring program websites, and dispensing medications in smaller and more frequent batches can help lower risk of misuse of the stimulant. Furthermore, knowing whether someone has a past SUD might also help in choosing between treatment approaches: if they have a past history of recovering from a particular treatment (e.g., a medication, a particular psychotherapeutic approach, 12-step work, etc.), their eating problem might be more likely to respond to something similar. Finally, as one might imagine, ED or FA with comorbid SUD are more vulnerable in many areas than those without SUD; in particular those with comorbid SUD have even higher reward sensitivity, more difficulty engaging in goal-directed activity, lower self-directedness, higher anxiety, higher impulsivity and poorer executive function, more depression and PTSD, more harm avoidance, and less access to emotion regulation skills (e.g., acceptance) than those with problematic eating alone [5, 32, 54].

12.4.2 ED History

It is also essential to screen for a history of dangerous levels of restrictive or avoidant behavior around food in the distant past or recently and to ask about a history of purging or other compensatory behaviors. Utilizing a validated restraint scale could be a helpful supplement to clinical history [53]. If the history is positive, the next step is to determine as best as possible whether the restricting or bingeing came first. If the restrictive behavior came first, that might indicate a heightened concern that the restrictive aspect of their eating problem is primary. One aim in screening for EDs is to look for "false FA positives" and enhance specificity and sensitivity of our diagnostic efforts [32]. Dietary restraint can be a primary contributor of "noise" in the FA signal, meaning excessive levels of dietary restraint will lead to bingeing and experiences around food that mimic FA [32]. Asking about which came first, the FA symptoms and bingeing or the restriction may be helpful in narrowing down the diagnosis between a primary FA and primary ED, and treatment recommendations can come from that [32].

A history of higher levels of food avoidance, restriction, and compensatory behavior might indicate that an abstinence-based nutritional approach to treatment (Chap. 13) would be high risk. In those reporting concerning restrictive and compensatory behavior, a softer or modified-abstinence approach might be best, as "abstinence-talk" could be triggering and dangerous, and/or abstinence-based approaches might best be abandoned and traditional eating disorder treatment approaches utilized [32]. In addition to severe and concerning restrictive and/or compensatory past or present behavior, related psychopathology (e.g., chronic dieting and severe body dissatisfaction) might indicate the need for a traditional ED treatment approach [32].

12.4.3 Obesity History and Related Health Concerns

Obviously, determining weight and body mass index and assessing for comorbidities associated with obesity and other negative weight-related consequences are essential components of all FA assessments. This would include getting a detailed history about prior weight loss attempts and successes, weight gain and maintenance histories, and a detailed history of prior treatments and programs tried for weight loss and adherence challenges. Information obtained from asking these kinds of questions will especially come into play when determining the risk-benefit ratios for an abstinence-based nutritional approach. For example, those with higher levels of obesity or comorbidity might incline someone with FA towards diving headfirst into an abstinence-based approach without first trying more standard approaches.

12.4.4 Psychiatric Comorbidity

Obesity, EDs, and FA are associated with higher rates of depression, anxiety, ADHD, personality disorders, early life adversity, and trauma [32] (Chap. 6). High FA scores should alert providers to the heightened possibility of these kinds of comorbidities. Assessing for comorbid psychiatric diagnoses as you would do with any ED or obesity patient is still always warranted (Chaps. 2 and 3), and appropriate treatment of these disorders could significantly improve binging, promote weight loss, and reduce FA symptoms [32].

12.5 Conclusion

In summary, it is important to assess for FA using the YFAS at a minimum and screen for related comorbidities, both to assure accurate diagnosis and to optimize treatment planning.

References

1. Lacroix E, von Ranson KM. Prevalence of social, cognitive, and emotional impairment among individuals with food addiction. Eat Weight Disord. 2021;26(4):1253–8.
2. Lin CY, Cheung P, Imani V, Griffiths MD, Pakpour AH. The mediating effects of eating disorder, food addiction, and insomnia in the association between psychological distress and being overweight among Iranian adolescents. Nutrients. 2020;12(5):1371.
3. Burrows T, Kay-Lambkin F, Pursey K, Skinner J, Dayas C. Food addiction and associations with mental health symptoms: a systematic review with meta-analysis. J Hum Nutr Diet. 2018;31(4):544–72.
4. Burrows T, Skinner J, McKenna R, Rollo M. Food addiction, binge eating disorder, and obesity: is there a relationship? Behav Sci (Basel). 2017;7(3):54.
5. Jimenez-Murcia S, Aguera Z, Paslakis G, Munguia L, Granero R, Sanchez-Gonzalez J, et al. Food addiction in eating disorders and obesity: analysis of clusters and implications for treatment. Nutrients. 2019;11(11):2633.
6. Kiyici S, Koca N, Sigirli D, Aslan BB, Guclu M, Kisakol G. Food addiction correlates with psychosocial functioning more than metabolic parameters in patients with obesity. Metab Syndr Relat Disord. 2020;18(3):161–7.
7. Adams RC, Sedgmond J, Maizey L, Chambers CD, Lawrence NS. Food addiction: implications for the diagnosis and treatment of overeating. Nutrients. 2019;11(9):2086.
8. Chao AM, Shaw JA, Pearl RL, Alamuddin N, Hopkins CM, Bakizada ZM, et al. Prevalence and psychosocial correlates of food addiction in persons with obesity seeking weight reduction. Compr Psychiatry. 2017;73:97–104.
9. Burrows T, Hides L, Brown R, Dayas CV, Kay-Lambkin F. Differences in dietary preferences, personality and mental health in Australian adults with and without food addiction. Nutrients. 2017;9(3):285.
10. Burrows T, Collins R, Rollo M, Leary M, Hides L, Davis C. The feasibility of a personality targeted intervention for addictive overeating: FoodFix. Appetite. 2021;156:104974.
11. Wiedemann AA, Carr MM, Ivezaj V, Barnes RD. Examining the construct validity of food addiction severity specifiers. Eat Weight Disord. 2021;26:1503–9.
12. Sarkar S, Kochhar KP, Khan NA. Fat addiction: psychological and physiological trajectory. Nutrients. 2019;11(11):2785.
13. Granero R, Hilker I, Aguera Z, Jimenez-Murcia S, Sauchelli S, Islam MA, et al. Food addiction in a Spanish sample of eating disorders: DSM-5 diagnostic subtype differentiation and validation data. Eur Eat Disord Rev. 2014;22(6):389–96.
14. Nicolau J, Romerosa JM, Rodriguez I, Sanchis P, Bonet A, Arteaga M, et al. Associations of food addiction with metabolic control, medical complications and depression among patients with type 2 diabetes. Acta Diabetol. 2020;57(9):1093–100.
15. Meule A, Gearhardt AN. Food addiction in the light of DSM-5. Nutrients. 2014;6(9):3653–71.
16. Gearhardt AN, Corbin WR, Brownell KD. Development of the Yale Food Addiction Scale Version 2.0. Psychol Addict Behav. 2016;30(1):113–21.

17. Pursey KM, Stanwell P, Gearhardt AN, Collins CE, Burrows TL. The prevalence of food addiction as assessed by the Yale Food Addiction Scale: a systematic review. Nutrients. 2014;6(10):4552–90.
18. Penzenstadler L, Soares C, Karila L, Khazaal Y. Systematic review of food addiction as measured with the Yale Food Addiction Scale: implications for the food addiction construct. Curr Neuropharmacol. 2019;17(6):526–38.
19. Gearhardt AN, White MA, Masheb RM, Morgan PT, Crosby RD, Grilo CM. An examination of the food addiction construct in obese patients with binge eating disorder. Int J Eat Disord. 2012;45(5):657–63.
20. Smith DG, Robbins TW. The neurobiological underpinnings of obesity and binge eating: a rationale for adopting the food addiction model. Biol Psychiatry. 2013;73(9):804–10.
21. Meule A, von Rezori V, Blechert J. Food addiction and bulimia nervosa. Eur Eat Disord Rev. 2014;22(5):331–7.
22. de Vries SK, Meule A. Food addiction and bulimia nervosa: new data based on the Yale Food Addiction Scale 2.0. Eur Eat Disord Rev. 2016;24(6):518–22.
23. Granero R, Jimenez-Murcia S, Gearhardt AN, Aguera Z, Aymami N, Gomez-Pena M, et al. Validation of the Spanish version of the Yale Food Addiction Scale 2.0 (YFAS 2.0) and clinical correlates in a sample of eating disorder, gambling disorder, and healthy control participants. Front Psychiatry. 2018;9:208.
24. Fauconnier M, Rousselet M, Brunault P, Thiabaud E, Lambert S, Rocher B, et al. Food addiction among female patients seeking treatment for an eating disorder: prevalence and associated factors. Nutrients. 2020;12(6):1897.
25. Gearhardt AN, Boswell RG, White MA. The association of "food addiction" with disordered eating and body mass index. Eat Behav. 2014;15(3):427–33.
26. Romero X, Aguera Z, Granero R, Sanchez I, Riesco N, Jimenez-Murcia S, et al. Is food addiction a predictor of treatment outcome among patients with eating disorder? Eur Eat Disord Rev. 2019;27(6):700–11.
27. Ivezaj V, White MA, Grilo CM. Examining binge-eating disorder and food addiction in adults with overweight and obesity. Obesity. 2016;24(10):2064–9.
28. Schulte EM, Wadden TA, Allison KC. An evaluation of food addiction as a distinct psychiatric disorder. Int J Eat Disord. 2020;53(10):1610–22.
29. Davis C, Carter JC. Compulsive overeating as an addiction disorder. A review of theory and evidence. Appetite. 2009;53(1):1–8.
30. Gearhardt AN, White MA, Masheb RM, Grilo CM. An examination of food addiction in a racially diverse sample of obese patients with binge eating disorder in primary care settings. Compr Psychiatry. 2013;54(5):500–5.
31. Ivezaj V, Wiedemann AA, Lawson JL, Grilo CM. Food addiction in sleeve gastrectomy patients with loss-of-control eating. Obes Surg. 2019;29(7):2071–7.
32. Wiss D, Brewerton T. Separating the signal from the noise: how psychiatric diagnoses can help discern food addiction from dietary restraint. Nutrients. 2020;12(10):2937.
33. Hilker I, Sanchez I, Steward T, Jimenez-Murcia S, Granero R, Gearhardt AN, et al. Food addiction in bulimia nervosa: clinical correlates and association with response to a brief psychoeducational intervention. Eur Eat Disord Rev. 2016;24(6):482–8.
34. Ben-Porat T, Weiss R, Sherf-Dagan S, Rottenstreich A, Kaluti D, Khalaileh A, et al. Food addiction and binge eating during one year following sleeve gastrectomy: prevalence and implications for postoperative outcomes. Obes Surg. 2021;31(2):603–11.
35. Ivezaj V, Wiedemann AA, Grilo CM. Food addiction and bariatric surgery: a systematic review of the literature. Obes Rev. 2017;18(12):1386–97.
36. Tinghino B, Lugoboni F, Amatulli A, Biasin C, Bramani Araldi M, Cantiero D, et al. The FODRAT study (FOod addiction, DRugs, Alcohol and Tobacco): first data on food addiction prevalence among patients with addiction to drugs, tobacco and alcohol. Eat Weight Disord. 2021;26(2):449–55.
37. Burrows T, Verdejo-Garcia A, Carter A, Brown RM, Andrews ZB, Dayas CV, et al. Health professionals' and health professional trainees' views on addictive eating behaviours: a cross-sectional survey. Nutrients. 2020;12(9):2860.
38. Gordon EL, Ariel-Donges AH, Bauman V, Merlo LJ. What is the evidence for "food addiction?" A systematic review. Nutrients. 2018;10(4):477.
39. Schulte EM, Gearhardt AN. Associations of food addiction in a sample recruited to be nationally representative of the United States. Eur Eat Disord Rev. 2018;26(2):112–9.
40. Lin YS, Tung YT, Yen YC, Chien YW. Food addiction mediates the relationship between perceived stress and body mass index in Taiwan young adults. Nutrients. 2020;12(7):1951.
41. Bourdier L, Fatseas M, Maria AS, Carre A, Berthoz S. The psycho-affective roots of obesity: results from a French study in the general population. Nutrients. 2020;12(10):2962.
42. Davis C. A commentary on the associations among "food addiction", binge eating disorder, and obesity: overlapping conditions with idiosyncratic clinical features. Appetite. 2017;115:3–8.
43. Hauck C, Weiss A, Schulte EM, Meule A, Ellrott T. Prevalence of "food addiction" as measured with the Yale Food Addiction Scale 2.0 in a representative German sample and its association with sex, age and weight categories. Obes Facts. 2017;10(1):12–24.
44. Meule A. A critical examination of the practical implications derived from the food addiction concept. Curr Obes Rep. 2019;8(1):11–7.

45. Brunault P, Ducluzeau PH, Bourbao-Tournois C, Delbachian I, Couet C, Reveillere C, et al. Food addiction in bariatric surgery candidates: prevalence and risk factors. Obes Surg. 2016;26(7):1650–3.
46. Goldman RL, Canterberry M, Borckardt JJ, Madan A, Byrne TK, George MS, et al. Executive control circuitry differentiates degree of success in weight loss following gastric-bypass surgery. Obesity. 2013;21(11):2189–96.
47. Long CG, Blundell JE, Finlayson G. A systematic review of the application and correlates of YFAS-diagnosed "food addiction" in humans: are eating-related "addictions" a cause for concern or empty concepts? Obes Facts. 2015;8(6):386–401.
48. Nunes-Neto PR, Kohler CA, Schuch FB, Solmi M, Quevedo J, Maes M, et al. Food addiction: prevalence, psychopathological correlates and associations with quality of life in a large sample. J Psychiatr Res. 2018;96:145–52.
49. Gearhardt AN, Corbin WR, Brownell KD. Preliminary validation of the Yale Food Addiction Scale. Appetite. 2009;52(2):430–6.
50. Lin Z, Qu S. Legend of weight loss: a crosstalk between the bariatric surgery and the brain. Obes Surg. 2020;30(5):1988–2002.
51. Parnarouskis L, Schulte EM, Lumeng JC, Gearhardt AN. Development of the highly processed food withdrawal scale for children. Appetite. 2020;147:104553.
52. Schulte EM, Smeal JK, Lewis J, Gearhardt AN. Development of the highly processed food withdrawal scale. Appetite. 2018;131:148–54.
53. Bryant EJ, Rehman J, Pepper LB, Walters ER. Obesity and eating disturbance: the role of TFEQ restraint and disinhibition. Curr Obes Rep. 2019;8(4):363–72.
54. Claudat K, Brown TA, Anderson L, Bongiorno G, Berner LA, Reilly E, et al. Correlates of co-occurring eating disorders and substance use disorders: a case for dialectical behavior therapy. Eat Disord. 2020;28(2):142–56.

How to Treat Food Addiction from a Nutritional Perspective: Consideration of Diet and Abstinence

13

13.1 Nutritional Approaches and Consideration of Abstinence

As discussed, FA is a valid construct, particularly as it relates to foods high in added sweeteners, fats, and refined ingredients (Chap. 11) [1, 2]. Many of those that believe in FA suggest that treatment should involve reducing intake of or abstaining completely from "addictive" foods (e.g., foods that prime the reward system, trigger craving, cause positive (from euphoric effects) and negative (from soothing effects) conditioning, have a more rapid effect on reward circuits, adversely affect appetite and satiety regulating homeostatic mechanisms, reduce the ability to feel full from any foods, etc.) [2–7]. These are also foods that tend to be high in fat or sugar, high in salt, and highly processed and easily/rapidly absorbed (Chap. 11).

If there is a rule of thumb for what abstinence might look like in FA, or what foods might best be avoided in a general way, it will be to reduce significantly or abstain from these more addictive foods (Chap. 11). There are reasons to believe that completely eliminating these foods would be of benefit for health and recovery. In fact, some experts suggest that sugar is a toxin, and the World Health Organization recommends significantly limiting intake of sugar for all people for general well-being [8, 9], and reduction of sugary drink consumption is also associated with obesity prevention [10].

Examples of typically problematic foods (Chap. 11, Table 11.1) might include chocolate, ice cream, French fries, pizza, cookies, chips, cake, sugar beverages, and sugar cereals [2, 11–13]. A combination of sweet and fat has been proposed as being especially associated with addictive symptoms in humans [1, 14]. High sodium may be another important target [15]. Processed and refined foods are more palatable by design and generally wise to avoid across the board [16]. The use of the glycemic index, protein, and/or fat content in weight loss diets has produced varied and non-definitive results (Chap. 2), but it still might be wise to avoid those foods with high glycemic indexes [17–20], given what we know about the strong reinforcing effects of rapid blood glucose elevation on reward circuits (Chap. 8).

Some also or instead suggest focusing on significantly reducing or abstaining from individual trigger foods [2] or particular problem foods that the individual tends to overeat and crave [2, 3, 21, 22]. One related way to help people simplify their dietary approaches would be to help them choose a focus on between fat and sugar addiction [23]. Also relatedly, some researchers have proposed three of highly palatable foods, high fat and sodium, high fat and sugar, and high sugar and sodium (defined by percent calories coming from each of the categories) [15], and developed a

C. E. Wilcox, *Food Addiction, Obesity, and Disorders of Overeating*,
https://doi.org/10.1007/978-3-030-83078-6_13

"hyperpalatable (HP) food" numerical scoring system to determine whether a food fits or doesn't fit into one of these three categories. This might be utilized and referenced to develop a diet to suggest to people with FA (e.g., avoid all foods that score highly in their particular trigger category), although it may not be a practical approach in the long run. The Yale Food Addiction Scale (YFAS) addressed food as a whole (not based on macronutrient content). A helpful questionnaire to develop next would be one to help patients identify which foods are most problematic for them.

A low carbohydrate ketogenic diet, which is essentially a one-size-fits-all abstinence-based approach, has been found to reduce reward, lower appetite, and increase satiety. In one small observational study, a low-carbohydrate ketogenic diet was initiated by three patients with obesity and comorbid binge eating and FA symptoms [18, 20, 24]. All patients tolerated the diet (macronutrient proportion: 10% carbohydrate, 30% protein, and 60% fat; at least 1200 calories/day) for 6–7 months without adverse events and reported significant reductions in binge eating episodes and FA symptoms including cravings and lack of control. Patients also lost 10–24% of their body weight and maintained gains in weight and binge eating up to 9–17 months after initiation [18, 20, 24].

In a study using a more individualized approach and focusing on food quantities, Vidmar and colleagues [2, 10, 21, 22] recently examined a FA model-based weight loss intervention phone app in a small group of obese adolescents which involved abstaining from "problem foods" (problem foods defined as foods they had cravings for or difficulty resisting). While weight loss was comparable to a standard weight loss intervention control group, the "abstinence" group had higher retention rates [10, 21, 22], and the app was more cost-effective (only two in-person visits and 12 contact hours total with mostly text and phone calls). A larger trial is now underway [2, 21, 22]. The food plan in this study involved staged withdrawal from problem foods (two problem foods at a time at 10-day intervals), then staged withdrawal from daytime (starting at a certain time of day, then progressively expanding the window) eating, and finally from excessive amounts of food consumed at meals reducing amounts in 2% increments.

12-step groups vary in their suggestions (abstaining from personal trigger foods and/or committing to 3–4 meals a day "with nothing in between" are commonly suggested in Overeaters Anonymous (OA), whereas Food Addicts Anonymous encourages fixed food plans for all members). The primary goal of 12-step program engagement for substance use disorder (SUD) and "compulsive overeating" is abstinence. For food, what that means is often defined by the individual in collaboration with their sponsor [10, 25, 26]. Although these approaches have come under scrutiny because success rates have not been well documented and out of concerns that they might lead to ED development (Chaps. 4 and 5), they also haven't been studied well [2]. Nevertheless, many individuals struggling with overeating report that applying an abstinence model helped them to control their eating [10, 25, 26]. If a more rigorous program is preferred by a patient, the provider should screen carefully for restrictive behavior prior to initiating and follow weights and disordered eating behaviors carefully [2, 27].

For patients to discover what foods are triggers for them, they could be instructed to keep a food journal. In this journal, they can list all foods they eat, paying attention to foods and patterns of eating that precede addictive eating or loss of control, and emotional responses to foods including improved mood, or increased cravings. This might help determine which of the approaches outlined above will be best suited for the individual patient.

13.2 Related Tips

13.2.1 Increase Satiety and Brain Health-Promoting Foods

In addition to avoiding the aforementioned highly palatable or triggering foods in particular, it's important for patients with FA to not get excessively hungry and get adequate intake of brain health-promoting foods. Satiety-promoting foods (Chap. 11, Table 11.1) include protein, fiber, and whole grains [19]. Foods that are high in dietary protein and high in fiber increase satiety and encourage weight loss [7, 28–30]. Studies have reported that foods that are high in dietary protein tend to increase the perception of satiety are less liked than low-protein foods [7, 31] and produce an increase in sensory-specific satiety (meaning they don't trigger immediate craving and overeating), compared to low-protein foods [7, 32]. Indeed, absorbed foods that might contain sucrose or fructose but that have high fiber contents (e.g., fruit) may not be prone to causing brain changes that lead to conditioning and binge use or overconsumption because fiber limits rapid absorption [9, 33, 34] (Chap. 9).

One commercial diet deserves mention here: https://www.drfuhrman.com/get-started/quick-start. This diet requires abstaining from many food groups and could be experienced as extreme for some patients. However, the website has a nice summary about foods to include that may have beneficial antioxidant effects and which might also promote satiety and brain recovery. It also suggests minimizing two macronutrients (carbohydrate, fat) and increasing various micronutrients. However, this approach has not been formally studied, and it is probably safer and less expensive to stick with nutritional recommendations that are less restrictive until we have more data to support the safety of these kinds of popular culture-based diets.

Furthermore, it is important to reverse nutrient deficiencies. Nutrient deficiencies can negatively impact mood (which could in turn increase craving for relief of negative mood) [35] and addictive behavior via dopaminergic mechanisms such as drug-seeking [35] and so will likely increase FA behavior too. Indeed, amino acids such as tryptophan, phenylalanine, and tyrosine are important for production of neurotransmitters such as serotonin, dopamine, and noradrenaline. Cofactors such as magnesium, zinc, chromium, selenium, folate, B12, lithium, and n-3 polyunsaturated fat are also important to replenish [35]. These nutrient deficiencies can be reversed with multivitamins but even more effective is to increase their intake through food that is rich in these components.

Antioxidants are also emphasized by some practitioners and experts [35, 36] (https://www.drfuhrman.com/get-started/quick-start). Recall that reactive oxygen radicals trigger inflammation, and this feeds into addictive behavior (Chap. 9). An antioxidant-rich diet reduces the experience of hunger and food intake suggesting that antioxidants may be able to reverse some of the deficits in the reward system that perpetuate obesity [36]. Antioxidant therapy has been shown to reverse impulsive behavior in general, as well [36]. An antioxidant and pro-oxidant food ratio of 2:3 per meal is the ideal nutritional ratio for good health and ideal weight in normal weight individuals, and a ratio of 3:4 is ideal for obese individuals because of their state of chronic oxidative stress, and inflammation is posited to be needed to promote recovery from obesity [36]. Additionally, N-acetyl cysteine (NAC) is an antioxidant that has some weak evidence for minimizing habit formation (e.g., conditioning) caused by L-Dopa, indicating that it might be able to help reduce compulsive use of HP foods and their power to usurp behavior and undermine weight loss attempts [37].

Finally, preliminary work supporting the potentially important role gut microbiota could play in food addiction via effects on brain reward circuitry (as we discussed in Chap. 10) has indicated probiotic supplementation might be useful. In one study probiotics administration significantly reduced weight, improved eating behavior, and decreased serum level of neuropeptide-Y compared to the placebo group [38].

13.2.2 Do Not Over-restrict Calorie Intake

Over-restriction is recognized by ED specialists worldwide as a major contributor to bingeing behavior and ultimately binge eating disorder (BED) and other EDs. In Alcoholics Anonymous one of the first things a "newcomer" learns is the acronym "HALT" suggesting that one should not get too "hungry, angry, lonely, or tired." During recovery from all additions, it is imperative not to get excessively hungry. The same advice should hold true for recovery from FA [3]. Patients should be reminded that although the long-term goal may be weight loss, that abstinence is designed to reduce hedonic overeating, e.g., to reduce the eating behavior that goes above one's homeostatic needs. Although weight loss will likely follow, and although in most people some calorie restriction may be safe, excessive starvation will undermine their attempts to get stable and may trigger bingeing [3, 10]. Promoting abstinence from certain foods as outlined above should not include restricting access to healthy foods [3, 10].

In support of these suggestions, recall how hunger and calorie restriction increases food cue reactivity and several other addictive processes in animal and human models (Chap. 9). Yo-yo dieting primes the reward system [39, 40]. Deprivation lowers the threshold for activation of reward pathways and increases the stress response, increasing sensitivity to both drugs of abuse and food as well as their conditioned cues, potentially increasing consumption, reinforcement, and future consumption of (due to conditioning) both drugs and food [35, 41–43].

That said, it's important to mention the other side that several studies have shown how caloric restriction might actually improve brain health and particularly cognition [44]. Whether this applies to impulse control or in people with FA is not yet clear. Furthermore, rapid weight loss has not been found to predict worse outcomes, in some studies: one trial showed that larger initial weight loss during energy-restricting diets was associated with better long-term outcomes [10, 45], although cause and effect is unclear in this study because it was not prospective and randomized. Finally, there is growing evidence about the general health benefits of intermittent fasting [46] (also discussed in Chap. 2).

Likely clinical practice will involve individually tailored treatment and a bit of trial and error. If there is excessive bingeing, backing off on calorie restriction for a while might help someone get back on track, and then increasing restriction could be tried again. For whom more rapid initial weight loss is safe and for whom it is not will involve detailed assessment (Chap. 12) and careful following.

13.2.3 Realize that Craving Will Diminish with Time in Recovery

Craving is, of course, both a withdrawal symptom and a result of conditioning [47–49]. As previously discussed, across different substances (including food), the experience of craving and its cognitive and neural mechanisms are largely similar [10]. Indeed, withdrawal symptoms may increase in the short term, which results in greater conditioned cue reactivity and greater craving. For example, when trait chocolate cravers (who had normal weight) were instructed to refrain from eating chocolate-containing foods (but to maintain regular consumption of all other foods), they reported more intense chocolate craving after 2 weeks [10, 50]. As a result, many people with FA may experience, in the first few weeks of abstinence from a trigger food or a group of foods, strong desires to resume eating their trigger foods, and in the context of these cravings, their brains search for and latch on to any number of justifications to do so. These justifications can completely undermine what felt like a firm commitment, just days prior, and will take people off-course [2].

While short-term deprivation increases cravings for avoided foods, long-term restriction results in reduction of food cravings that can facilitate extinction of conditioned responses [2, 51]. When examining the effects of weight loss interventions in obesity, food cravings tend to decrease during energy-restricting diets over time [10, 52, 53]. And the decrease in cravings is selective for the types of food avoided: cravings for high-carbohydrate foods selectively decreased during a low-carbohydrate diet, while cravings for fatty foods decreased during a low-fat diet [10, 54].

Neuroimaging work in humans also indicates that cue reactivity can be extinguished over time and the ability of drug or emotional cues to trigger craving also diminishes. Before starting a diet, individuals with high YFAS scores had greater activation in reward regions of the brain in response to food cues. After maintaining a prescribed diet of 1600 kcal/day (50% carbohydrates, 30% fats, and 20% proteins) for 3 months, individuals with high YFAS scores compared to those with low YFAS scores had brains that were indistinguishable from one another (i.e., the differences between those with FA and without were no longer present) [55, 56]. Another study showed that activation to food cues reduced in medial prefrontal cortex and other cortical areas from before to after 12 weeks of a nutritional and behavioral program in which participants replaced high-calorie foods with high bulk low-calorie foods [57, 58]. Greater activation in the nucleus accumbens at study entry, indicating reward sensitivity, predicted less weight loss over the 12-week program [57, 58].

In alcohol use disorder (AUD), as well, abstinence has been found to breed more abstinence and promote positive brain changes [59]. Abstinence from problem foods will likely ultimately do the same for people with FA. Interventional strategies that successfully reduce craving for and consumption of alcohol, tobacco, etc. can likely be applied to reduce craving for and consumption of food as well [10, 60, 61] to increase chances of success for getting more abstinence time (Chap. 14). With time in recovery, people can be reassured that things will get better and that they will experience the extinguishing of the food cue conditioning and reduced impulsivity and the process will naturally build on itself in a cyclical beneficial way [62]. People should know that although their cravings may increase initially, they will get better over time. It might be useful to suggest they consider the first month of abstinence as an experiment, to test the hypothesis that the cravings and dysphoria will likely pass. If it doesn't pass after a certain period of time, they can, at that point, reassess their approach.

13.2.4 Abstinence Is Not Absolute: Avoid All-or-Nothing Thinking

Although abstention from problematic foods is ideal, the idea of complete abstinence from certain food items may not be accurate from a nutritional or neurochemical point of view in the same way that it is for substances of abuse. If one's goal is to abstain completely from sugar, how to carry this out is not entirely clear, since fruit and vegetables also contain glucose, for example [10]. Moreover, it's much easier to "slip" accidentally with food. Humans eat several times a day, and there is a lot of opportunity to eat a problem food without realizing it. For example, individuals who try to avoid eating sugar may still (inadvertently) consume some foods that contain sugar or, at least, other forms of carbohydrates [10].

Tailor-made hybrid models between inclusive and exclusive approaches have been useful according to some experts. These approaches usually require some trial-and-error and are best done under the supervision of an registered dietitian and a psychiatrist/psychotherapist who understands EDs, FA, SUDs, and the associations with other psychiatric diagnoses described herein [2].

In addition, it's important to remember that individual differences exist and need to be taken into account in food plan development [21, 22]. Although fat, sugar, and highly processed foods are certainly the most likely culprits for most FA, it's important to tailor food plans to the individual. Although, for some, complete abstinence might work best, it might also not be practical for others, especially in the long term, given the complexity of food and its intense cultural interweaving. Also, what is "addictive" to one person might not be a problem for another. The definition of abstinence in relation to food will likely not be the same from one person to the next.

13.2.5 Is It Better to Start More Extreme or Use a Graded Approach During Initiation?

Some approaches suggest making a rapid more extreme change in eating such as is seen with adopting a ketogenic diets [18, 20, 24], whereas others have been tested more graded approaches [21, 22, 63]. Until more research is done, it is not clear which approach is most useful and for which people. Relatedly, identifying the problem foods can be difficult. It might be wise to ask people to be overinclusive on what they abstain from and, once stabilized, slowly work back in foods they're not sure about, until they start to lose stability around eating again. On the one hand, the world is full of food; it's a challenge to abstain from certain foods, especially with food being so tied to socialization (even more so than liquor). On the other hand, abstinence might bring relief faster than a slow taper. The 12-step programs talk about surrendering to the program, which for people with FA might involve surrendering to a food plan. And when people achieve sobriety in the early days of recovery, they often report a "pink cloud" which reinforces future abstinence. The confidence and freedom from craving and obsession really feels good and might argue for a more rapid change initially.

In SUD treatment, either total abstinence or substance use reduction, a "harm-reduction" approach (decreasing substance use to a level that is non-problematic [64]), is considered reasonable treatment strategies. In SUD treatment, harm reduction might work for some people, but many people end up ultimately choosing abstinence because it's so much easier.

13.2.6 Track Progress

Many weight management programs suggest tracking food intake or weight over time, which has been shown to improve outcomes. This might also be helpful in FA. However, in FA treatment, the goal is also to reduce the symptoms of FA (the sense of loss of control, craving, negative consequences of use, etc.). Remember the goals of behavior and dietary change are to enhance overall well-being and function. Patients might also consider tracking peace of mind, self-esteem, or personal sense of self-control to assess if what they're doing with their diet and other self-care is helping or harming them over time. Thus, encouraging them to consider these as equally if not more important than weight loss or abstinence may be best, in the long run.

13.3 How to Incorporate FA Treatment into ED Treatment Programming

As we've mentioned there is great concern that the "abstinence model" might be taken too far by some individuals with ED or predisposed to ED and that FA-based nutritional approaches might increase bingeing, ED risk, resurgence of dormant ED, or worsening ED symptoms [2]. As a general rule, the ED treatment culture is not highly supportive of the FA model for these reasons. It has been argued that abstinence models may be ineffective or—as they may reinforce problematic dietary restriction—even be hazardous, particularly in individuals with bulimia and BED [10, 65]. As reviewed in previous chapters (Chaps. 3 and 5), whether restriction and/or dieting causes bingeing and obesity in all people and how to identify those more vulnerable to restriction induced ED or obesity is still not clear.

Current practice in cognitive behavior therapy (CBT)-based ED treatment programs aim to reduce dysfunctional dieting and restraint of any kind (including attempting to abstain from certain foods) in favor of emphasizing regular eating patterns with flexible and moderate food consumption and no forbidden foods [10] which arguably refutes the FA model [65, 66]. In fact, this specific nutritional aspect of CBT-based ED treatment may be of great benefit for many patients who binge eat. For example, a reduction in dietary restraint has been shown to moderate the increased effectiveness of CBT on binge eating in a sample of patients with bulimia [66, 67].

The truth is that an abstinence-based nutritional approach might be helpful for some and harmful for others [2], and at this point we don't know for whom it is best to choose which. How to tailor nutritional recommendations for people with comorbid FA and ED may come down to three things. The first is the importance of doing a risk-benefit analysis. Potential harms of including an abstinence approach to eating are high for a patient with severe bulimia, but potential harms of not identifying and treating FA in someone with obesity is also high [2]. The second important issue is that providers shoud screen for restrictive patterns, which, if present, may indicate a greater risk of adverse outcomes from an abstinence-based approach. The assessment process is absolutely key (Chap. 12). Failure to consider restrictive eating patterns is an important criticism of FA that has led many ED professionals to reject the construct altogether [2]. The third is to recognize and identify impulsivity and cue reactivity as part of the eating pathology. Existing treatments sometimes fail to recognize impulsivity and susceptibility to environmental cues as key parts of the eating pathology [2, 68, 69]. If recognized, and if identified to be a bigger problem than, say, over-restriction, then an FA nutritional approach may prove more effective.

It will be very challenging, in residential settings especially, to implement divergent nutritional strategies where patients might compare food plans with one another [2], running the risk of exacerbating restrict-binge-purge patterns. How can one give conflicting messages to a patient one is treating, especially when a message of restriction might trigger other patients in the program, leading to potentially dangerous consequences? Some authors recommend that if an ED is present in addition to FA, clinicians should first provide more standard evidence-based treatments for the ED to see if the FA resolves [2, 70]. Indeed, studies suggest that FA most likely improves with ED treatment. For example, FA symptoms resolved when bulimia nervosa (BN) symptoms remitted [2, 70, 71] in a study using non-abstinence-based eating disorder treatment interventions. Also recall from Chap. 11 the animal studies that show that providing sugar and fat intermittently causes more addictive brain changes than continuous access animal models, which would imply that bingeing itself may be a cause of FA and a primary treatment target, avoiding restrictive approaches [72].

If a standard evidence-based ED treatment paradigm is ineffective, then an FA approach can be attempted next. When food alters dopamine circuitry, efforts by people with FA to moderate food intake while still eating "addictive" foods can make "intuitive eating" feel impossible, and the common ED paradigm which favors an "all foods fit" or "no bad foods" approach [2, 73] might trigger people with FA. In studies of OA, individuals struggling with overeating report that applying an abstinence model helped them to control their eating [10, 25, 26]. If an FA approach is deemed potentially useful, treatment of the FA might best be done in outpatient settings, or in settings designed for FA treatment, and progress can be supervised by clinicians and nutritionists experienced in EDs, SUDs, impulsivity treatment, and the FA concept [2] as well as medical personnel to watch for safety issues, in case dangerous bingeing or purging commences. Several residential and home-based intensive programs exist currently in the United States (SHiFT Recovery by Acorn – https://foodaddiction.com; COR – https://www.theretreat.org/programs/weekend-retreats/cor-retreats).

For obese patients with ED and FA, it may be wise to refer to an obesity clinic which utilizes behavioral weight loss therapy. A systematic review and meta-analysis found that structured and professionally run obesity treatments are associated with reduced ED prevalence, risk, and symptoms in children [2, 74].

Some would suggest that if some binging occurs following an attempt at abstinence should not lead to immediate cessation of the food plan. Saying that an abstinence approach is ineffective because people binge when they finally eat sweets is like saying that abstinence from alcohol is ineffective because those with AUD binge after taking the first drink [2, 11]. Failure to consider the possibility of increased craving and bingeing impulses during the first weeks of abstinence due to withdrawal is an important criticism of those that unilaterally say that if abstinence triggers binging, they should not try abstinence again [2, 10, 11].

It will also be important to distinguish between flexible and rigid restraint [2, 10, 75]. In some cases, restraint is related to a lower body weight, better weight regulation, and a better diet quality. In others, restraint predicts poor diet, overeating, and obesity [2, 27]. Relatedly, it is key to remember that abstinence doesn't mean semi-starvation. Removing particular food groups from a person's food plan should also be accompanied by an equal degree of emphasis on increasing healthy foods, adequate micronutrient, protein and fiber intake, and minimizing excessive calorie restriction and hunger.

Whether or not ED treatment providers accept the term "FA," avoiding foods that trigger their own overconsumption to the best of their ability, deliberate inclusion of health-promoting foods, and many of the behavioral, lifestyle, and medication interventions that we will go over in Chap. 14 (which target impulsivity and habitual patterns of responding, depression and anxiety management, developing coping mechanisms, enhancing positive social connections, addressing cognitive distortions such as justifications, as well as neuromodulation, cognitive training, encouraging adequate sleep and exercise, and medication) can still be considered for some patients with ED, especially those with comorbid obesity [2, 3], and these interventions do not contradict standard ED treatment approaches (Chap. 14, Table 14.1).

13.4 What to Do with "Normal Weight" FA Patients?

Is it ever wise to suggest an abstinence-based approach in someone who doesn't need to lose weight for health reasons (e.g., with a normal body mass index)? The jury is still out on this, but FA is associated with distress even if the person is of normal weight and is often related to feelings of loss of control. Perhaps assessing body image distortions could be helpful here, and if the goal is about weight maintenance rather than loss, and if the target symptom is loss of control rather than weight, then in combination with increasing healthy foods and eating adequate calories, and trialling an abstinence approach and some of the additional suggestions reviewed in the next section might be appropriate. More studies are needed, however, to confirm this.

13.5 Conclusion

Many dietary recommendations have been made regarding FA treatment; however none have been extensively studied. Given that many approaches appear to be useful for some, but maybe not all FA patients, it is important to individualize treatment. Some recommendations, which appear to make good nutritional sense such as avoiding or limiting HP foods, including more whole grains and fiber in one's diet are probably safe to suggest to most FA patients. Treatment should be individualized, taking into account a patient's comorbidities, especially noting the presence of EDs and how particular diets may affect those. It is also important to take individual preferences into account. More research in this area is needed to further our ability to target particular recommendations to individual patients.

References

1. Gordon EL, Ariel-Donges AH, Bauman V, Merlo LJ. What is the evidence for "food addiction?" A systematic review. Nutrients. 2018;10(4):477.
2. Wiss D, Brewerton T. Separating the signal from the noise: how psychiatric diagnoses can help discern food addiction from dietary restraint. Nutrients. 2020;12(10):2937.
3. Treasure J, Leslie M, Chami R, Fernandez-Aranda F. Are trans diagnostic models of eating disorders fit for purpose? A consideration of the evidence for food addiction. Eur Eat Disord Rev. 2018;26(2):83–91.
4. Gearhardt AN, Corbin WR, Brownell KD. Preliminary validation of the Yale Food Addiction Scale. Appetite. 2009;52(2):430–6.
5. Gearhardt AN, Corbin WR, Brownell KD. Development of the Yale Food Addiction Scale Version 2.0. Psychol Addict Behav. 2016;30(1):113–21.
6. Sclafani A. Gut-brain nutrient signaling. Appetition vs. satiation. Appetite. 2013;71:454–8.
7. Onaolapo AY, Onaolapo OJ. Food additives, food and the concept of "food addiction": is stimulation of the brain reward circuit by food sufficient to trigger addiction? Pathophysiology. 2018;25(4):263–76.
8. Rodda SN, Booth N, Brittain M, McKean J, Thornley S. I was truly addicted to sugar: a consumer-focused classification system of behaviour change strategies for sugar reduction. Appetite. 2020;144:104456.
9. Lustig RH, Schmidt LA, Brindis CD. Public health: the toxic truth about sugar. Nature. 2012;482(7383):27–9.
10. Meule A. A critical examination of the practical implications derived from the food addiction concept. Curr Obes Rep. 2019;8(1):11–7.
11. Ifland J, Preuss HG, Marcus MT, Rourke KM, Taylor W, Theresa Wright H. Clearing the confusion around processed food addiction. J Am Coll Nutr. 2015;34(3):240–3.

12. Ifland JR, Preuss HG, Marcus MT, Rourke KM, Taylor WC, Burau K, et al. Refined food addiction: a classic substance use disorder. Med Hypotheses. 2009;72(5):518–26.
13. Schulte EM, Avena NM, Gearhardt AN. Which foods may be addictive? The roles of processing, fat content, and glycemic load. PLoS One. 2015;10(2):e0117959.
14. Markus CR, Rogers PJ, Brouns F, Schepers R. Eating dependence and weight gain; no human evidence for a "sugar-addiction" model of overweight. Appetite. 2017;114:64–72.
15. Fazzino TL, Rohde K, Sullivan DK. Hyper-palatable foods: development of a quantitative definition and application to the US food system database. Obesity. 2019;27(11):1761–8.
16. Guise S. Mini habits for weight loss: stop dieting. Form new habits. Change your lifestyle without suffering. Selective Entertainment LLC; 2016.
17. San-Cristobal R, Navas-Carretero S, Martinez-Gonzalez MA, Ordovas JM, Martinez JA. Contribution of macronutrients to obesity: implications for precision nutrition. Nat Rev Endocrinol. 2020;16(6):305–20.
18. Carmen M, Safer DL, Saslow LR, Kalayjian T, Mason AE, Westman EC, et al. Treating binge eating and food addiction symptoms with low-carbohydrate Ketogenic diets: a case series. J Eat Disord. 2020;8:2.
19. Sievenpiper JL. Low-carbohydrate diets and cardiometabolic health: the importance of carbohydrate quality over quantity. Nutr Rev. 2020;78(Suppl 1):69–77.
20. Sethi Dalai S, Sinha A, Gearhardt AN. Low carbohydrate ketogenic therapy as a metabolic treatment for binge eating and ultraprocessed food addiction. Curr Opin Endocrinol Diabetes Obes. 2020;27(5):275–82.
21. Vidmar AP, Pretlow R, Borzutzky C, Wee CP, Fox DS, Fink C, et al. An addiction model-based mobile health weight loss intervention in adolescents with obesity. Pediatr Obes. 2019;14(2):e12464.
22. Vidmar AP, Salvy SJ, Pretlow R, Mittelman SD, Wee CP, Fink C, et al. An addiction-based mobile health weight loss intervention: protocol of a randomized controlled trial. Contemp Clin Trials. 2019;78:11–9.
23. Sarkar S, Kochhar KP, Khan NA. Fat addiction: psychological and physiological trajectory. Nutrients. 2019;11(11):2785.
24. Di Rosa C, Lattanzi G, Taylor SF, Manfrini S, Khazrai YM. Very low calorie ketogenic diets in overweight and obesity treatment: effects on anthropometric parameters, body composition, satiety, lipid profile and microbiota. Obes Res Clin Pract. 2020;14(6):491–503.
25. Rodriguez-Martin BC, Gallego-Arjiz B. Overeaters anonymous: a mutual-help fellowship for food addiction recovery. Front Psychol. 2018;9:1491.
26. Russell-Mayhew S, von Ranson KM, Masson PC. How does overeaters anonymous help its members? A qualitative analysis. Eur Eat Disord Rev. 2010;18(1):33–42.
27. Bryant EJ, Rehman J, Pepper LB, Walters ER. Obesity and eating disturbance: the role of TFEQ restraint and disinhibition. Curr Obes Rep. 2019;8(4):363–72.
28. Larsen TM, Dalskov SM, van Baak M, Jebb SA, Papadaki A, Pfeiffer AF, et al. Diets with high or low protein content and glycemic index for weight-loss maintenance. N Engl J Med. 2010;363(22):2102–13.
29. Schoeller DA, Buchholz AC. Energetics of obesity and weight control: does diet composition matter? J Am Diet Assoc. 2005;105(5 Suppl 1):S24–8.
30. Luhovyy BL, Akhavan T, Anderson GH. Whey proteins in the regulation of food intake and satiety. J Am Coll Nutr. 2007;26(6):704S–12S.
31. Johnson J, Vickers Z. Factors influencing sensory-specific satiety. Appetite. 1992;19(1):15–31.
32. Sivertsen HK, Ueland O, Westad F. Development of satiating and palatable high-protein meat products by using experimental design in food technology. Food Nutr Res. 2010;54:5114.
33. Laliberte M, Mccabe RE, Taylor V. The cognitive behavioral workbook for weight management. Raincoast Books; 2009.
34. Wu WC, Inui A, Chen CY. Weight loss induced by whole grain-rich diet is through a gut microbiota-independent mechanism. World J Diabetes. 2020;11(2):26–32.
35. Jeynes KD, Gibson EL. The importance of nutrition in aiding recovery from substance use disorders: a review. Drug Alcohol Depend. 2017;179:229–39.
36. Tobore TO. Towards a comprehensive theory of obesity and a healthy diet: the causal role of oxidative stress in food addiction and obesity. Behav Brain Res. 2020;384:112560.
37. Gibson AS, Keefe KA, Furlong TM. Accelerated habitual learning resulting from L-dopa exposure in rats is prevented by N-acetylcysteine. Pharmacol Biochem Behav. 2020;198:173033.
38. Narmaki E, Borazjani M, Ataie-Jafari A, Hariri N, Doost AH, Qorbani M, et al. The combined effects of probiotics and restricted calorie diet on the anthropometric indices, eating behavior, and hormone levels of obese women with food addiction: a randomized clinical trial. Nutr Neurosci. 2020:1–13.
39. Wilcox CE. Binge eating disorder. American Physician Institute; 2019. Available from: CMEtoGo.com.
40. Sinha R. Role of addiction and stress neurobiology on food intake and obesity. Biol Psychol. 2018;131:5–13.
41. Aitken TJ, Greenfield VY, Wassum KM. Nucleus accumbens core dopamine signaling tracks the need-based motivational value of food-paired cues. J Neurochem. 2016;136(5):1026–36.
42. Carr KD. Chronic food restriction: enhancing effects on drug reward and striatal cell signaling. Physiol Behav. 2007;91(5):459–72.
43. Volkow ND, Wang GJ, Fowler JS, Tomasi D, Telang F. Addiction: beyond dopamine reward circuitry. Proc Natl Acad Sci U S A. 2011;108(37):15037–42.
44. Grigolon RB, Brietzke E, Trevizol AP, McIntyre RS, Mansur RB. Caloric restriction, resting metabolic

rate and cognitive performance in non-obese adults: a post-hoc analysis from CALERIE study. J Psychiatr Res. 2020;128:16–22.

45. Casazza K, Brown A, Astrup A, Bertz F, Baum C, Brown MB, et al. Weighing the evidence of common beliefs in obesity research. Crit Rev Food Sci Nutr. 2015;55(14):2014–53.
46. de Cabo R, Mattson MP. Effects of intermittent fasting on health, aging, and disease. N Engl J Med. 2019;381(26):2541–51.
47. Addolorato G, Leggio L, Abenavoli L, Gasbarrini G. Neurobiochemical and clinical aspects of craving in alcohol addiction: a review. Addict Behav. 2005;30(6):1209–24.
48. Anton RF. What is craving? Models and implications for treatment. Alcohol Res Health. 1999;23(3):165–73.
49. Heinz A, Lober S, Georgi A, Wrase J, Hermann D, Rey ER, et al. Reward craving and withdrawal relief craving: assessment of different motivational pathways to alcohol intake. Alcohol Alcohol. 2003;38(1):35–9.
50. Richard A, Meule A, Friese M, Blechert J. Effects of chocolate deprivation on implicit and explicit evaluation of chocolate in high and low trait chocolate cravers. Front Psychol. 2017;8:1591.
51. Meule A. The psychology of food cravings: the role of food deprivation. Curr Nutr Rep. 2020;9(3):251–7.
52. Kahathuduwa CN, Binks M, Martin CK, Dawson JA. Extended calorie restriction suppresses overall and specific food cravings: a systematic review and a meta-analysis. Obes Rev. 2017;18(10):1122–35.
53. Oustric P, Gibbons C, Beaulieu K, Blundell J, Finlayson G. Changes in food reward during weight management interventions – a systematic review. Obes Rev. 2018;19(12):1642–58.
54. Martin CK, Rosenbaum D, Han H, Geiselman PJ, Wyatt HR, Hill JO, et al. Change in food cravings, food preferences, and appetite during a low-carbohydrate and low-fat diet. Obesity. 2011;19(10):1963–70.
55. Guzzardi MA, Garelli S, Agostini A, Filidei E, Fanelli F, Giorgetti A, et al. Food addiction distinguishes an overweight phenotype that can be reversed by low calorie diet. Eur Eat Disord Rev. 2018;26(6):657–70.
56. Gordon EL, Lent MR, Merlo LJ. The effect of food composition and behavior on neurobiological response to food: a review of recent research. Curr Nutr Rep. 2020;9(2):75–82.
57. Murdaugh DL, Cox JE, Cook EW 3rd, Weller RE. fMRI reactivity to high-calorie food pictures predicts short- and long-term outcome in a weight-loss program. Neuroimage. 2012;59(3):2709–21.
58. Schlogl H, Horstmann A, Villringer A, Stumvoll M. Functional neuroimaging in obesity and the potential for development of novel treatments. Lancet Diabetes Endocrinol. 2016;4(8):695–705.
59. Wilcox CE, Dekonenko CJ, Mayer AR, Bogenschutz MP, Turner JA. Cognitive control in alcohol use disorder: deficits and clinical relevance. Rev Neurosci. 2014;25:1–24.
60. May J, Andrade J, Kavanagh DJ, Feeney GF, Gullo MJ, Statham DJ, et al. The craving experience questionnaire: a brief, theory-based measure of consummatory desire and craving. Addiction. 2014;109(5):728–35.
61. Appelhans BM, French SA, Pagoto SL, Sherwood NE. Managing temptation in obesity treatment: a neurobehavioral model of intervention strategies. Appetite. 2016;96:268–79.
62. Clasen MM, Riley AL, Davidson TL. Hippocampal-dependent inhibitory learning and memory processes in the control of eating and drug taking. Curr Pharm Des. 2020;26(20):2334–52.
63. Wiss DA, Avena N, Rada P. Sugar addiction: from evolution to revolution. Front Psych. 2018;9:545.
64. Marlatt GA. The controlled-drinking controversy. A commentary. Am Psychol. 1983;38(10):1097–110.
65. Wilson GT. Eating disorders, obesity and addiction. Eur Eat Disord Rev. 2010;18(5):341–51.
66. Adams RC, Sedgmond J, Maizey L, Chambers CD, Lawrence NS. Food addiction: implications for the diagnosis and treatment of overeating. Nutrients. 2019;11(9):2086.
67. Wilson GT, Fairburn CC, Agras WS, Walsh BT, Kraemer H. Cognitive-behavioral therapy for bulimia nervosa: time course and mechanisms of change. J Consult Clin Psychol. 2002;70(2):267–74.
68. Manasse SM, Espel HM, Schumacher LM, Kerrigan SG, Zhang F, Forman EM, et al. Does impulsivity predict outcome in treatment for binge eating disorder? A multimodal investigation. Appetite. 2016;105:172–9.
69. Bergh C, Callmar M, Danemar S, Holcke M, Isberg S, Leon M, et al. Effective treatment of eating disorders: results at multiple sites. Behav Neurosci. 2013;127(6):878–89.
70. Hilker I, Sanchez I, Steward T, Jimenez-Murcia S, Granero R, Gearhardt AN, et al. Food addiction in bulimia nervosa: clinical correlates and association with response to a brief psychoeducational intervention. Eur Eat Disord Rev. 2016;24(6):482–8.
71. Meule A, von Rezori V, Blechert J. Food addiction and bulimia nervosa. Eur Eat Disord Rev. 2014;22(5):331–7.
72. Blanco-Gandia MC, Minarro J, Rodriguez-Arias M. Common neural mechanisms of palatable food intake and drug abuse: knowledge obtained with animal models. Curr Pharm Des. 2020;26(20):2372–84.
73. Freeland-Graves JH, Nitzke S, Academy of Nutrition and Dietetics. Position of the academy of nutrition and dietetics: total diet approach to healthy eating. J Acad Nutr Diet. 2013;113(2):307–17.
74. Jebeile H, Gow ML, Baur LA, Garnett SP, Paxton SJ, Lister NB. Treatment of obesity, with a dietary component, and eating disorder risk in children and adolescents: a systematic review with meta-analysis. Obes Rev. 2019;20(9):1287–98.
75. Linardon J. The relationship between dietary restraint and binge eating: examining eating-related self-efficacy as a moderator. Appetite. 2018;127:126–9.

14 Clinical Applications of the Food Addiction Concept

14.1 Treatment Overview

As discussed in Chap. 4, there is a pressing need for more efficacious, tolerable, and safe treatments for people with obesity and binge eating. In Chap. 5 we introduced several areas of current ongoing controversy about FA, but argued there are many reasons to hope that applying this concept will improve clinical outcomes. In Chap. 13, nutritional interventions to help people with FA were discussed. Here we will discuss non-nutritional interventions for FA treatment, many of which are derived from SUD treatment principles. Table 14.1 summarizes what we will be discussing in detail in the rest of this chapter.

SUD are associated with a lifelong (albeit diminishing with time in recovery) risk of relapse. This is because the brain, which has been damaged by chronic use and conditioning, takes time to heal. Treatment goals involve minimizing negative affect states, reducing substance and environmental cue reactivity, preventing habitual responding, and improving impulse control. Like in SUD, treatment of FA will involve long-term maintenance of brain health.

SUD are often treated with medications to reduce withdrawal symptoms, but much more importantly, medications are utilized to reduce relapse risk in the long term by re-balancing the brain reward and impulse control system. Examples of medications that work via some or all of these mechanisms for SUD include naltrex-

Table 14.1 Overview of treatment recommendations

Psychoeducation	Decreases self-blame, stigma, and reluctance to accept evidence-based medications
Psychosocial interventions	Cognitive behavioral therapy Behavioral weight management Motivational interviewing Mindfulness-based therapies DBT/ACT targeting emotion regulation Body image work
Sleep, Exercise	Improves impulse control Enhances mood Promotes recovery from FA
Medications	Naltrexone/bupropion SR Topiramate/phentermine Bupropion Lisdexamfetamine Naltrexone Topiramate Zonisamide Selective serotonin reuptake inhibitors Liraglutide
Treatment of underlying psychiatric disorders	Medications Evidence-based therapies
Self-help groups/12-step/Other support	Overeaters anonymous, food addicts anonymous, intensive outpatient or residential treatment program (SHiFT recovery by acorn for e.g.), sponsor or dietitian/ nutritionist for food plan development and accountability
TMS	On the horizon, stay tuned
Surgery	Bariatric surgery

C. E. Wilcox, *Food Addiction, Obesity, and Disorders of Overeating*,
https://doi.org/10.1007/978-3-030-83078-6_14

one, acamprosate, topiramate, and disulfiram for alcohol use disorder; varenicline, bupropion, and nicotine replacement therapy for nicotine use disorder; and methadone, buprenorphine, and naltrexone for opioid use disorder [1]. Evidence-based psychosocial interventions for SUD (provided in either group or individual formats) include cognitive behavior therapy (CBT), mindfulness-based (MB) relapse prevention, interventions which improve emotion regulation such as dialectical behavior therapy (DBT), and acceptance and commitment therapy (ACT), 12-step facilitation approaches, and motivational interviewing [2] (see Appendix for extensive list of useful therapy manuals).

Notably, many of the evidence-based interventions for SUD are already adapted for and being utilized to treat obesity and EDs (Chaps. 2 and 3), which provides further reason to believe that many might also prove beneficial for the treatment of FA. However, there has been little treatment research on FA, so most of these recommendations are speculative and need further formal study in randomized clinical trials before widespread deployment.

The transdiagnostic model for ED treatment assumes that all EDs will respond to a similar therapeutic approach [3–7], and this assumption has led providers to assume that the approaches utilized for anorexia and bulimia will also work for binge eating disorder (BED), which was only recently included in the *Diagnostic and Statistical Manual* (DSM). However, it is not known whether ED approaches are best for all cases of BED and bulimia nervosa, especially where FA symptoms predominate or in people who also have obesity [3–7]. An alternate approach, outlined in one recent paper [4], argues that people with FA should utilize an abstinence-based nutritional approach (Chap. 13) (which would not be encouraged in a typical ED treatment program) and should also have the following three focuses during treatment: (1) reduction of habitual responding (e.g., conditioning based food cues) and impulsivity through psychotherapy, cognitive training techniques, and medications; (2) diminishment of negative reinforcement based behaviors (e.g., emotional eating) by reducing negative affect and increasing coping skills and alternate behaviors and social connection; and (3) reduction of compensatory behaviors such as vomiting or excessive exercise with psychoeducation and coping mechanisms skills training. This model directly speaks to what we extensively discussed in Chap. 8 regarding the underlying neurobiological causes of FA-like behavior.

In addition to abstinence, interventional strategies that successfully reduce craving for and consumption of alcohol, tobacco, and illicit drugs will also likely reduce craving for and compulsive consumption of food [8–10].

14.2 Supplemental Programmatic Elements Which Might Be Useful for Treatment of FA

14.2.1 Psychoeducation: FA Is a Brain-Based Disorder

Patients with FA and their providers should understand that the overeating is not due to character weakness or a problem of "willpower" but is rooted in brain chemistry. They should also understand how some of the suggested treatments would be expected to work, mechanistically, as this may enhance adherence to a particular dietary recommendation or medication. For example, knowing that sugar causes craving and loss of control via a biological cascade of events outside of one's control may help someone to stay on track with a commitment not to eat sugar. Understanding that it's not just about the calories, but that particular palatable foods may lead to loss of control of eating in some people, could motivate people to stay away from those particular foods and enhance their chances of success.

A brain-based explanation of SUD is often referred to as the disease-based model of addiction and is known to decrease stigma and self-blame [6, 11–13]. Patients can be educated utilizing materials such as Figs. 7.1 and 7.2 (Chap. 7) to explain the neurobiological underpinnings of addictive behavior. Such models of understanding may also benefit people with obesity and binge eating, in addition to FA [6, 14–16]. This is important in light of the fact that shame worsens mood, and therefore recovery outcomes, since increasing negative affect can trigger increased emotional eating for self-soothing. Indeed, studies show that fear of being stigmatized predicts worsening FA status, maladaptive eating behaviors, stress, and weight gain [3, 17, 18]. However, it is also posited that biological explanations might reduce self-efficacy and might undermine someone's motivation to reduce calorie intake or change their eating patterns [6, 15, 19]. At this point it is not yet known what effects emphasizing the neurobiology might have on individual perceptions, attitudes, and behavior in FA, but based on the effects of such psychoeducation in SUD, it will likely be recommended [6].

Recall, from Chap. 4 the low acceptability among providers and the public of medications for obesity treatment [20]. Widespread psychoeducation regarding the neurobiology of overeating may also increase providers' inclination to suggest evidence-based medication treatments and patients to accept such suggestions. Indeed, physicians are, in general, less likely to believe in brain-based aspects of SUD than attorneys, showing physicians may have more stigmatizing beliefs than others, which is an obvious problem that should be addressed through increased provider education [13].

14.2.2 Psychosocial Interventions

There are numerous manuals available to guide providers in the application of evidence-based psychosocial interventions for SUDs, EDs, and psychiatric comorbidities (Appendix).

14.2.2.1 CBT

CBT is a therapeutic approach extensively informed by research for the treatment of EDs, obesity, and SUD, alike [7]. Generally, CBT interventions ask patients to critically evaluate the thoughts, feelings, and behaviors that result in maladaptive eating and then to modify them, helping patients to recognize potential triggers and develop appropriate coping strategies [7]. CBT for SUD, obesity, and ED targets irrational beliefs and cognitive distortions, focuses on identification of and use of effective coping skills, and emphasizes identifying and avoiding triggers (environmental, food/substance cue-related, and emotional triggers) [6, 21, 22]. CBT for ED differs from that utilized for SUD and obesity, however, in that CBT for EDs also includes a non-abstinence-based, all-foods-included nutritional component as previously discussed.

In FA or FA-like patients, CBT-approaches will likely prove useful. One study examined 47 internet sources to extract the CBT-like strategies endorsed by self-perceived sugar addicts. Actional strategies that reportedly worked for the participants included avoidance, meal consumption-planning, environmental restructuring, professional and social support, addressing underlying issues, and urge management, among others [3, 23]. Another group has developed a mobile health CBT-based strategy which includes CBT therapeutic components and also involves a staged food withdrawal from problem foods and between-meal or excessive eating, and it is described in detail in Chap. 13 [24]. Others have proposed a body-focused repetitive behavior (BFRB) approach for FA adapted from treatment utilized for other compulsive disorders such as nail-biting, skin picking, and hair pulling [25]. BFRB therapies incorporate distractions, competing behaviors, triggers avoidance, relaxation methods, aversion techniques, and distress tolerance. Adding action-based CBT components improved the weight loss more than just the sensory-based CBT components in the BFRB approach for FA, and weight loss was maintained for 5 months afterwards [25].

Another CBT-like approach, which hasn't been formally studied but which could be integrated in to CBT for FA, emphasizes the roles of attentional bias (excessive focus on food or emotional cues), temporal discounting (undervaluing future rewards), and the cold-hot empathy gap (when individuals are in a "hot," motivated state they overestimate the degree to which they will value a reward, in comparison to a non-motivated, neutral, "cold" state). This approach suggests distinguishing between temptation resistance strategies aimed at overcoming temptation while it is experienced and temptation prevention strategies that seek to avoid or minimize exposure to tempting stimuli since inhibiting habitual cue-driven behaviors during a "hot" state is much more difficult and requires prospective thinking to identify and avoid exposure to foods that may challenge future self-control [10, 26]. The latter kind of strategy places emphasis on minimizing temptation through stimulus control (removing tempting food from the home), scheduling and planning, time locking safes, or even financial contracting (punishment strategy) or social contracting (publicly committing to the goal) [10], and it dovetails well with abstinence-based nutritional approaches. The treatment plan (what foods to abstain from, how to reduce exposure to triggering simuli) can be decided upon when someone is ideally in a "cold state" and cognitive functions are intact.

14.2.2.2 Behavioral Weight Management

In addition to CBT, behavioral weight management (Chap. 2) shows promise in several uncontrolled studies for FA. For example, a 14-week group lifestyle modification program including caloric reduction significantly reduced addictive eating behaviors in one study [3, 27]. A 6-week integrative group for weight management in another study reduced FA from pre to post and utilized strategies such as mindful eating, keeping a food diary, carrying out an exercise plan, regular weigh-ins, and planning for social eating [3, 28].

14.2.2.3 Motivational Interviewing (MI)

MI is extensively utilized in SUD to motivate change in behavior [8, 29]. Indeed, it may help for FA as well, although it has not been hugely successful in obesity, in general [30]. In one study, a person-centered MI-based intervention was delivered in three sessions via telehealth to individuals with FA and obesity or overweight called "FoodFix." This intervention was associated with a reduction in energy intake from "non-core foods" (i.e., foods with added or high amounts of salt, sugar, and/or fat) compared with the waitlist control intervention, but both the active and control groups showed reductions in Yale Food Addiction Scale (YFAS) scores [31].

14.2.2.4 Psychotherapy to Reduce Negative Affect States, Improve Emotion Regulation, and Address Alexithymia

Several bodies of work indicate that emotional eating (or eating to self-sooth, the basis of negative reinforcement-driven eating) may be more resistant to change and extinction compared to external (food-cue driven) eating [32, 33]. For example, 4 years after a diet intervention, scores on emotional eating had hardly changed in both the male and the female patients with diabetes type 2, whereas scores on external eating had declined significantly in the female patients [33]. This might indicate a need for people with FA and emotional eating to do more extensive work on emotion regulation and deeper psychological issues. Such work may involve efforts to teach people how to recognize their own emotions, since "difficulty identifying feelings" (alexithymia) was associated with emotional eating and may mediate the relationship between depression and emotional eating [33]. Other emotion regulation-focused psychotherapeutic strategies such as DBT and ACT might be particularly useful for people who struggle with emotional eating, but more work needs to be done in this area to confirm.

14.2.2.5 Mindfulness-Based (MB) Approaches

MB interventions and emotion regulation-based strategies, like DBT and ACT, which incorporate mindfulness are helpful in SUD, ED, and obesity populations (reviewed in Chaps. 2 and 3) but have not been formally studied in FA. Lower interoceptive awareness was found to be associated with FA in an ED population, indicating that more work on mindful eating and becoming aware of internal hunger and satiety cues might prove useful in this population [34]. Furthermore, impulsivity is a major contributor to FA, and mindfulness work has been shown to improve impulse control in numerous populations [35]. These interventions can be utilized now and should be studied in people with FA.

14.2.2.6 Body Image Work

Body image work may also prove important in FA treatment, when relevant. Shape/weight overvaluation is associated with BED and bulimia [3, 36–38]. Relatedly, those with heightened body image disturbance are more likely to engage in dietary restraint [3, 37], which may contribute to bingeing as well as FA symptoms [3]. However, weight loss might be the most effective way to improve body image in individuals with FA [39].

14.2.3 Importance of Sleep

As described in Chap. 9, adequate sleep is important for improvement in mood, executive function, impulse control, and recovery from both SUD and disorders of overeating. Patients with sleep disturbance should be counseled to adopt sleep hygiene techniques and, if prescribed, take sleeping supplements. Melatonin may especially be helpful, and some early work indicates that it may have secondary utility in reducing adiposity [40]. In fact, setmelanotide is a melanocortin-4 receptor agonist under study for obesity treatment [41]. Getting adequate exercise, which improves sleep in people with a variety of psychiatric illness [42], should be recommended. Patients with difficulty sleeping and FA might also benefit from CBT for insomnia [43].

14.2.4 Importance of Exercise

Clearly, exercise is important for treatment of obesity, and it can reduce appetite, increase calories burned, and slightly increase resting metabolic rate as discussed in Chap. 2. However, there is growing evidence that exercise will likely be key for FA treatment for other reasons including its beneficial effects on dysphoria and negative affect [44] and impulse control [45] the latter of which may be mediated by restoring type 2 and type 3 dopamine receptors (D2) in the dorsal striatum (Chaps. 7 and 8) [46]. More studies are needed in this area as well.

14.2.5 Importance of Getting Psychiatric and Psychological Care

As we discussed in Chap. 6, FA is associated with and likely made worse by a variety of psychiatric comorbidities, including major depressive disorder (MDD), bipolar disorder, anxiety disorders, attention deficit hyperactivity disorder (ADHD), post-traumatic stress disorder (PTSD), and personality disorders. Since many studies show that stress and negative affect can drive habitual behaviors via negative reinforcement [47], and that impulsivity can contribute to loss of control of eating, treatment of FA should involve aggressive assessment for and management of these comorbid disorders. Evidence-based psychotherapies such as CBT, ACT, DBT, other emotion regulation trainings, MB interventions, interpersonal psychotherapy (IPT), and psychodynamic therapy can be utilized. Furthermore, psychiatric evaluation for possible pharmacotherapeutic management of an underlying disorder should always be considered. Medications targeting these comorbidities and evidence-based treatments are key.

Failure to recognize and treat PTSD and other trauma-based sequelae is a major contributor to poor outcomes in the treatment of EDs and obesity and is also believed to play a big role in some people FA as well which we have discussed in more detail in Chap. 6 [48]. Multiple studies indicate childhood maltreatment predicts FA which then predicts obesity [48]. This link is also likely maintained through negative reinforcement learning and connected to emotional eating [47]. Evidence-based trauma therapies such as exposure therapy or trauma-focused CBT may be useful for these individuals for reducing FA symptoms, although this has not been directly studied.

14.2.6 Neuromodulation Techniques

There has been recent explosion in research on and use of non-convulsive (e.g., not electroconvulsive therapy) brain stimulation techniques for the treatment of a variety of psychiatric disorders. This includes a growing body of work exploring their potential for reducing craving and addictive behavior [49, 50]. The most commonly applied stimulation method clinically is repetitive transcranial magnetic stimulation (rTMS), although transcranial direct current stimulation, vagal nerve stimulation, and even deep brain stimulation are being studied for obesity and BED, too [7, 51]. rTMS is Food and Drug Association (FDA)-approved for the treatment of several disorders [MDD, obsessive compulsive disorder (OCD)] using more than one approach [49, 50], and it is a safe way to focally affect brain activation [51]. rTMS is used in awake participants and is therefore minimally disruptive, associated with minimal side effects, and is quite safe when used appropriately within guidelines [7, 49, 50, 52–54]. rTMS works via a number of potential mechanisms to alter neural activity, including by increasing connectivity and increasing dopamine function for example [7, 8, 55, 56]. rTMS studies have primarily focused on stimulating the (usually left) dorsolateral prefrontal cortex (DLPFC), to enhance cognitive control. Some rTMS studies are now starting to explore other targets such as the anterior cingulate cortex (ACC) and cerebellum [57]. Moreover, deep rTMS, which allows for access to deeper brain structures in a noninvasive way, is being studied for other psychiatric disorders and may one day prove useful for reduction of drug and food cravings, since the circuitry involved in regulating feeding tend to be deeper (the insula striatum and hypothalamus are inaccessible with standard rTMS coils) [49, 50].

When applied to the DLPFC, rTMS has been shown to effectively reduce cravings for cigarettes, alcohol, and other drugs of abuse, especially when applied for multiple sessions, and may be useful for drug use reduction in cocaine and nicotine use disorders [49, 50]. The DLPFC is an area involved extensively in inhibitory control, and stimulation of this region may act to boost self-control, potentially by increasing dopamine release in the caudate nucleus, which rTMS has been shown to do [7].

rTMS is also currently being investigated for its potential to reduce food craving and consumption [7] and shows promise for this purpose too. Application of rTMS to DLPFC reduces self-reported food craving and appetite in single and multi-session format [6, 51, 56, 58, 59]. For example, rTMS to the left DLPFC did not affect cue-induced craving for palatable foods, whereas there was an increase in craving in the sham group [7, 60]. Most definitively, a randomized controlled trial of rTMS delivered to the left DLPFC was effective in decreasing food intake and facilitating weight loss in obese patients, suggesting that rTMS could be an effective treatment option for obesity and FA [61].

14.2.7 12-Step Programs and Other Support

Studies show that Alcoholics Anonymous (AA) and Narcotic Anonymous (NA) attendance predicts abstinence for individuals with alcohol and other SUD [62, 63]. 12-step programs are believed to work as a consequence of the fellowship and community-building, an increased sense of goal directedness and structure, use of more effective coping skills (often learned through sponsorship and step work), engagement in sober activities, and increased self-efficacy and hope [64]. Increased spirituality and reduction in depression are also important mechanisms by which these programs promote recovery [65–67]. Providers are encouraged to recommend AA and NA to people in recovery to promote better functioning and reduced substance use in individuals with SUD. 12-step facilitation is an established evidence-based treatment for SUD that focuses on getting people engaged in AA or NA [68].

The Overeaters Anonymous (OA) organization is a 12-step-based program that promotes the central belief that obesity is a symptom of "compulsive overeating," an addictive-like illness with physical, emotional, and spiritual components [3, 7, 8, 69, 70]. Individuals are required to acknowledge that compulsive overeating is beyond their willpower to overcome alone, and, to control their food intake, overeaters are encouraged to adopt a food plan and surrender to a "higher power." "Food Addicts Anonymous" (another 12-step program affiliated with OA) is similar, but has a more rigid, one-sized-fits-all food plan [3, 7, 8, 69, 70]. The primary goal of 12-step program treatment for "compulsive overeating" is abstinence, like in NA and AA. Abstinence is definable by the overeater in OA in collaboration with their sponsor (and might involve three meals a day and up to two snacks "with nothing in between" or avoiding particular trigger foods) or by adherence to a uniform food plan for Food Addicts Anonymous [3, 7, 8, 69, 70]. Just like AA and NA, OA and FA involve group meetings for individuals to share their feelings and experiences [3, 7, 8, 69, 70].

Unlike AA, very little research into the efficacy of OA has been done [7]. Some individuals struggling with overeating report that applying an abstinence model helped them to control their eating [8, 69, 70]. But little is known about the long-term success (and possible adverse effects) of such an approach. In a study of 60 women, 12-step self-help groups for compulsive eating have been shown to reduce anxiety and depression, but not FA [3]. Larger, long-term studies are needed.

That said, OA and related programs may serve many of the needs of the person with FA and support many of the recommendations made in this chapter and Chap. 13. Going to a meeting can provide distraction and replace a counterproductive behavior (e.g., bingeing or eating a palatable food) with a more productive one. Animal studies show that environmental enrichment reduces food seeking and taking in rats [71]: "keeping busy" is an oft-cited coping mechanism by many people in recovery from SUD. Reducing loneliness, isolation, and shame, all of which can fuel obesity, BE, FA, and other addictions [72–75], may be another benefit of 12-step participation. As discussed earlier, overweight and obesity are associated with higher shame and guilt and a preference for isolative activities [7, 76]. This social isolation can subsequently exacerbate overeating, creating a vicious cycle [77, 78]. With engagement in a fellowship of people with similar struggles, and with increased support and socialization, one would expect to see a reduction in the shame and isolation, breaking this vicious cycle.

There are numerous additional resources which patients can access to obtain increased structure and support. For example, a virtual intensive outpatient and a residential treatment program are available through SHiFT Recovery by Acorn (www.foodaddicion.com) and food addiction recovery retreats are available through COR (https://cormn.org). Many people with FA find it almost impossible to develop a food plan and stick with it without outside support from a sponsor or dietitian/nutritionist: the "addict brain" fights hard to keep less helpful foods (foods that are both craved and that trigger the disease) in the food plan, ultimately sabotaging attempts to stay abstinent, whereas the "eating disorder" brain over-restricts caloric intake. Sponsor- and dietitian/nutritionist-involvement can help the person with FA find that middle ground between succumbing to justifications/rationalizations to overeat versus over restricting which can then trigger binge eating.

14.2.8 Medications

There are a number of evidence-based pharmacotherapeutic treatments for obesity, BED, and bulimia nervosa (Chaps. 2 and 3), albeit with some downfalls (Chap. 4), working via several important addiction-based mechanisms (Chap. 10) (see Table 2.1). Early work is starting to show these medicines also reduce FA symptoms. For example, an open-label trial on the efficacy and tolerability of naltrexone/bupropion SR for treating altered eating behaviors and weight loss in BED showed a significant and similar weight loss (approximately 8%) and reductions in YFAS scores for both a group of people with obesity plus BED and BED alone [79].

For people with FA, it is wise to chose pharmacotherapies approved both for the treatment of

BED and obesity that target reward, conditioning, negative reinforcement and impulse control mechanisms. For example, topiramate and possibly zonisamide likely act by reducing cue reactivity and global impulse control; naltrexone (in naltrexone/bupropion) may reduce cue reactivity, food elicited pleasure/liking, and improve impulse control, especially during exposure to impulsivity during opioid release; stimulants like bupropion, lisdexamfetamine, and phentermine (in topiramate/phentermine) likely also improve impulse control; selective serotonin reuptake inhibitors likely reduce and anxiety and depression symptoms; and glucagon-like peptide 1 agonists (e.g., liraglutide) act on primary homeostatic appetitive mechanisms but may also have direct effects on addiction/reward circuitry like pleasure from food and cue reactivity [1, 3, 6, 41, 79–84]. Any of these medicines would be reasonable first-line choices in FA, although one may be more suited to one patient over another based on individual vulnerabilities, such as emotion regulation, food cue-induced reactivity, impulse control difficulties, depression or anxiety, or sensitivity to just a taste of pleasurable food. One can also make medication choices based on the patient's medical history, keeping in mind side effect profiles and medical or psychiatric contraindications [84] (Table 2.1).

Whether stimulants are safe to prescribe to people with FA is not yet known, and these medications should be used with caution. Bupropion/naltrexone and phentermine/topiramate contain stimulants (bupropion and phentermine both have stimulant activity) and are approved for long-term weight management [6, 41, 81, 85]. Lisdexamfetamine is also approved for BED and promotes weight loss. On the one hand, one would surmise that since stimulants (especially lisdexamfetamine and bupropion) reduce impulsivity and enhance prefrontal activity in some people [86, 87], they would be useful in addictive disorders. However, stimulants also have high addictive potential, and, as we have seen in Chap. 6, and addiction transfer is not uncommon. Prescribed long acting stimulants are used in stimulant use disorder treatment [88] but have not been found to be highly effective in other drug use disorders like alcohol or nicotine use disorders [89], perhaps because they prime the reward system. Research is needed to test long-term outcomes of these medicines in people with especially severe FA symptomatology. One study found that a stimulant appetite suppressant that enhanced dopamine functioning was not effective in adults who screened positive for FA on the YFAS compared with controls [90]. Further work to investigate for whom stimulants are most helpful and for whom they are most harmful is needed. Of the stimulants, bupropion is probably the least addictive and most safe for use in FA populations, with the caveat that it is contraindicated in patients with concurrent purging behaviors. Also, recall that any expected potential health benefits from the modest weight loss during treatment with stimulants, like lisdexamfetamine and phentermine, are likely nullified by their adverse cardiovascular effects (heart rate and blood pressure elevations), and, therefore, from a cardiovascular perspective, many professionals are of the opinion that stimulants have a net negative effect on health outcomes.

Future work could also consider exploring the utility of already approved medicines like prazosin [91, 92] in people with comorbid PTSD (for which prazosin is often prescribed) and FA, or anti-obesity medicines like glucagon like-1 (GLP-1) agonists that also enhance hippocampal functioning may show promise in treatment of SUD's via improved hippocampal functioning and other reward-based mechanisms [41, 93–95].

14.2.9 Bariatric Surgery

Bariatric surgery appears to be an effective treatment for FA [96]. Recall that bariatric surgery is indicated and highly effective for people with severe obesity, inducing significant weight loss in the majority of patients, and that the weight loss is more often than not maintained over years [97] (Chap. 2). Surgery-induced weight loss is also associated with remission of FA symptoms [98–100]. In one study, the proportion of individuals meeting criteria for a FA diagnosis reduced to 2% post-surgery from 32% pre-surgery [97, 100]. Another long-term follow-up study found that the rates of FA reduced from 58% to 7% at 6 months although there was some rebound in FA rates later on, with rates of FA up to 14% at 12 months after surgery [97, 101]. A third study also showed some evidence of FA resurgence after long-term follow-up: FA was identified in 41% and BE in 48% of individuals before sleeve gastrectomy (all FA patients also had BE), and at month 3, FA was seen in 10% of patients and at month 6, 7%. However, at month 12, 29% of patients met FA criteria again. BE, however, was still lower than baseline at all time points (17% at month 12) [96]. The group of women with FA had lower weight loss outcomes and a higher average body mass index (BMI) at month 12 as well [96, 102].

Several scientific studies have uncovered possible mechanisms for the beneficial effect of surgery on FA symptoms which we review in Chap. 10 in detail. In brief, surgery causes reversal of dopamine receptor downregulation in the striatum and hyperreactivity to food cues, restores the brain-gut-microbiome axis imbalance, and dampens excessive dopamine release to sweet consumption and food reward.

14.3 Subtyping and FA Treatment Matching

Obesity is increasingly recognized as a heterogeneous condition [103, 104], and experts believe that there are likely many different reasons why people gain excess weight. The same is likely true of BED and bulimia nervosa [39]. One important theme in obesity and ED research is to better identify and understand possible subtypes [103–106] which could then segue into studies to identify which treatments work best in which subtypes, in order to match treatments to the individual's particular needs [103, 104, 106, 107]. Indeed there is great variability in the degree of weight change in obesity and ED clinical trials [39, 103, 104], with some individuals gaining and others losing large amounts of weight, and by doing mean effects, rather than identifying subgroups more likely to respond, current analyses are potentially masking hidden benefits of our treatments. This push to identify subtypes is in line with efforts to utilize more "precision-medicine" across all fields [108, 109].

14.3.1 Within-FA Treatment Matching

One possible way to look for treatment matching effects is to explore whether or not different subgroups exist within the population of those with an FA diagnosis. Subgroups could be defined by co-occuring disorders, or by traits and vulnerabilites (e.g. by those more driven by food cues versus negative affect versus those with impulsivity issues). Indeed, we can probably already start making some of our management decisions in this way. For example, we can choose medicines based on comorbidities as discussed above. If someone has comorbid depression or anxiety, we could prescribe a selective serotonin reuptake inhibitor; if they have comorbid alcohol use disorder, we might prescribe topiramate or zonisamide; if they have comorbid ADHD, we might prescribe lisdexamfetamine or bupropion; if they have comorbid PTSD, we might prescribe prazosin; or if the person with FA is obese or has type II diabetes, we might prescribe a GLP-1 agonist. Although rTMS is not approved for the treatment of obesity or EDs, in the case of someone with treatment-resistant MDD or OCD (two diagnoses for which there are commonly utilized FDA-approved rTMS stimulation protocols [49, 50]) who also has comorbid FA, we could be more inclined to refer for rTMS treatment. For those that are especially sensitive to the effects of food cues, abstinence (which will promote faster extinguising of conditioning), and naltrexone or topiramate (which reduce the power of cues to trigger food-seeking) might be especially useful. For those that struggle with negative reinforcement based eating or comfort eating, SSRIs, interpersonal therapy, social support and sleep might be especially useful. For those that go through severe food withdrawal, time "clean" might be strongly encouraged. For those with high levels of impulsivity, exercise, sleep, medications like lisdexamfetamine, bupropion and topiramate (which are known to improve impulse control), and psychotherapies like DBT and ACT may be good to emphasize.

An intriguing recent study identified three subtypes of FA [98]: a dysfunctional group, Cluster 1, characterized by the highest ED severity and psychopathology, for which authors propose treatment focused on ED symptomatology and FA only secondarily; Cluster 2 with better levels of functioning, but the highest levels of FA for which authors proposed treatment could target FA aggressively, focusing on reward related processes and conditioning, perhaps encouraging a more restrictive food plan; and Cluster 3 with a high prevalence of obesity but more grazing behavior than bingeing for whom authors suggested that focusing on reduction in BMI first might then lead to reductions in FA and craving and/or that this group could be a surgery target [98].

Another recent article examined external eating (cue-driven and dependent on positive reinforcement mechanisms) and emotional eating (related to negative reinforcement), modeling these as different constructs [33]. This may, incidentally, map onto a growing body of work in the alcohol literature by researchers examining motivations for drinking and which shows that those that drink for reward may be in a separate category from those who drink for relief of negative affect and out of habit (the latter two motivations overlap) [110]. This categorization is likely to apply in FA. For example, in other work in FA, authors found that impulsivity contributes directly to external eating, whereas depression and alexithymia as well as impulsivity contributed to emotional eating [33]. Furthermore, weight loss resulted in reductions in external eating over time, but emotional eating did not remit [33, 111, 112]. It is also theorized that the alexithymia may contribute to impulsive overeating via an additional inability to read visceral sensations [33]. These findings would imply that people who suffer from emotional eating should engage in some deeper therapy work and work to help them identify their emotions and/or consider psychiatric evaluation for medication treatment to reduce risk of relapse, whereas those with external eating might best focus on weight loss, avoiding foods and triggers. Both might benefit from medications or interventions (e.g., exercise) that reduce impulsivity.

Another subgroup within FA populations might be those with a history of trauma or high levels of stress. Studies show that food addiction is a mediator of psychological distress [113] or perceived stress [114] and BMI. FA is also a mediator of early life adversity (ELA) on obesity, [3, 115–117]. These findings would indicate that targeting FA as soon as it develops holds promise for people with stress and trauma as it could prevent obesity later on. Early intervention for ELA may prevent obesity since usually the FA and obesity develop later in life or the trauma might be a target of treatment that could help reduce BMI. The same kinds of relationships are seen for ED symptoms in that childhood maltreatment, especially physical neglect and physical abuse, was associated with higher global ED severity scores, and this effect was mediated by FA scores [118]. This would imply that targeting FA in people with a history of trauma early could prevent ED development and/or might also reduce ED symptoms in those who have already developed it [119, 120] and further emphasizes the importance of providing trauma treatment to prevent and promote recovery from obesity and EDs and FA alike.

Finally, female gender was a predictor of severe food addiction, and high reward sensitivity was significantly associated with more severe FA symptoms in females [98, 121]. This is consistent with what's seen in females with SUD deemed "telescoping" which is believed in part to be due to estrogen enhancing dopaminergic activity (and therefore conditioning process etc.). Theoretically women could require more attention to dopamine-mediated processes such as reward and conditioning, and treatments targeting these processes over others might be useful.

14.3.2 Using FA as a Treatment Matching Variable for Patients with Obesity and BE

FA started off as a concept to explain a potential subtype of obesity [98, 120, 122, 123] that might provide more information than the presence or absence of a comorbid BED or bulimia nervosa diagnosis. And using the presence of FA to identify a subtype of obesity which might be more responsive to treatment with addiction-like models including abstinence-based approaches and brain-based interventions holds promise. Those with a diagnosis of FA might be more susceptible to highly processed foods, too [124]. Although not yet studied, people with FA would also be expected to respond to MI more than those without, given the robust effects of MI in SUD populations. Although BED did not moderate outcome to MI (which was less effective than nutritional psychoeducation) [30], one wonders if FA diagnosis might. Unfortunately, very little has been done in this area, and more research is needed. There are no studies (clinical trials) looking at food addiction as a predictor of outcome to particular diets, psychosocial interventions, or medications. FA also seems like an excellent potential matching variable for studies looking at the effects of more restrictive diets on treatment outcomes in individuals with BED and obesity to answer questions about in whom a more restrictive diet is safe and in whom it is not.

A few studies do deserve mention, however, showing poorer response to treatment with those with FA in response to standard treatment. One study showed that women with FA had less favorable weight loss outcomes and BMI post sleeve gastrectomy at year one [96, 102]. In another study, FA was found to be a mediator in the relationship between ED severity and treatment outcome [125] indicating that those with higher FA symptoms were less likely to respond to the standard ED treatment provided in that study. Finally in an intervention study among women with bulimia, those with higher FA severity at baseline were less likely to obtain abstinence from binge-purge episodes following treatment [3, 126]. If nothing else, it is clear that patients with FA should potentially be watched more closely and given more intensive initial intervention than those without.

14.4 Conclusion

There is currently a paucity of research into non-nutritional treatment of patients with FA. However, there is a growing body of preliminary evidence to support a number of possible treatment options, many of which have been borrowed or adapted from current treatments for SUDs, EDs, and obesity. Additionally, combining several treatment modalities may provide additive or synergistic benefit to selective patients. Considering an individual patient's unique symptoms and comorbidities will provide practitioners guidance in determining the best course of treatment for their patients.

References

1. Wilcox CE, Bogenschutz MB. Psychopharmacologies for alcohol and drug use disorders. In: McCrady BS, Epstein EE, editors. Addictions: a comprehensive guidebook. 2nd ed. New York: Oxford University Press; 2013. p. 526–50.
2. Center for Substance Abuse Treatment. Groups and substance abuse treatment. In: Substance abuse treatment: group therapy, Treatment improvement protocol (TIP) series, No. 41. Rockville: Substance Abuse and Mental Health Services Administration (US); 2005. Available from: https://www.ncbi.nlm.nih.gov/books/NBK64223/.
3. Wiss D, Brewerton T. Separating the signal from the noise: how psychiatric diagnoses can help discern food addiction from dietary restraint. Nutrients. 2020;12(10):2937.
4. Treasure J, Leslie M, Chami R, Fernandez-Aranda F. Are trans diagnostic models of eating disorders fit for purpose? A consideration of the evidence for food addiction. Eur Eat Disord Rev. 2018;26(2):83–91.
5. Carter A, Hardman CA, Burrows T. Food addiction and eating addiction: scientific advances and their clinical, social and policy implications. Nutrients. 2020;12(5):1485.
6. Carter A, Hendrikse J, Lee N, Yucel M, Verdejo-Garcia A, Andrews ZB, et al. The neurobiology of "food addiction" and its implications for obesity treatment and policy. Annu Rev Nutr. 2016;36:105–28.
7. Adams RC, Sedgmond J, Maizey L, Chambers CD, Lawrence NS. Food addiction: implications for the diagnosis and treatment of overeating. Nutrients. 2019;11(9):2086.
8. Meule A. A critical examination of the practical implications derived from the food addiction concept. Curr Obes Rep. 2019;8(1):11–7.
9. May J, Andrade J, Kavanagh DJ, Feeney GF, Gullo MJ, Statham DJ, et al. The craving experience questionnaire: a brief, theory-based measure of consummatory desire and craving. Addiction. 2014;109(5):728–35.
10. Appelhans BM, French SA, Pagoto SL, Sherwood NE. Managing temptation in obesity treatment: a neurobehavioral model of intervention strategies. Appetite. 2016;96:268–79.

11. Meurk C, Fraser D, Weier M, Lucke J, Carter A, Hall W. Assessing the place of neurobiological explanations in accounts of a family member's addiction. Drug Alcohol Rev. 2016;35(4):461–9.
12. Dackis C, O'Brien C. Neurobiology of addiction: treatment and public policy ramifications. Nat Neurosci. 2005;8(11):1431–6.
13. Avery JJ, Avery JD, Mouallem J, Demner AR, Cooper J. Physicians' and attorneys' beliefs and attitudes related to the brain disease model of addiction. Am J Addict. 2020;29(4):305–12.
14. Latner JD, Puhl RM, Murakami JM, O'Brien KS. Food addiction as a causal model of obesity. Effects on stigma, blame, and perceived psychopathology. Appetite. 2014;77:77–82.
15. Pearl RL, Lebowitz MS. Beyond personal responsibility: effects of causal attributions for overweight and obesity on weight-related beliefs, stigma, and policy support. Psychol Health. 2014;29(10):1176–91.
16. Sikorski C, Luppa M, Kaiser M, Glaesmer H, Schomerus G, Konig HH, et al. The stigma of obesity in the general public and its implications for public health – a systematic review. BMC Public Health. 2011;11:661.
17. Meadows A, Higgs S. Internalized weight stigma and the progression of food addiction over time. Body Image. 2020;34:67–71.
18. Puhl RM, Himmelstein MS, Pearl RL. Weight stigma as a psychosocial contributor to obesity. Am Psychol. 2020;75(2):274–89.
19. Lee NM, Carter A, Owen N, Hall WD. The neurobiology of overeating. Treating overweight individuals should make use of neuroscience research, but not at the expense of population approaches to diet and lifestyle. EMBO Rep. 2012;13(9):785–90.
20. Gadde KM, Atkins KD. The limits and challenges of antiobesity pharmacotherapy. Expert Opin Pharmacother. 2020;21(11):1319–28.
21. Fairburn CG. Overcoming binge eating, second edition: the proven program to learn why you binge and how you can stop. New York: The Guilford Press; 2013.
22. Lanza PV, Garcia PF, Lamelas FR, Gonzalez-Menendez A. Acceptance and commitment therapy versus cognitive behavioral therapy in the treatment of substance use disorder with incarcerated women. J Clin Psychol. 2014;70:644–57.
23. Rodda SN, Booth N, Brittain M, McKean J, Thornley S. I was truly addicted to sugar: a consumer-focused classification system of behaviour change strategies for sugar reduction. Appetite. 2020;144:104456.
24. Vidmar AP, Pretlow R, Borzutzky C, Wee CP, Fox DS, Fink C, et al. An addiction model-based mobile health weight loss intervention in adolescents with obesity. Pediatr Obes. 2019;14(2):e12464.
25. Pretlow RA, Stock CM, Roeger L, Allison S. Treatment of the sensory and motor components of urges to eat (eating addiction?): a mobile-health pilot study for obesity in young people. Eat Weight Disord. 2020;25(6):1779–87.
26. Seligman ME, Railton P, Baumeister RF, Sripada C. Navigating into the future or driven by the past. Perspect Psychol Sci. 2013;8(2):119–41.
27. Chao AM, Wadden TA, Tronieri JS, Pearl RL, Alamuddin N, Bakizada ZM, et al. Effects of addictive-like eating behaviors on weight loss with behavioral obesity treatment. J Behav Med. 2019;42(2):246–55.
28. Miller-Matero LR, Brescacin C, Clark SM, Troncone CL, Tobin ET. Why WAIT? Preliminary evaluation of the weight assistance and intervention techniques (WAIT) group. Psychol Health Med. 2019;24(9):1029–37.
29. Hettema JE, Hendricks PS. Motivational interviewing for smoking cessation: a meta-analytic review. J Consult Clin Psychol. 2010;78(6):868–84.
30. Barnes RD, Ivezaj V, Martino S, Pittman BP, Grilo CM. Back to basics? No weight loss from motivational interviewing compared to nutrition psychoeducation at one-year follow-up. Obesity. 2017;25(12):2074–8.
31. Burrows T, Collins R, Rollo M, Leary M, Hides L, Davis C. The feasibility of a personality targeted intervention for addictive overeating: FoodFix. Appetite. 2021;156:104974.
32. van Strien T, Ouwens MA. Effects of distress, alexithymia and impulsivity on eating. Eat Behav. 2007;8(2):251–7.
33. Ouwens MA, van Strien T, van Leeuwe JF. Possible pathways between depression, emotional and external eating. A structural equation model. Appetite. 2009;53(2):245–8.
34. Fauconnier M, Rousselet M, Brunault P, Thiabaud E, Lambert S, Rocher B, et al. Food addiction among female patients seeking treatment for an eating disorder: prevalence and associated factors. Nutrients. 2020;12(6):1897.
35. Janssen L, Kan CC, Carpentier PJ, Sizoo B, Hepark S, Schellekens MPJ, et al. Mindfulness-based cognitive therapy v. treatment as usual in adults with ADHD: a multicentre, single-blind, randomised controlled trial. Psychol Med. 2019;49(1):55–65.
36. Forrest LN, Jacobucci RC, Grilo CM. Empirically determined severity levels for binge-eating disorder outperform existing severity classification schemes. Psychol Med. 2020:1–11.
37. Andres A, Saldana C. Body dissatisfaction and dietary restraint influence binge eating behavior. Nutr Res. 2014;34(11):944–50.
38. Thompson KJ. Body image, eating disorders and obesity: an integrative guide for assessment and treatment. Washington, DC: American Psychological Association; 2000.
39. Pacanowski CR, Mason TB, Crosby RD, Mitchell JE, Crow SJ, Wonderlich SA, et al. Weight change over the course of binge eating disorder treatment: relationship to binge episodes and psychological factors. Obesity. 2018;26(5):838–44.
40. Genario R, Cipolla-Neto J, Bueno AA, Santos HO. Melatonin supplementation in the management

of obesity and obesity-associated disorders: a review of physiological mechanisms and clinical applications. Pharmacol Res. 2021;163:105254.
41. Coulter AA, Rebello CJ, Greenway FL. Centrally acting agents for obesity: past, present, and future. Drugs. 2018;78(11):1113–32.
42. Lederman O, Ward PB, Firth J, Maloney C, Carney R, Vancampfort D, et al. Does exercise improve sleep quality in individuals with mental illness? A systematic review and meta-analysis. J Psychiatr Res. 2019;109:96–106.
43. van der Zweerde T, Bisdounis L, Kyle SD, Lancee J, van Straten A. Cognitive behavioral therapy for insomnia: a meta-analysis of long-term effects in controlled studies. Sleep Med Rev. 2019;48:101208.
44. Schuch FB, Stubbs B. The role of exercise in preventing and treating depression. Curr Sports Med Rep. 2019;18(8):299–304.
45. Lambez B, Harwood-Gross A, Golumbic EZ, Rassovsky Y. Non-pharmacological interventions for cognitive difficulties in ADHD: a systematic review and meta-analysis. J Psychiatr Res. 2020;120:40–55.
46. Robertson CL, Ishibashi K, Chudzynski J, Mooney LJ, Rawson RA, Dolezal BA, et al. Effect of exercise training on striatal dopamine D2/D3 receptors in methamphetamine users during behavioral treatment. Neuropsychopharmacology. 2016;41(6):1629–36.
47. Koob GF, Powell P, White A. Addiction as a coping response: hyperkatifeia, deaths of despair, and COVID-19. Am J Psychiatry. 2020;177(11):1031–7.
48. Wiss DA, Brewerton TD. Adverse childhood experiences and adult obesity: a systematic review of plausible mechanisms and meta-analysis of cross-sectional studies. Physiol Behav. 2020;223:112964.
49. Wilcox CE. Non-convulsive neurostimulation for the treatment of psychiatric disorders part I: FDA-approved treatments. American Physician Institute; 2020. Available from: CMEToGo.com.
50. Wilcox CE. Non-convulsive neurostimulation for the treatment of psychiatric disorders part II: emerging treatments. American Physician Institute; 2020. Available from: CMEToGo.com.
51. Val-Laillet D, Aarts E, Weber B, Ferrari M, Quaresima V, Stoeckel LE, et al. Neuroimaging and neuromodulation approaches to study eating behavior and prevent and treat eating disorders and obesity. Neuroimage Clin. 2015;8:1–31.
52. Maizey L, Allen CP, Dervinis M, Verbruggen F, Varnava A, Kozlov M, et al. Comparative incidence rates of mild adverse effects to transcranial magnetic stimulation. Clin Neurophysiol. 2013;124(3):536–44.
53. Rossi S, Hallett M, Rossini PM, Pascual-Leone A, Safety of TMS Consensus Group. Safety, ethical considerations, and application guidelines for the use of transcranial magnetic stimulation in clinical practice and research. Clin Neurophysiol. 2009;120(12):2008–39.
54. Taylor R, Galvez V, Loo C. Transcranial magnetic stimulation (TMS) safety: a practical guide for psychiatrists. Australas Psychiatry. 2018;26(2):189–92.
55. Feil J, Zangen A. Brain stimulation in the study and treatment of addiction. Neurosci Biobehav Rev. 2010;34(4):559–74.
56. Hall PA, Vincent CM, Burhan AM. Non-invasive brain stimulation for food cravings, consumption, and disorders of eating: a review of methods, findings and controversies. Appetite. 2018;124:78–88.
57. Wilcox CE, Clifford J, Ling J, Mayer AR, Bigelow R, Bogenschutz MP, et al. Stroop-related cerebellar and temporal activation is correlated with negative affect and alcohol use disorder severity. Brain Imaging Behav. 2020;14:586–98.
58. Wilcox CE. Binge eating disorder. American Physician Institute; 2019. Available from: CMEtoGo.com.
59. Kinasz KR, Ross DA, Cooper JJ. Eat to live or live to eat? The neurobiology of appetite regulation. Biol Psychiatry. 2017;81(9):e73–e5.
60. Uher R, Yoganathan D, Mogg A, Eranti SV, Treasure J, Campbell IC, et al. Effect of left prefrontal repetitive transcranial magnetic stimulation on food craving. Biol Psychiatry. 2005;58(10):840–2.
61. Kim SH, Chung JH, Kim TH, Lim SH, Kim Y, Lee YA, et al. The effects of repetitive transcranial magnetic stimulation on eating behaviors and body weight in obesity: a randomized controlled study. Brain Stimul. 2018;11(3):528–35.
62. Kelly JF, Stout RL, Magill M, Tonigan JS, Pagano ME. Mechanisms of behavior change in alcoholics anonymous: does Alcoholics Anonymous lead to better alcohol use outcomes by reducing depression symptoms? Addiction. 2010;105(4):626–36.
63. Tonigan JS, Toscova R, Miller WR. Meta-analysis of the literature on Alcoholics Anonymous: sample and study characteristics moderate findings. J Stud Alcohol. 1996;57(1):65–72.
64. Donovan DM, Ingalsbe MH, Benbow J, Daley DC. 12-step interventions and mutual support programs for substance use disorders: an overview. Soc Work Public Health. 2013;28(3–4):313–32.
65. Tonigan JS. Spirituality and alcoholics anonymous. South Med J. 2007;100(4):437–40.
66. Tonigan JS. Alcoholics anonymous outcomes and benefits. Recent Dev Alcohol. 2008;18:357–72.
67. Wilcox CE, Pearson MR, Tonigan JS. Effects of long-term AA attendance and spirituality on the course of depressive symptoms in individuals with alcohol use disorder. Psychol Addict Behav. 2015;29(2):382–91.
68. MATCH. Matching alcoholism treatments to client heterogeneity: project MATCH posttreatment drinking outcomes. J Stud Alcohol. 1997;58(1):7–29.
69. Rodriguez-Martin BC, Gallego-Arjiz B. Overeaters anonymous: a mutual-help fellowship for food addiction recovery. Front Psychol. 2018;9:1491.
70. Russell-Mayhew S, von Ranson KM, Masson PC. How does overeaters anonymous help its members? A qualitative analysis. Eur Eat Disord Rev. 2010;18(1):33–42.
71. Grimm JW, Sauter F. Environmental enrichment reduces food seeking and taking in rats: a review. Pharmacol Biochem Behav. 2020;190:172874.

72. Sun Y, Li Y, Bao Y, Meng S, Sun Y, Schumann G, et al. Brief report: increased addictive internet and substance use behavior during the COVID-19 pandemic in China. Am J Addict. 2020;29(4):268–70.
73. Rolland B, Haesebaert F, Zante E, Benyamina A, Haesebaert J, Franck N. Global changes and factors of increase in caloric/salty food intake, screen use, and substance use during the early COVID-19 containment phase in the general population in France: survey study. JMIR Public Health Surveill. 2020;6(3):e19630.
74. Cherikh F, Frey S, Bel C, Attanasi G, Alifano M, Iannelli A. Behavioral food addiction during lockdown: time for awareness, time to prepare the aftermath. Obes Surg. 2020;30(9):3585–7.
75. Van de Graaf RC, Hofstra L. Obesity and covid-19: the role of the food industry. BMJ. 2020;370:m2813.
76. Hayden-Wade HA, Stein RI, Ghaderi A, Saelens BE, Zabinski MF, Wilfley DE. Prevalence, characteristics, and correlates of teasing experiences among overweight children vs. non-overweight peers. Obes Res. 2005;13(8):1381–92.
77. Neumark-Sztainer D, Falkner N, Story M, Perry C, Hannan PJ, Mulert S. Weight-teasing among adolescents: correlations with weight status and disordered eating behaviors. Int J Obes Relat Metab Disord. 2002;26(1):123–31.
78. Pretlow RA. Addiction to highly pleasurable food as a cause of the childhood obesity epidemic: a qualitative Internet study. Eat Disord. 2011;19(4):295–307.
79. Carbone EA, Caroleo M, Rania M, Calabro G, Staltari FA, de Filippis R, et al. An open-label trial on the efficacy and tolerability of naltrexone/bupropion SR for treating altered eating behaviours and weight loss in binge eating disorder. Eat Weight Disord. 2021;26:779–88.
80. Hutson PH, Balodis IM, Potenza MN. Binge-eating disorder: clinical and therapeutic advances. Pharmacol Ther. 2018;182:15–27.
81. Vetter ML, Faulconbridge LF, Webb VL, Wadden TA. Behavioral and pharmacologic therapies for obesity. Nat Rev Endocrinol. 2010;6(10):578–88.
82. Rubio G, Martinez-Gras I, Manzanares J. Modulation of impulsivity by topiramate: implications for the treatment of alcohol dependence. J Clin Psychopharmacol. 2009;29(6):584–9.
83. Maisel NC, Blodgett JC, Wilbourne PL, Humphreys K, Finney JW. Meta-analysis of naltrexone and acamprosate for treating alcohol use disorders: when are these medications most helpful? Addiction. 2013;108(2):275–93.
84. Khalil H, Ellwood L, Lord H, Fernandez R. Pharmacological treatment for obesity in adults: an umbrella review. Ann Pharmacother. 2020;54(7):691–705.
85. Jung J, Fugh-Berman A. Marketing messages in continuing medical education (CME) modules on binge-eating disorder (BED). J Am Board Fam Med. 2020;33(2):240–51.
86. Brady KT, Gray KM, Tolliver BK. Cognitive enhancers in the treatment of substance use disorders: clinical evidence. Pharmacol Biochem Behav. 2011;99(2):285–94.
87. Spencer RC, Devilbiss DM, Berridge CW. The cognition-enhancing effects of psychostimulants involve direct action in the prefrontal cortex. Biol Psychiatry. 2015;77(11):940–50.
88. Moeller FG, Schmitz JM, Herin D, Kjome KL. Use of stimulants to treat cocaine and methamphetamine abuse. Curr Psychiatry Rep. 2008;10(5):385–91.
89. Joos L, Goudriaan AE, Schmaal L, Fransen E, van den Brink W, Sabbe BG, et al. Effect of modafinil on impulsivity and relapse in alcohol dependent patients: a randomized, placebo-controlled trial. Eur Neuropsychopharmacol. 2013;23(8):948–55.
90. Davis C, Levitan RD, Kaplan AS, Kennedy JL, Carter JC. Food cravings, appetite, and snack-food consumption in response to a psychomotor stimulant drug: the moderating effect of "food-addiction". Front Psychol. 2014;5:403.
91. Hicks C, Sabino V, Cottone P. The alpha-1 adrenergic receptor antagonist prazosin reduces binge-like eating in rats. Nutrients. 2020;12(6):1569.
92. Wilcox CE, Tonigan JS, Bogenschutz MP, Clifford J, Bigelow R, Simpson T. A randomized, placebo-controlled, clinical trial of prazosin for the treatment of alcohol use disorder. J Addict Med. 2018;12(5):339–45.
93. Clasen MM, Riley AL, Davidson TL. Hippocampal-dependent inhibitory learning and memory processes in the control of eating and drug taking. Curr Pharm Des. 2020;26(20):2334–52.
94. Farr OM, Sofopoulos M, Tsoukas MA, Dincer F, Thakkar B, Sahin-Efe A, et al. GLP-1 receptors exist in the parietal cortex, hypothalamus and medulla of human brains and the GLP-1 analogue liraglutide alters brain activity related to highly desirable food cues in individuals with diabetes: a crossover, randomised, placebo-controlled trial. Diabetologia. 2016;59(5):954–65.
95. Hernandez NS, Schmidt HD. Central GLP-1 receptors: novel molecular targets for cocaine use disorder. Physiol Behav. 2019;206:93–105.
96. Ben-Porat T, Weiss R, Sherf-Dagan S, Rottenstreich A, Kaluti D, Khalaileh A, et al. Food addiction and binge eating during one year following sleeve gastrectomy: prevalence and implications for postoperative outcomes. Obes Surg. 2021;31(2):603–11.
97. Sarkar S, Kochhar KP, Khan NA. Fat addiction: psychological and physiological trajectory. Nutrients. 2019;11(11):2785.
98. Jimenez-Murcia S, Aguera Z, Paslakis G, Munguia L, Granero R, Sanchez-Gonzalez J, et al. Food addiction in eating disorders and obesity: analysis of clusters and implications for treatment. Nutrients. 2019;11(11):2633.
99. Murray SM, Tweardy S, Geliebter A, Avena NM. A longitudinal preliminary study of addiction-like

responses to food and alcohol consumption among individuals undergoing weight loss surgery. Obes Surg. 2019;29(8):2700–3.
100. Pepino MY, Stein RI, Eagon JC, Klein S. Bariatric surgery-induced weight loss causes remission of food addiction in extreme obesity. Obesity. 2014;22(8):1792–8.
101. Sevincer GM, Konuk N, Bozkurt S, Coskun H. Food addiction and the outcome of bariatric surgery at 1-year: prospective observational study. Psychiatry Res. 2016;244:159–64.
102. Ivezaj V, Wiedemann AA, Grilo CM. Food addiction and bariatric surgery: a systematic review of the literature. Obes Rev. 2017;18(12):1386–97.
103. Higgins GA, Sellers EM, Fletcher PJ. From obesity to substance abuse: therapeutic opportunities for 5-HT2C receptor agonists. Trends Pharmacol Sci. 2013;34(10):560–70.
104. Higgins GA, Zeeb FD, Fletcher PJ. Role of impulsivity and reward in the anti-obesity actions of 5-HT2C receptor agonists. J Psychopharmacol. 2017;31(11):1403–18.
105. Blundell JE, Dulloo AG, Salvador J, Fruhbeck G, EASO SAB Working Group on BMI. Beyond BMI--phenotyping the obesities. Obes Facts. 2014;7(5):322–8.
106. Field AE, Camargo CA Jr, Ogino S. The merits of subtyping obesity: one size does not fit all. JAMA. 2013;310(20):2147–8.
107. Ziauddeen H, Fletcher PC. Is food addiction a valid and useful concept? Obes Rev. 2013;14(1):19–28.
108. Dishman E. Precision medicine. 2018. https://www.nih.gov/precision-medicine-initiative-cohort-program. Accessed 2018.
109. Bearden CE, Thompson PM. Emerging global initiatives in neurogenetics: the enhancing neuroimaging genetics through meta-analysis (ENIGMA) consortium. Neuron. 2017;94(2):232–6.
110. Grodin EN, Bujarski S, Venegas A, Baskerville WA, Nieto SJ, Jentsch JD, et al. Reward, relief and habit drinking: initial validation of a brief assessment tool. Alcohol Alcohol. 2019;54(6):574–83.
111. Forman EM, Shaw JA, Goldstein SP, Butryn ML, Martin LM, Meiran N, et al. Mindful decision making and inhibitory control training as complementary means to decrease snack consumption. Appetite. 2016;103:176–83.
112. Van Strien T, Van de Laar FA. Intake of energy is best predicted by overeating tendency and consumption of fat is best predicted by dietary restraint: a 4-year follow-up of patients with newly diagnosed type 2 diabetes. Appetite. 2008;50(2–3):544–7.
113. Lin YS, Tung YT, Yen YC, Chien YW. Food addiction mediates the relationship between perceived stress and body mass index in Taiwan young adults. Nutrients. 2020;12(7):1951.
114. Lin CY, Cheung P, Imani V, Griffiths MD, Pakpour AH. The mediating effects of eating disorder, food addiction, and insomnia in the association between psychological distress and being overweight among Iranian adolescents. Nutrients. 2020;12(5):1371.
115. Romano KA, Heron KE, Amerson R, Howard LM, MacIntyre RI, Mason TB. Changes in disordered eating behaviors over 10 or more years: a meta-analysis. Int J Eat Disord. 2020;53(7):1034–55.
116. Elsenburg LK, Smidt N, Liefbroer AC. The longitudinal relation between accumulation of adverse life events and body mass index from early adolescence to young adulthood. Psychosom Med. 2017;79(3):365–73.
117. Elsenburg LK, van Wijk KJE, Liefbroer AC, Smidt N. Accumulation of adverse childhood events and overweight in children: a systematic review and meta-analysis. Obesity. 2017;25(5):820–32.
118. Bou Khalil R, Sleilaty G, Richa S, Seneque M, Iceta S, Rodgers R, et al. The impact of retrospective childhood maltreatment on eating disorders as mediated by food addiction: a cross-sectional study. Nutrients. 2020;12(10):2969.
119. Cope EC, Gould E. New evidence linking obesity and food addiction. Biol Psychiatry. 2017;81(9):734–6.
120. Sinha R. Role of addiction and stress neurobiology on food intake and obesity. Biol Psychol. 2018;131:5–13.
121. Loxton NJ, Tipman RJ. Reward sensitivity and food addiction in women. Appetite. 2017;115:28–35.
122. Gearhardt AN, Boswell RG, White MA. The association of "food addiction" with disordered eating and body mass index. Eat Behav. 2014;15(3):427–33.
123. Ferrario CR. Food addiction and obesity. Neuropsychopharmacology. 2017;42(1):361.
124. Seid H, Rosenbaum M. Low carbohydrate and low-fat diets: what we don't know and why we should know it. Nutrients. 2019;11(11):2749.
125. Romero X, Aguera Z, Granero R, Sanchez I, Riesco N, Jimenez-Murcia S, et al. Is food addiction a predictor of treatment outcome among patients with eating disorder? Eur Eat Disord Rev. 2019;27(6):700–11.
126. Hilker I, Sanchez I, Steward T, Jimenez-Murcia S, Granero R, Gearhardt AN, et al. Food addiction in bulimia nervosa: clinical correlates and association with response to a brief psychoeducational intervention. Eur Eat Disord Rev. 2016;24(6):482–8.

Part VI

Research Possibilities

15 Emerging Treatments and Areas for Future Research

15.1 Emerging Treatments for Disordered Eating

15.1.1 Neurostimulation

In addition to repetitive transcranial magnetic stimulation (rTMS; Chap. 14), there are several non-convulsive neurostimulation techniques that are under study for the treatment of addictive disorders, obesity, and EDs associated with binge eating that hold promise for the treatment of FA. Transcranial direct current stimulation (tDCS) is one of these techniques, and it has received growing attention for the treatment of a wide variety of psychiatric and neurologic disorders. Like rTMS, tDCS is applied to awake participants, induces few side effects, and is generally considered to be safe [1–6]. Also similar to rTMS, tDCS works via a number of potential mechanisms to alter neural activity, including by increasing connectivity, and increasing dopamine function, for example, and studies have primarily focused on stimulation of the dorsolateral prefrontal cortex (PFC) to enhance cognitive control [3, 5–7]. Unlike rTMS, tDCS is still primarily just a research tool, and not yet approved for treatment of any disorders, since definitive efficacy has not yet been established [3, 5, 6]. However, tDCS is believed to involve a more appropriately matched sham condition than TMS especially when participants receive active stimulation for a short initial period [3].

There is a large and growing body of research demonstrating the promising potential of tDCS to reduce impulsivity and craving in substance use and related disorders, particularly with stimulation of the dorsolateral PFC [3]. However, more research to determine the most effective protocols for treatment are needed before it will be deployed into clinical practice [8].

tDCS also shows some promise for obesity treatment and might reduce craving for sweets and food intake [3, 8–18]. One study found a significant increase in cue-induced craving, measured before and after stimulation in the sham condition, but a significant reduction in craving and a reduction in food intake during an ad libitum eating phase in the active treatment group [11, 14]. However, metanalyses have shown mixed results, with a more recent one including eight studies, finding no effect on craving [3, 8, 19, 20]. Longer and more numerous tDCS sessions than has been tested may increase effects (as is seen with rTMS), and more research is probably still warranted [8].

Deep brain stimulation (DBS) is a surgical technique that is FDA approved for the treatment of refractory depression and obsessive compulsive disorder, and it has been proposed for use in the treatment of EDs and obesity [9, 21]. In animal studies, lateral hypothalamic stimulation typically leads to appetite stimulation and weight gain, while ventromedial hypothalamic stimulation typically leads to appetite reductions and

C. E. Wilcox, *Food Addiction, Obesity, and Disorders of Overeating*,
https://doi.org/10.1007/978-3-030-83078-6_15

weight loss, but it has not been demonstrated to be effective in human trials (Chap. 1, Fig. 1.1) [9]. Therefore, given the invasiveness and potential for risk, and the fact that safety and efficacy have not yet been demonstrated, more research would need to be done before this will be deployed into clinical practice [9, 22].

Vagus nerve stimulation is approved for the treatment of depression and is under-study for both relapse prevention and detoxification in SUD [1, 2]. Vagus nerve signaling has been found to be reduced in obesity [1, 2], and vagus nerve stimulators are theorized to offer some benefit for obesity and binge eating as well [9, 22], although this has not yet been formally studied.

Finally, although rTMS holds promise for treatment of disordered eating and overeating (Chap. 14), more research is needed to establish the ideal brain regions and stimulation parameters for FA, obesity, and ED treatment. Additional approaches could include targeting cerebellum or more deeper structures and longer or more frequent sessions or by applying stimulation just after triggering symptoms (e.g., craving, with a food cue)—an approach which has been piloted in other disorders like post-traumatic stress disorder with some success [1, 2, 9, 21, 23, 24]. One other interesting proposal under study involves integrating virtual reality with neurostimulation using a symptom-triggering approach [25]. Finally, it has been suggested that there be more research integrating functional magnetic resonance imaging (fMRI) with rTMS to improve the accuracy of neuroanatomical targets and confirm the effect of treatment on intended brain circuits [9].

15.1.2 Real-Time fMRI (Rt-fMRI) Neurofeedback Training

Neurofeedback training is a noninvasive method that can be used to alter neural plasticity and is under study for the treatment of several psychiatric and neurologic disorders. When used during fMRI, it provides participants with real-time feedback of their own brain's response to certain cues or other stimuli, to allow them to then be able to learn how to increase or decrease their response, so that they may gain volitional control over specific brain regions and downstream behaviors [9, 21, 22]. In the study of SUDs, neurofeedback training typically involves increasing activity in control regions, such as the PFC, and decreasing activity in regions associated with craving, such as the anterior cingulate (ACC) [3]. One study found that decreasing activity in the ACC with rt-fMRI neurofeedback was also correlated with decreased nicotine craving in smokers [3]. These kinds of interventions also hold promise for the treatment of FA and overeating in general, as people could be taught to volitionally downregulate neural activity in brain regions responsible for the perception of hunger and food craving, and increase activity in regions involved in behavioral control [26]. Neurofeedback training during fMRI is now being studied in obesity, and it is also being tested in combination with cognitive reappraisal training (involves cognitive reframing of stimuli and situations) and other emotion regulation techniques in individuals with binge eating [3, 9, 21, 22, 27–31]. There is also hope that electroencephalography (EEG) might be a useful substitute for fMRI for feedback provision, important in that EEG is more widely available and less expensive [3].

15.1.3 Cognitive Training

As we've discussed in Chaps. 6 and 8, hedonic eating is triggered by sensory food-related cues, or stressful stimuli, and heightened food cue reactivity in vulnerable people leads to more robust feeding responses and reduced ability to inhibit these habitual inclinations to overeat [3, 21]. Substance use and SUD are driven by similar processes as hedonic overeating (Chaps. 6 and 7).

In the context of SUD, cognitive trainings, such as those that address approach, attentional, and affective biases to drug-related cues, otherwise known as cognitive bias modification trainings, or trainings that target impulsivity globally or in relation to drug cues, otherwise known as inhibitory control trainings, are designed to help people recover. However, in the clinical realm, these trainings have had only mixed success in SUD; attempts to refine the interventions to improve their effectiveness are still underway [3, 32, 33].

Trainings such as these are under development and study to modify eating behavior too, for example, for obesity treatment, and show promise [3, 7, 9, 33–39]. For example, one study found that participants were three times more likely to select fruit over a granola bar after receiving evaluative conditioning training where positive (relative to negative or neutral) words and images were paired with images of fruit [3, 40]. Similarly, another showed that participants were more likely to select fruit over an unhealthy snack when snack images were repeatedly paired with negative body images compared to a blank screen [3, 41]. Tasks training response inhibition globally such as stop signal and go/no-go training [32] and to food stimuli, specifically, are also showing encouraging effects across a range of eating-related behaviors including food consumption, food choices, and even weight loss [3, 42, 43].

Several other nuanced approaches that act within the same cognitive systems are under development and study. For example, virtual reality cue exposure and emotional regulation video game training are being studied and improved upon [32]. Another research group has developed an intervention to target impairments in delay discounting, by training patients to engage in episodic future thinking (EFT), which emphasizes the importance of considering future consequences of actions today. Inclusion of a health goal with EFT may promote healthy decisions and result in positive behavior changes [44]. Habit reversal training utilized in treatment of other disorders such as ticks and stuttering [45, 46] is being piloted in eating disordered populations. Finally, trainings that incorporate cognitive reappraisal strategies, such as altering ones thinking about how good a food looks to eat to thinking of the long-term health consequences of eating unhealthy food when viewing images of such foods, are also being developed and have been found to regulate appetitive responses to highly palatable foods and increase inhibitory PFC and decrease reward region (ventral striatum, amygdala) activation during fMRI [9, 47]. No doubt more will be known and available in the cognitive-training realm in the near future for FA and overeating disorders treatment, but like with SUD successful use for treating clinical populations has not yet been established.

15.1.4 Emerging Pharmacotherapies

In light of increasing research indicating that FA exists, and its underlying neural mechanisms (Chaps. 8 and 9), there are numerous emerging potential medications—some of which are already approved for the treatment of other disorders and need studies to determine whether they are also effective for FA, others which are not yet FDA-approved for use in humans—but are important in that they show great promise for FA and other disorders associated with overeating.

Medications which affect the cannabinoid system need further study (Chaps. 1 and 9) including peripheral cannabinoid type 1 receptor (CB1) antagonists [48–50], central CB1 antagonists [51], and peripheral cannabinoid type 2 receptor (CB2) agonists [50]. Leptin partial agonists also show promise for greater food intake suppression, reduce, and may reduce leptin resistance importantly in leptin receptor containing anorexigenic proopiomelanocortin (POMC) neurons of the hypothalamic arcuate nucleus [48, 49]. Recall that lorcaserin, a 5HT2C receptor agonist, was effective for promoting weight loss and smoking cessation, but was taken off the market due to causing cancer; new 5HT2C agonists are now under development in the wake of lorcaserin [52, 53]. Medications with anti-inflammatory and/or macrophage inhibiting effects (e.g., ibudilast and other phosphodiesterase modulators, minocycline, salsalate, other cytokine therapies) deserve further attention for treatment of FA and overeating [50]. Atomoxetine and other dopamine (DA) and norepinephrine (NE) reuptake inhibitors that might reduce impulse control need further exploration for FA as well; atomoxetine has been found to be somewhat useful in BED, for example [54], and tesofensine, a potent triple reuptake inhibitor (serotonin, NE, DA) is in phase III trials for obesity [55]. Psychedelics are also getting increasing attention for the treatment of a variety of psychiatric disorders and may have positive effects on depression and substance use [56], as well as improving well-being scores in EDs [57]. Medications targeting various aspects of the homeostatic system are at various stages of development for the treatment of obesity and other forms of overeating and include melanocortin type 4 receptor agonists (setmelanotide) [50, 55] medications targeting the PPAR receptors [50, 58], ghrelin antagonists [59] or anti-ghrelin vaccines [50], orexin receptor antagonists [54], and numerous other gut-neuropeptides [60]. Finally, several other medication classes that are helpful in SUD treatment deserve further study in FA, such as the alpha-1 antagonists prazosin and doxazosin [61]; GABA-B receptor antagonists, which may improve impulse control [54]; and finally varenicline, which reduces both nicotine and alcohol use and acts on the cholinergic system [58, 62–66].

15.1.5 Emerging Natural Supplements

Although there is a massive amount of research into alterative or "natural" supplements for obesity, BED, and FA, a few in particular deserve special mention in light of what we know about brain mechanisms behind FA. For one, melatonin [67, 68] by stimulating the MCR4 receptor can reduce appetite and reward responsivity. Second, probiotics and other gut-brain-microbiome interventions [69–73] and interventions to alter the ratios between antioxidant and pro-oxidant food ratios (recall, an antioxidant and pro-oxidant food ratio of 2:3 per meal is the ideal nutritional ratio) [74] are especially interesting potential interventions which can reduce inflammatory processes in the gut and brain, thereby reducing homeostatic and hedonic drives to eat; they influence both the rapidity of absorption of glucose and lipids (thereby reducing conditioning effects) and have direct beneficial effects on brain function (Chap. 9). Antioxidants might also prevent habit learning through DA release reduction [75]. Finally, there is emerging data about the potential beneficial role on weight and hedonic overeating of increasing dietary flavenoids [76], oleoylethanolamide (which is a satiety signal inhibiting food intake through the involvement of central noradrenergic and oxytocinergic neurons) [77], and a nutrigenomic dopamine agonist to reduce "reward deficiency syndrome" [78].

15.2 Other Areas for Future Research for Disorders of Overeating

15.2.1 Treatment Matching Research

An important area of research across many fields of medicine and mental health treatment is in the area of "treatment matching." Treatment matching involves using patient profiles and characteristics, or objective markers such as blood levels or neuroimaging findings, to individualize treatments, choose between several available treatment options and optimize therapeutic regimens for patients. If we know for whom a treatment is more likely to work best, this will increase effect sizes of treatments in clinical trials, and patients will experience better results.

15.2.1.1 Treatment Matching in Overeaters

There is an infinite amount of research that can be done in this area given the multifactorial etiologies of obesity, BED and FA, and heterogeneity of clinical presentations [52, 53]. However, a few interesting concepts will be mentioned here that might be higher on the list of areas to explore.

One set of contrasts that might prove useful for subtyping individuals who have obesity, BED, and/or FA comes from a study which found that external eating (cue-driven, reward eating, for positive reinforcement) is distinct from emotional eating (negative affect driven, relief eating, for negative reinforcement) and that external eating may be more strongly related to impulsivity whereas emotional eating is more strongly linked to depression [79]. Treatment targeting (say) external eating might aim to reduce impulsivity and cue reactivity, whereas treatment targeting someone with emotional eating might aim to target depressive symptoms more aggressively. Studies to test this hypothesis are needed.

In another provocative study, naltrexone was found to block the effects of morphine on impulsivity but had no effect on global impulsivity per se [54, 80]. This leads to questions about for whom a μ opioid receptor antagonist might work best. One might hypothesize from this that μ opioid agonists, like food or morphine, can trigger impulsivity, which then feeds forward to cause further and further overconsumption of itself and loss of control. It would be interesting to study whether or not μ opioid blockers might work best in people who report feeling triggered to overeat when they eat one or several tastes of palatable food (anecdotally, people report feeling that eating itself is a trigger that causes more craving that can spiral into a binge). Future research might work to define this trait better and then see if it might be utilized as a treatment matching variable for naltrexone studies.

Many experts posit that genotyping might one day prove useful to predict response to particular diets [81–83]. Particular genotypes might identify people who have a tendency towards inflammatory responses to certain foods or people with particular DA receptor profiles, which could further guide macronutrient compositions of recommended diets. More work should be done to test these hypotheses [84].

Also, many believe that fMRI holds promise for predicting response to particular treatments [9, 26]. For example, people who have greater reactivity to food cues might be especially responsive to fMRI-neurofeedback approaches, cognitive trainings focused on attentional or approach bias reduction, or medications (e.g., topiramate) that might work in the brain (e.g., glutamate AMPA antagonist) to block neural systems responsible for cue-elicited approach behavior [9, 26, 33, 52, 53]. Food cue reactivity testing with fMRI could also be utilized to help an individual identify their own problem foods.

Finally, a recently published study in people with FA and/or obesity, BED, or bulimia identified three separate clusters of people: those whose overeating was by driven by a combination of ED and FA, those who suffered primarily from FA, or those with primarily obesity [33]. Based on these emergent subgroupings, the authors of the study went on to further suggest that each group might best be served with treatments targeting their particular vulnerabilities, the primarily FA group with a dietary approach focused on reducing intake of high-fat and high-sugar foods and food cue reactivity, the primarily obese group with weight loss treatment, and the group with both ED and FA to more traditional ED treatment, and focus on psychiatric and psychological dysfunction. The utility of this clustering approach to treatment matching and for improving clinical outcomes should be explored in future work.

Finally, identifying for whom stimulant medications would be most useful for treatment of the various types of overeating needs to be studied more rigorously. Recall the study showing that people with FA did worse on methylphenidate (which increases DA function) than those without, from the standpoint of appetite and cravings [85] (Chap. 14). Furthermore, there's reason to be concerned that people with a history of addiction might be more susceptible to develop a stimulant use disorder due to prescription of these medications.

15.2.1.2 Treatment Matching Using FA as a Matching Variable

At the most obvious level, and already discussed in Chaps. 13 and 14, we argue strongly that a FA diagnosis should be explored as a potential treatment matching variable within all overeaters. Indeed, someone who overeats for primarily hedonic reasons will be much more likely to respond to treatments targeting these systems, whereas someone who overeats due to imbalanced homeostatic systems will likely respond more robustly to medicines targeting homeostatic mechanisms like leptin resistance. Treatments which would be more likely to work in FA over other types of disordered eating syndromes include abstinence-based nutritional approaches, interventions which reduce reward-sensitivity and improve emotion regulation, and treatments targeting impulse control, for example. Treatments which are known to work in SUD (like motivational interviewing, varenicline, topiramate, or prazosin) might be more likely to work in people with FA as well.

Studies that utilize fMRI to distinguish people with FA-like brain patterns (e.g., alterations in in hedonic, emotional, or cognitive control networks) from those without (e.g., changes in homeostatic brain regions) can inform hypothesis development for future treatment matching research, too. For example, sibutramine (a medication which has since been taken off the market, but acts on serotonergic and NE circuits) did not affect activation in the ventral striatum but did affect activation in the hypothalamus, which also predicted degree of weight change during 2 weeks of treatment, indicating that this medicine was acting primarily on the hypothalamic (e.g., homeostatic) appetitive control system [26]. A hypothesis from this might be that those with greater activation in the hypothalamus to food cues might be more responsive to sibutramine and/or that people with overeating due to hypothalamic mechanisms might be more likely to respond to this treatment than those whose overeating is purely reward-based, for example.

15.3 Other FA-Specific Research Needs

There is still a huge amount of research that needs to be done on FA, specifically. Below we will mention some of these areas, which have to do with diagnosis, etiology, public health, and treatment.

15.3.1 FA Diagnosis

In this textbook we have reviewed an extensive amount of evidence, both clinical and neuroscientific, that FA represents a distinct phenomenon from established EDs such as bulimia nervosa or BED. Still, it's still unclear whether FA and BED are separate enough constructs to warrant a separate diagnostic category in human populations, and more research in this area is needed. Further, if they are indeed truly distinguishable, more tools are needed (scales, diagnostic criteria) to help clinicians distinguish one category of patient from the other [86]. Future studies are needed to further examine and establish orthogonal diagnostic criteria specific to FA [87]. This will be especially important in light of the risks of dietary restraint triggering disordered eating in some people [88] discussed below more.

15.3.2 FA Etiology

In terms of identifying the mechanisms of FA, there are several areas that need more research. Perhaps the most important one from a treatment perspective is that more information on the role of restrained eating in the development of FA is needed. Do yo-yo diets trigger FA, and if so, in whom? How about other types of restrictive eating, such as eliminating certain types of food, like sugar or white flower, from the diet (which would be a potential treatment approach for FA)? This will directly inform whether or not the development of abstinence-like diets are wise and for whom [88].

Second, the story about DA and its role in FA, and how alterations in DA signaling lead to and perpetuate FA-like behavior, is still somewhat unclear, and in some cases the literature is contradictory (Chaps. 8 and 9). For example, both hypersensitive DA systems (which will lead to greater reward sensitivity, greater acute conditioning effects, motor sensitization, cross-sensitization, addiction transfer, and binge consumption) and downregulated or hypoactive dopamine systems as often marked by low type 2 dopamine receptor (DRD2) density in the striatum but also blunted DA release to reward (both of which will lead to tolerance, increased anhedonia/reward deficiency, reduced pleasure from natural rewards, increased impulsivity) are described to underlie addictive behavior around substances of abuse and highly palatable (HP) food (Chaps. 7 and 8). The literature is not entirely clear on when (at which stage of the addiction process), where (in which brain regions), and how [e.g., via the DRD2, DA transporter (DAT), or type 1 dopamine (DRD1) receptor] these changes might be influencing behavior. Indeed, not all studies have shown reduced DRD2 expression in the striatum in FA [89]. This is especially important in light of the fact that stimulant medications could theoretically be useful in FA treatment by reducing impulsivity via their actions on priming both DA and NE circuitry in cases where DA hypofunction is the cause, or it could be harmful, promoting addiction and/or excessively sensitizing the DA system [85]. Understanding how hypofunction and hyperfunction play into the FA picture more clearly would be useful for further identifying treatments and making treatment matching hypotheses.

15.3.3 Nutritional Approaches for FA Treatment

More research is needed to identify the ideal dietary recommendations for people who meet diagnostic thresholds for FA. In particular, the usefulness of abstinence models in the treatment of EDs and obesity needs to be rigorously tested in future studies. A large prospective study of individuals meeting criteria for FA separated into a restricted diet group (excluding, say, identified trigger foods) and a non-diet group (including all challenging foods) would be informative, timely, and warranted [88]. However, there are numerous more subtle areas of further exploration that need to be ironed out in this subject area as well.

For one, if an abstinence approach works best, what are the best food items to recommend people abstain from? Should it be personalized or the same for all-comers? If personalized, and targeting trigger foods, or that which the individual is conditioned to seek, how to best identify those trigger foods? Or would it be best to identify or subgroup based on macronutrient composition of the addictive element in the food? There have already been calls for research into questionnaires to help classify patients into these kinds of subcategories, as some posit that addressing fat addiction separate from sugar addiction might prove useful [7, 81]. Or is it simply the case that, in the end, maybe all people with FA are more sensitive to all HP foods [7]? One interesting series of studies have begun to try to classify and score different foods in terms of their inflammatory potentials (and their effects on levels of, e.g., interleukin-6, C-reactive protein, tumor necrosis factor a receptor 2, and cancer risk) and further work into how these index scores might impact FA risk and behavior could one day prove useful in developing a one-size-fits-all FA diet [90, 91], given what we know about the effects of inflammation on hedonic, emotional, and cognitive control brain circuits (Chap. 9).

If abstinence approaches are found to be more effective, the next series of studies might focus on ways to improve a patient's motivation to try an abstinence-based approach and to promote longer-term adherence to diets, given issues of HP food being more pervasively intertwined in our culture than substances and necessary for survival, making dietary change especially challenging. How (inpatient, residential, outpatient), and by whom (primary care, nutritionists, psychiatrists), should abstinence diets be implemented to maximize long-term success? One key way that FA would be expected to differ from SUDs is that a person cannot abstain from eating completely in a similar manner as abstaining from taking drugs [92], which might make abstinence approaches doubly challenging, so and how to address that and support patients through treatment will be an essential area of research.

It will be essential to study, as well, how to best tailor dietary recommendations for patients with comorbid EDs. For whom are abstinence approaches safe, given the supposed risk of restrictive eating on development and persistence of BED and bulimia? Once we have a better understanding about how to best distinguish FA from ED during diagnosis may help, but it will likely prove more complex than this, as abstinence-based approaches can also reduce ED symptoms (Chap. 13) and people often end up meeting criteria for both ED and FA (Chaps. 6 and 12). Identifying an individual's trigger foods, and recommending abstinence from them, alone, might prove more useful (having a softer approach) for people with ED [81]. Similarly, emphasizing the fact that abstinence does not mean caloric restriction (caloric restriction will trigger hedonic craving and lead to bingeing) will also be important in these patients (Chaps. 9 and 14). More research to identify clinical predictors of response to abstinence-based approaches (e.g., studying whether specific elements in a patient's history about dieting and restrictive behaviors predict outcomes) could reveal useful information for providers [93].

Furthermore, it will be essential to ask questions in research studies about what treating should do clinicians do with normal-weight FA. FA and binge eating can cause significant distress even in the absence of causing weight gain and its associated medical consequences. But how to help these people is not clear. Should clinicians focus on body image and discourage abstinence-based approaches, given the risk that it might trigger restrictive behavior around food and ED? Or will this group have a risk of going on to develop obesity, and would FA-like nutritional approaches prevent obesity and related mental health problems?

Finally, a separate mention of intermittent fasting is deserved, given its growing popularity. Studies into the health benefits of intermittent fasting are increasingly promising from the standpoint of physical health [94] (Chap. 2). Intermittent fasting is beneficial for a variety of organ systems in animal and human models and may improve metabolic syndrome, neurodegenerative disorder presentation, cancer risk and recovery, and lifespan [93, 94]. Modest effects on appetite may be seen too [71, 94] (Chap. 2). All these health benefits may be acting via ketogenesis or via direct effects through oxidative stress and inflammation. Even caloric restriction, alone [93], may be useful for several of these metrics, too. However, it is not yet clear for whom intermittent fasting will prove safe in the long-run and for whom will it trigger binge eating and weight gain. It is also not known if it could hurt or help treat FA. In one small study, alternate day fasting [95] actually was found to reduce binge eating, but this was not limited to patients who had BED, and it was a single-group design.

15.3.4 Treatment of HP Food Withdrawal

As discussed in previous chapters, sudden cessation of highly processed or HP food intake can result in a clinical withdrawal syndrome in both animals and humans, and there is already in existence a self-report scale (ProWS) for clinical use to measure the amount or severity of HP food withdrawal [96, 97]. However, the original validation study for this particular questionnaire was performed in individuals who had been trying to diet, and the questions were retrospective, and so the possibility that some of the symptoms were due to a caloric deficit cannot be ruled out [92, 96]. Thus, future research is warranted to track ProWS symptoms prospectively and compare withdrawal symptoms that occur when highly processed HP foods are removed from the diet with and without simultaneously introducing caloric restriction. Once the withdrawal syndrome is confirmed and its accurate measurement in humans and animals validated further, we can then investigate treatments, for example, with medications that might reduce the discomfort associated with withdrawal and make the transition to abstinence-based diets easier.

15.3.5 Psychosocial Interventions for FA Treatment

More research into mechanisms by which the current psychotherapies for weight loss and ED treatment work, and/or research to optimize and identify the active ingredients in cognitive training paradigms, are in order. Furthermore, as we discussed above, treatment matching research, to identify for whom a particular type of therapy works best for FA symptom reduction, are in order. Furthermore, more research into whether motivational interviewing (MI) might work in FA would be of high priority; whereas MI has not yet been shown to have efficacy beyond standard interventions for weight loss (Chaps. 2 and 14), it is highly effective in SUD and could be very helpful motivating people to try an abstinence-based approach. Contingency management is a therapy that grants patients rewards of monetary value, or money proper, for abstinence time and is effective especially for the treatment of stimulant use disorder; it deserves study for FA treatment as well [21].

Another important priority is to more definitively explore the efficacy of Overeaters Anonymous (OA). The growing literature on Alcoholics Anonymous (AA) indicates that AA works and provides numerous mechanisms about how it might be promoting recovery (Chap. 14). For FA and other types of overeating, it is unclear whether the 12-step approach is helpful, and it will be key to ask in future studies whether OA meeting attendance or sponsorship promotes recovery. If so, how is it working, and for whom does it work best? Does it work for obesity treatment and/or BED without FA? What about Food Addicts Anonymous? There are numerous forms of self-help support groups for individuals with addictive eating on an online search; however a study found that only 3 of 13 involved credentialed health professionals [98, 99].

15.3.6 Public Health, Stigma, Self-Efficacy, and FA

Finally, it is important to determine whether public health interventions aimed at reducing our population's exposure to highly processed, high-sugar, and high-fat foods might reduce the risk of FA development along with reducing the risk of obesity and BED. Such interventions may indeed prove helpful, because more difficulty accessing these kinds of foods might reduce out of control eating and weight gain and, as a result, subsequently reduce chronic dieting and/or binge eating. On the other hand, chronic dieting due to expectations of excessive thinness might be a trigger for FA development too, as existing ED treatments would suggest [88]. If excessive focus on thinness (rather than excess exposure to HP foods) is the major cause of FA, then public health interventions to reduce exposure to HP foods wouldn't have a huge beneficial effect on FA rates. This remains to be studied.

Whether growing acceptance of the concept of FA will have a beneficial or negative impact on weight-related externalized or internalized stigma is still not clear. While FA might reduce externalized stigma, it may increase internalized stigma, early studies show [88, 100]. Furthermore, more widespread belief that certain food products can be addictive may increase the population's support for policies intended to curb their use [88, 100], as well as support of individual patients by family and friends who want to attempt an abstinence-based nutritional plan.

Finally, questions have been raised regarding the effects of neurobiological explanation of obesity or FA on patients' sense of self-efficacy and eating/weight outcomes. Studies exploring this question could also inform policy makers about the utility of spreading the concept of FA from a public health perspective too (Chap. 5).

15.4 Conclusion

In summary, the evidence for FA is growing, and it is becoming more and more clear that the construct is valid and has utility for the treatment of people and for improving well-being, physical health, and mental health. That said, there is a large amount of research yet to be done to clarify the best way to diagnose the disorder, to establish valid measurement tools, to identify efficacious treatments, and to determine for whom particular treatments are more likely to work best. With more investigation in these areas, it is entirely possible that FA might be considered more seriously for inclusion in future versions of the DSM, reflecting knowledge gained in the areas of genetic, physiological, and neurobiological, clinical, epidemiological, and public health research [101].

References

1. Wilcox CE. Non-convulsive neurostimulation for the treatment of psychiatric disorders part I: FDA-approved treatments. American Physician Institute; 2020. Available from: CMEToGo.com.
2. Wilcox CE. Non-convulsive neurostimulation for the treatment of psychiatric disorders part II: emerging treatments. American Physician Institute; 2020. Available from: CMEToGo.com.
3. Adams RC, Sedgmond J, Maizey L, Chambers CD, Lawrence NS. Food addiction: implications for the diagnosis and treatment of overeating. Nutrients. 2019;11(9):2086.
4. Matsumoto H, Ugawa Y. Adverse events of tDCS and tACS: a review. Clin Neurophysiol Pract. 2017;2:19–25.
5. Feil J, Zangen A. Brain stimulation in the study and treatment of addiction. Neurosci Biobehav Rev. 2010;34:559–74.
6. Hall PA, Vincent CM, Burhan AM. Non-invasive brain stimulation for food cravings, consumption, and disorders of eating: a review of methods, findings and controversies. Appetite. 2018;124:78–88.
7. Meule A. A critical examination of the practical implications derived from the food addiction concept. Curr Obes Rep. 2019;8(1):11–7.
8. Chen J, Qin J, He Q, Zou Z. A meta-analysis of transcranial direct current stimulation on substance and food craving: what effect do modulators have? Front Psych. 2020;11:598.
9. Val-Laillet D, Aarts E, Weber B, Ferrari M, Quaresima V, Stoeckel LE, et al. Neuroimaging and neuromodulation approaches to study eating behavior and prevent and treat eating disorders and obesity. Neuroimage Clin. 2015;8:1–31.
10. Kekic M, McClelland J, Campbell I, Nestler S, Rubia K, David AS, et al. The effects of prefrontal cortex transcranial direct current stimulation (tDCS) on food craving and temporal discounting in women with frequent food cravings. Appetite. 2014;78:55–62.
11. Fregni F, Orsati F, Pedrosa W, et al. Transcranial direct current stimulation of the prefrontal cortex modulates the desire for specific foods. Appetite. 2008;51:34–41.
12. Goldman RL, Borckardt JJ, Frohman HA, O'Neil PM, Madan A, Campbell LK, et al. Prefrontal cortex transcranial direct current stimulation (tDCS) temporarily reduces food cravings and increases the self-reported ability to resist food in adults with frequent food craving. Appetite. 2011;56(3):741–6.
13. Ljubisavljevic M, Maxood K, Bjekic J, Oommen J, Nagelkerke N. Long-term effects of repeated prefrontal cortex transcranial direct current stimulation (tDCS) on food craving in normal and overweight young adults. Brain Stimul. 2016;9(6):826–33.
14. Lapenta OM, Sierve KD, de Macedo EC, Fregni F, Boggio PS. Transcranial direct current stimulation modulates ERP-indexed inhibitory control and reduces food consumption. Appetite. 2014;83:42–8.
15. Ray MK, Sylvester MD, Helton A, Pittman BR, Wagstaff LE, McRae TR 3rd, et al. The effect of expectation on transcranial direct current stimulation (tDCS) to suppress food craving and eating in individuals with overweight and obesity. Appetite. 2019;136:1–7.
16. Ray MK, Sylvester MD, Osborn L, Helms J, Turan B, Burgess EE, et al. The critical role of cognitive-based trait differences in transcranial direct current stimulation (tDCS) suppression of food craving and eating in frank obesity. Appetite. 2017;116:568–74.
17. Montenegro RA, Okano AH, Cunha FA, Gurgel JL, Fontes EB, Farinatti PT. Prefrontal cortex transcranial direct current stimulation associated with aerobic exercise change aspects of appetite sensation in overweight adults. Appetite. 2012;58(1):333–8.
18. Sedgmond J, Lawrence NS, Verbruggen F, Morrison S, Chambers CD, Adams RC. Prefrontal brain stimulation during food-related inhibition training: effects on food craving, food consumption and inhibitory control. R Soc Open Sci. 2019;6(1):181186.
19. Jansen JM, Daams JG, Koeter MW, Veltman DJ, van den Brink W, Goudriaan AE. Effects of non-invasive neurostimulation on craving: a meta-analysis. Neurosci Biobehav Rev. 2013;37(10 Pt 2):2472–80.
20. Lowe CJ, Vincent C, Hall PA. Effects of noninvasive brain stimulation on food cravings and consumption: a meta-analytic review. Psychosom Med. 2017;79(1):2–13.
21. Carter A, Hendrikse J, Lee N, Yucel M, Verdejo-Garcia A, Andrews ZB, et al. The neurobiology of "food addiction" and its implications for obesity treatment and policy. Annu Rev Nutr. 2016;36:105–28.
22. Kinasz KR, Ross DA, Cooper JJ. Eat to live or live to eat? The neurobiology of appetite regulation. Biol Psychiatry. 2017;81(9):e73–e5.
23. Isserles M, Shalev AY, Roth Y, Peri T, Kutz I, Zlotnick E, et al. Effectiveness of deep transcranial magnetic stimulation combined with a brief exposure procedure in post-traumatic stress disorder--a pilot study. Brain Stimul. 2013;6(3):377–83.
24. Wilcox CE, Clifford J, Ling J, Mayer AR, Bigelow R, Bogenschutz MP, et al. Stroop-related cerebellar and temporal activation is correlated with negative affect and alcohol use disorder severity. Brain Imaging Behav. 2020;14:586–98.
25. Stramba-Badiale C, Mancuso V, Cavedoni S, Pedroli E, Cipresso P, Riva G. Transcranial magnetic stimulation meets virtual reality: the potential of integrating brain stimulation with a simulative technology for food addiction. Front Neurosci. 2020;14:720.
26. Schlogl H, Horstmann A, Villringer A, Stumvoll M. Functional neuroimaging in obesity and the potential for development of novel treatments. Lancet Diabetes Endocrinol. 2016;4(8):695–705.

27. Dewiputri WI, Auer T. Functional magnetic resonance imaging (FMRI) neurofeedback: implementations and applications. Malays J Med Sci. 2013;20(5):5–15.
28. Frank S, Lee S, Preissl H, Schultes B, Birbaumer N, Veit R. The obese brain athlete: self-regulation of the anterior insula in adiposity. PLoS One. 2012;7(8):e42570.
29. Ihssen N, Sokunbi MO, Lawrence AD, Lawrence NS, Linden DEJ. Neurofeedback of visual food cue reactivity: a potential avenue to alter incentive sensitization and craving. Brain Imaging Behav. 2017;11(3):915–24.
30. Kohl SH, Veit R, Spetter MS, Gunther A, Rina A, Luhrs M, et al. Real-time fMRI neurofeedback training to improve eating behavior by self-regulation of the dorsolateral prefrontal cortex: a randomized controlled trial in overweight and obese subjects. Neuroimage. 2019;191:596–609.
31. Spetter MS, Malekshahi R, Birbaumer N, Luhrs M, van der Veer AH, Scheffler K, et al. Volitional regulation of brain responses to food stimuli in overweight and obese subjects: a real-time fMRI feedback study. Appetite. 2017;112:188–95.
32. Treasure J, Leslie M, Chami R, Fernandez-Aranda F. Are trans diagnostic models of eating disorders fit for purpose? A consideration of the evidence for food addiction. Eur Eat Disord Rev. 2018;26(2):83–91.
33. Jimenez-Murcia S, Aguera Z, Paslakis G, Munguia L, Granero R, Sanchez-Gonzalez J, et al. Food addiction in eating disorders and obesity: analysis of clusters and implications for treatment. Nutrients. 2019;11(11):2633.
34. Hardman CA, Rogers PJ, Etchells KA, Houstoun KV, Munafo MR. The effects of food-related attentional bias training on appetite and food intake. Appetite. 2013;71:295–300.
35. Kemps E, Tiggemann M, Orr J, Grear J. Attentional retraining can reduce chocolate consumption. J Exp Psychol Appl. 2014;20(1):94–102.
36. Schmitz F, Svaldi J. Effects of bias modification training in binge eating disorder. Behav Ther. 2017;48(5):707–17.
37. Werthmann J, Field M, Roefs A, Nederkoorn C, Jansen A. Attention bias for chocolate increases chocolate consumption--an attention bias modification study. J Behav Ther Exp Psychiatry. 2014;45(1):136–43.
38. Zhang S, Cui L, Sun X, Zhang Q. The effect of attentional bias modification on eating behavior among women craving high-calorie food. Appetite. 2018;129:135–42.
39. Brockmeyer T, Hahn C, Reetz C, Schmidt U, Friederich HC. Approach bias modification in food craving-a proof-of-concept study. Eur Eat Disord Rev. 2015;23(5):352–60.
40. Walsh EM, Kiviniemi MT. Changing how I feel about the food: experimentally manipulated affective associations with fruits change fruit choice behaviors. J Behav Med. 2014;37(2):322–31.
41. Hollands GJ, Prestwich A, Marteau TM. Using aversive images to enhance healthy food choices and implicit attitudes: an experimental test of evaluative conditioning. Health Psychol. 2011;30(2):195–203.
42. Preuss H, Pinnow M, Schnicker K, Legenbauer T. Improving inhibitory control abilities (ImpulsE)-a promising approach to treat impulsive eating? Eur Eat Disord Rev. 2017;25(6):533–43.
43. Chami R, Cardi V, Lawrence N, MacDonald P, Rowlands K, Hodsoll J, et al. Targeting binge eating in bulimia nervosa and binge eating disorder using inhibitory control training and implementation intentions: a feasibility trial. Psychol Med. 2020:1–10.
44. Athamneh LN, Stein MD, Lin EH, Stein JS, Mellis AM, Gatchalian KM, et al. Setting a goal could help you control: comparing the effect of health goal versus general episodic future thinking on health behaviors among cigarette smokers and obese individuals. Exp Clin Psychopharmacol. 2021;29:59–72.
45. Schlogl H, Kabisch S, Horstmann A, Lohmann G, Muller K, Lepsien J, et al. Exenatide-induced reduction in energy intake is associated with increase in hypothalamic connectivity. Diabetes Care. 2013;36(7):1933–40.
46. Bate KS, Malouff JM, Thorsteinsson ET, Bhullar N. The efficacy of habit reversal therapy for tics, habit disorders, and stuttering: a meta-analytic review. Clin Psychol Rev. 2011;31(5):865–71.
47. Boutelle KN, Knatz S, Carlson J, Bergmann K, Peterson CB. An open trial targeting food cue reactivity and satiety sensitivity in overweight and obese binge eaters. Cogn Behav Pract. 2017;24(3):363–73.
48. Hankir MK, Seyfried F. Partial leptin reduction: an emerging weight loss paradigm. Trends Endocrinol Metab. 2020;31(6):395–7.
49. Zhao S, Zhu Y, Schultz RD, Li N, He Z, Zhang Z, et al. Partial leptin reduction as an insulin sensitization and weight loss strategy. Cell Metab. 2019;30(4):706–19.e6.
50. O'Rourke RW. The pathophysiology of obesity and obesity-related disease. In: Nguyen N, Brethauer SA, Morton JM, Ponce J, Rosenthal RJ, editors. The ASMBS textbook of bariatric surgery. Cham: Springer; 2020.
51. Murphy T, Le Foll B. Targeting the endocannabinoid CB1 receptor to treat body weight disorders: a preclinical and clinical review of the therapeutic potential of past and present CB1 drugs. Biomolecules. 2020;10(6):855.
52. Higgins GA, Sellers EM, Fletcher PJ. From obesity to substance abuse: therapeutic opportunities for 5-HT2C receptor agonists. Trends Pharmacol Sci. 2013;34(10):560–70.
53. Higgins GA, Zeeb FD, Fletcher PJ. Role of impulsivity and reward in the anti-obesity actions of 5-HT2C receptor agonists. J Psychopharmacol. 2017;31(11):1403–18.
54. Hutson PH, Balodis IM, Potenza MN. Binge-eating disorder: clinical and therapeutic advances. Pharmacol Ther. 2018;182:15–27.

55. Coulter AA, Rebello CJ, Greenway FL. Centrally acting agents for obesity: past, present, and future. Drugs. 2018;78(11):1113–32.
56. Bogenschutz MP, Forcehimes AA, Pommy JA, Wilcox CE, Barbosa PC, Strassman RJ. Psilocybin-assisted treatment for alcohol dependence: a proof-of-concept study. J Psychopharmacol. 2015;29(3):289–99.
57. Spriggs MJ, Kettner H, Carhart-Harris RL. Positive effects of psychedelics on depression and wellbeing scores in individuals reporting an eating disorder. Eat Weight Disord. 2021;26:1265–70.
58. Onaolapo AY, Onaolapo OJ. Food additives, food and the concept of "food addiction": is stimulation of the brain reward circuit by food sufficient to trigger addiction? Pathophysiology. 2018;25(4):263–76.
59. Schalla MA, Stengel A. Pharmacological modulation of ghrelin to induce weight loss: successes and challenges. Curr Diab Rep. 2019;19(10):102.
60. Alexiadou K, Tan TM. Gastrointestinal peptides as therapeutic targets to mitigate obesity and metabolic syndrome. Curr Diab Rep. 2020;20(7):26.
61. Hicks C, Sabino V, Cottone P. The alpha-1 adrenergic receptor antagonist prazosin reduces binge-like eating in rats. Nutrients. 2020;12(6):1569.
62. Avena NM, Gold JA, Kroll C, Gold MS. Further developments in the neurobiology of food and addiction: update on the state of the science. Nutrition. 2012;28(4):341–3.
63. Ashare RL, McKee SA. Effects of varenicline and bupropion on cognitive processes among nicotine-deprived smokers. Exp Clin Psychopharmacol. 2012;20(1):63–70.
64. Austin AJ, Duka T, Rusted J, Jackson A. Effect of varenicline on aspects of inhibitory control in smokers. Psychopharmacology. 2014;231(18):3771–85.
65. Hays JT, Croghan IT, Schroeder DR, Ebbert JO, Hurt RD. Varenicline for tobacco dependence treatment in recovering alcohol-dependent smokers: an open-label pilot study. J Subst Abus Treat. 2011;40(1):102–7.
66. Hendrickson LM, Guildford MJ, Tapper AR. Neuronal nicotinic acetylcholine receptors: common molecular substrates of nicotine and alcohol dependence. Front Psych. 2013;4:29.
67. Tumentemur G, Altunkaynak BZ, Kaplan S. Is melatonin, leptin or their combination more effective on oxidative stress and folliculogenesis in the obese rats? J Obstet Gynaecol. 2020;40(1):116–27.
68. Genario R, Cipolla-Neto J, Bueno AA, Santos HO. Melatonin supplementation in the management of obesity and obesity-associated disorders: a review of physiological mechanisms and clinical applications. Pharmacol Res. 2021;163:105254.
69. Dong TS, Mayer EA, Osadchiy V, Chang C, Katzka W, Lagishetty V, et al. A distinct brain-gut-microbiome profile exists for females with obesity and food addiction. Obesity. 2020;28(8):1477–86.
70. Perrault L. Obesity in adults: etiology and risk factors. In: UpToDate [Internet]. Wolters Kluwer; 2018. Available from: www.uptodate.com.
71. Perrault L. Obesity in adults: dietary therapy. In: UpToDate [Internet]. Wolters Kluwer; 2021, [cited Jan 1, 2021]. Available from: www.updtodate.com.
72. Gupta A, Osadchiy V, Mayer EA. Brain-gut-microbiome interactions in obesity and food addiction. Nat Rev Gastroenterol Hepatol. 2020;17(11):655–72.
73. Narmaki E, Borazjani M, Ataie-Jafari A, Hariri N, Doost AH, Qorbani M, et al. The combined effects of probiotics and restricted calorie diet on the anthropometric indices, eating behavior, and hormone levels of obese women with food addiction: a randomized clinical trial. Nutr Neurosci. 2020:1–13.
74. Tobore TO. Towards a comprehensive theory of obesity and a healthy diet: the causal role of oxidative stress in food addiction and obesity. Behav Brain Res. 2020;384:112560.
75. Gibson AS, Keefe KA, Furlong TM. Accelerated habitual learning resulting from L-dopa exposure in rats is prevented by N-acetylcysteine. Pharmacol Biochem Behav. 2020;198:173033.
76. Rufino AT, Costa VM, Carvalho F, Fernandes E. Flavonoids as antiobesity agents: a review. Med Res Rev. 2021;41(1):556–85.
77. Romano KA, Heron KE, Amerson R, Howard LM, MacIntyre RI, Mason TB. Changes in disordered eating behaviors over 10 or more years: a meta-analysis. Int J Eat Disord. 2020;53(7):1034–55.
78. Downs BW, Blum K, Bagchi D, Kushner S, Bagchi M, Galvin JM, et al. Molecular neuro-biological and systemic health benefits of achieving dopamine homeostasis in the face of a catastrophic pandemic (COVID-19): a mechanistic exploration. J Syst Integr Neurosci. 2020;7:1–8.
79. Ouwens MA, van Strien T, van Leeuwe JF. Possible pathways between depression, emotional and external eating. A structural equation model. Appetite. 2009;53(2):245–8.
80. Pattij T, Schetters D, Janssen MC, Wiskerke J, Schoffelmeer AN. Acute effects of morphine on distinct forms of impulsive behavior in rats. Psychopharmacology. 2009;205(3):489–502.
81. Sarkar S, Kochhar KP, Khan NA. Fat addiction: psychological and physiological trajectory. Nutrients. 2019;11(11):2785.
82. Seid H, Rosenbaum M. Low carbohydrate and low-fat diets: what we don't know and why we should know it. Nutrients. 2019;11(11):2749.
83. Heber D, Carpenter CL. Addictive genes and the relationship to obesity and inflammation. Mol Neurobiol. 2011;44(2):160–5.
84. San-Cristobal R, Navas-Carretero S, Martinez-Gonzalez MA, Ordovas JM, Martinez JA. Contribution of macronutrients to obesity: implications for precision nutrition. Nat Rev Endocrinol. 2020;16(6):305–20.

85. Gordon EL, Ariel-Donges AH, Bauman V, Merlo LJ. What is the evidence for "food addiction?" A systematic review. Nutrients. 2018;10(4):477.
86. Schulte EM, Potenza MN, Gearhardt AN. Specific theoretical considerations and future research directions for evaluating addictive-like eating as a substance-based, food addiction: comment on Lacroix et al. (2018). Appetite. 2018;130:293–5.
87. Hauck C, Cook B, Ellrott T. Food addiction, eating addiction and eating disorders. Proc Nutr Soc. 2020;79(1):103–12.
88. Wiss D, Brewerton T. Separating the signal from the noise: how psychiatric diagnoses can help discern food addiction from dietary restraint. Nutrients. 2020;12(10):2937.
89. Domingo-Rodriguez L, Ruiz de Azua I, Dominguez E, Senabre E, Serra I, Kummer S, et al. A specific prelimbic-nucleus accumbens pathway controls resilience versus vulnerability to food addiction. Nat Commun. 2020;11(1):782.
90. Tabung FK, Smith-Warner SA, Chavarro JE, Wu K, Fuchs CS, Hu FB, et al. Development and validation of an empirical dietary inflammatory index. J Nutr. 2016;146(8):1560–70.
91. Turner-McGrievy GM, Wirth MD, Shivappa N, Dunn CG, Crimarco A, Hurley TG, et al. Impact of a 12-month Inflammation Management Intervention on the Dietary Inflammatory Index, inflammation, and lipids. Clin Nutr ESPEN. 2019;30:42–51.
92. Schulte EM, Wadden TA, Allison KC. An evaluation of food addiction as a distinct psychiatric disorder. Int J Eat Disord. 2020;53(10):1610–22.
93. Grigolon RB, Brietzke E, Trevizol AP, McIntyre RS, Mansur RB. Caloric restriction, resting metabolic rate and cognitive performance in non-obese adults: a post-hoc analysis from CALERIE study. J Psychiatr Res. 2020;128:16–22.
94. de Cabo R, Mattson MP. Effects of intermittent fasting on health, aging, and disease. N Engl J Med. 2019;381(26):2541–51.
95. Hoddy KK, Kroeger CM, Trepanowski JF, Barnosky AR, Bhutani S, Varady KA. Safety of alternate day fasting and effect on disordered eating behaviors. Nutr J. 2015;14:44.
96. Schulte EM, Smeal JK, Lewis J, Gearhardt AN. Development of the highly processed food withdrawal scale. Appetite. 2018;131:148–54.
97. Parnarouskis L, Schulte EM, Lumeng JC, Gearhardt AN. Development of the highly processed food withdrawal scale for children. Appetite. 2020;147:104553.
98. Burrows T, Collins R, Rollo M, Leary M, Hides L, Davis C. The feasibility of a personality targeted intervention for addictive overeating: FoodFix. Appetite. 2021;156:104974.
99. Burrows T, Verdejo-Garcia A, Carter A, Brown RM, Andrews ZB, Dayas CV, et al. Health professionals' and health professional trainees' views on addictive eating behaviours: a cross-sectional survey. Nutrients. 2020;12(9):2860.
100. Carter A, Hardman CA, Burrows T. Food addiction and eating addiction: scientific advances and their clinical, social and policy implications. Nutrients. 2020;12(5):1485.
101. Meule A, Gearhardt AN. Food addiction in the light of DSM-5. Nutrients. 2014;6(9):3653–71.

Recommended Readings

Depression & Anxiety

Manuals and Clinical Guides

Feeling Good: The New Mood Therapy – David D. Burns MD

Acceptance and Commitment Therapy for Anxiety Disorders: A Practitioner's Treatment Guide to Using Mindfulness, Acceptance, and Values-Based Behavior Change – Georg H. Eifert, John P. Forsyth

The Mindfulness and Acceptance Workbook for Depression: Using Acceptance and Commitment Therapy to Move Through Depression and Create a Life Worth Living – Kirk D. Strosahl, Patricia J. Robinson

Comprehensive Guide to Interpersonal Psychotherapy – Myrna Weissman, John Markowitz, Gerald Klerman

Mindfulness-Based Cognitive Therapy For Depression – Zindel Segal, Mark Williams, John Teasdale

Self-Help Books

Mind Over Mood, Second Edition: Change How You Feel by Changing the Way You Think, Edition 2 – Dennis Greenberger, Christine A. Padesky

Mastery of Your Anxiety and Panic/ Mastery of Your Anxiety and Worry – Michelle Craske

Mindfulness: An Eight-Week Plan for Finding Peace in a Frantic World – Mark Williams, Danny Penman

The Mindful Way Workbook: An 8-Week Program to Free Yourself From Depression and Emotional Distress – John Teasdale, Mark Williams, Zindel Segal

Post-Traumatic Stress Disorder

Cognitive Processing Therapy for PTSD, A Comprehensive Manual – Patricia Resick, Candice Monson, Kathleen Chard

The PTSD Workbook: Simple Effective Techniques for Overcoming Traumatic Stress Symptoms – Mary Beth Williams, Soili Poijula

Addiction/Substance Use Disorders

Twelve Step facilitation Manual – https://pubs.niaaa.nih.gov/publications/projectmatch/match01.pdf

Seeking Safety: A Treatment Manual for PTSD and Substance Abuse – Lisa M. Najavits

Relapse Prevention, Second Edition: Maintenance Strategies in the Treatment of Addictive Behaviors – G. Alan Marlatt, Dennis M. Donovan

Mindfulness Based Relapse Prevention: Mindfulness-Based Relapse Prevention for Addictive Behaviors: A Clinician's Guide – Neha Chawla and Sarah W. Bowen

Community Reinforcement Approach – https://archives.drugabuse.gov/sites/default/files/cra.pdf

Motivational Interviewing Preparing People for Change – William Miller, Stephen Rollnick

More Motivational Interviewing Resources – www.motivationalinterviewing.org

Substance Abuse Treatment Group Therapy a Treatment Improvement Protocol TIP 41 – www.samhsa.gov

Stopping Anxiety Medication (Therapist Guide and Patient Manual) – Michael Otto, Mark Pollack

The Addiction Recovery Skills Workbook: Changing Addictive Behaviors Using CBT, Mindfulness, and Motivational Interviewing Techniques – Suzette Glasner-Edwards

C. E. Wilcox, *Food Addiction, Obesity, and Disorders of Overeating*,
https://doi.org/10.1007/978-3-030-83078-6

Eating Disorders and Obesity

The Body Image Workbook – Thomas F. Cash

Manuals and Clinical Guides

Cognitive Behavior Therapy and Eating Disorders – Christopher Fairburn
Eating Disorders: A Guide to Medical Care and Complications – Philip Mehler, Arnold Anderson
Body Image, Eating Disorders and Obesity: An Integrative Guide for Assessment and Treatment – Kevin Thompson
The Gravity of Weight: A Clinical Guide to Weight Loss and Maintenance – Sylvia R. Karasu and T. Byram Karasu

Self-Help Books

Overcoming Binge Eating – Christopher Fairburn
Binge No More: Your Guide to Overcoming Disordered Eating – Joyce D. Nash

Behavioral Obesity Weight Loss Manuals

The Learn Program for Weight Management – KD Brownell
Look AHEAD Counselor Information – https://www.div12.org/wpcontent/uploads/2015/04/Look-AHEAD-Counselor-Information.pdf
Look AHEAD Counsellor Manual – https://www.div12.org/wpcontent/uploads/2015/04/Look-AHEAD-Counselor-Manual.pdf
Look AHEAD Session Outlines – https://www.div12.org/wpcontent/uploads/2015/04/Look-AHEAD-outline1.pdf
Look AHEAD Patient Materials – https://www.div12.org/wpcontent/uploads/2015/04/Look-AHEAD-Participant-Handouts.pdf
Look AHEAD: Planning Ahead for Life Events – https://www.div12.org/wpcontent/uploads/2015/04/Planning-Aheadfor-Life-Events.pdf
Diabetes Prevention Program Counselor Manual: Core Sessions – https://www.div12.org/wp-content/uploads/2015/04/DPP-Core-Counselor-Materials.pdf
Diabetes Prevention Program Counselor Manual: After Core Sessions – https://www.div12.org/wp-content/uploads/2015/04/DPP-Counselor-Materials-After-Core.pdf
Diabetes Prevention Program Patient Manual: Core Sessions – https://www.div12.org/wp-content/uploads/2015/04/DPP-Participant-Notebook-first-16--sessions.pdf
Diabetes Prevention Program Patient Manual: After Core Sessions https://dppos.bsc.gwu.edu/web/dppos/after-core
Diabetes Prevention Program Patient Manual: Optional – https://www.div12.org/wp-content/uploads/2015/04/DPP-Optional-Participant-Handouts.pdf
Diabetes Prevention Program Research Cognitive-Behavioral Treatment for Obesity: A Clinician's Guide – Cooper, Fairburn, & Hawker
Handbook of Obesity Treatment – Wadden & Stunkard
Lifestyle Manual for Youth & Adolescents – https://www.div12.org/wpcontent/uploads/2015/04/Lifestyle-Change-Youth-Manual.pdf
Lifestyle Manual for Family Support – https://www.div12.org/wpcontent/uploads/2015/04/Lifestyle-Change-Family-Support-Person-Manual.pdf
Lifestyle Change Logging Forms for Youth & Adolescents – https://www.div12.org/wp-content/uploads/2015/04/Lifestyle-Change-Lifestyle-Log.pdf
Lifestyle Posters for Youth & Adolescents – https://www.div12.org/wpcontent/uploads/2015/04/Lifestyle-Posters.pdf
Behavioral Treatment for Obesity | Society of Clinical Psychology – https://div12.org/treatment/behavioral-treatment-for-obesity

Self-Help Weight-Loss Books

The Cognitive Behavioral Workbook for Weight Management: A Step-by-Step Program Laliberte, McCabe, & Taylor
Mini Habits for Weight Loss: Stop Dieting. Form New Habits. Change Your Lifestyle Without Suffering – Stephen Guise
Allen Carr's Easy way to Quit Emotional Eating: Set Yourself Free from Binge-eating and Comfort-Eating – Allen Carr, John Dicey
Clearing your Path to Permanent Weight Loss: The Truth About Why You've Failed in the Past and What You Must Know to Succeed Now – Cookie Rosenblum
The Hunger Fix: The Three-Stage Detox and Recovery Plan for Overeating and Food Addiction – Pamela Peeke, Mariska van Aalst

Insomnia

Say Good Night to Insomnia – Gregg Jacobs
Cognitive Behavioral Treatment of Insomnia – Michael Perlis, Carla Jungquist, Michael Smith, Donn Posner

Emotion Regulation – Other

Skills Training Manual for Treating Borderline Personality Disorder – Marsha Linehan

General

https://div12.org/diagnoses/

Index

C. E. Wilcox, *Food Addiction, Obesity, and Disorders of Overeating*,
https://doi.org/10.1007/978-3-030-83078-6